T0296668

Veterinary Neuroanatomy
A Clinical Approach

For Elsevier
Commissioning Editor: Robert Edwards
Development Editor: Helen Leng
Project Manager: Julie Taylor
Designer/Design Direction: Stewart Larking
Illustration Manager: Jennifer Rose

Veterinary Neuroanatomy
A Clinical Approach

Christine Thomson
BVSc(Hons) PhD DipACVIM(Neurol) DipECVN

Associate Professor, Comparative Physiology and Anatomy,
Institute of Veterinary, Animal and Biomedical Sciences,
Massey University, Palmerston North, New Zealand

Caroline Hahn
BS DVM MSc PhD DipDCEIM DipECVN MRCVS

Senior Lecturer in Clinical Neurosciences,
Royal (Dick) School of Veterinary Studies,
University of Edinburgh, UK

With a contribution by
Craig Johnson
BVSc DVA DipECVA PhD MRCVS

Associate Professor in
Veterinary Neurophysiology, IVABS,
Massey University Veterinary School,
Palmerston North, New Zealand

Illustrations by
Quentin Roper
National Centre for Teaching and Learning,
Massey University, Palmerston North, New Zealand

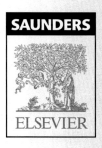

SAUNDERS

ELSEVIER

Edinburgh   London   New York   Oxford   Philadelphia   St Louis   Sydney   Toronto   2012

SAUNDERS
ELSEVIER

© 2012 Elsevier Ltd All rights reserved.

ISBN 9780702034824

British Library Cataloguing in Publication Data
A catalogue record for this book is available from the British Library

Library of Congress Cataloging in Publication Data
A catalog record for this book is available from the Library of Congress

Notices
Knowledge and best practice in this field are constantly changing. As new research and experience broaden our understanding, changes in research methods, professional practices, or medical treatment may become necessary.

Practitioners and researchers must always rely on their own experience and knowledge in evaluating and using any information, methods, compounds, or experiments described herein. In using such information or methods they should be mindful of their own safety and the safety of others, including parties for whom they have a professional responsibility.

With respect to any drug or pharmaceutical products identified, readers are advised to check the most current information provided (i) on procedures featured or (ii) by the manufacturer of each product to be administered, to verify the recommended dose or formula, the method and duration of administration, and contraindications. It is the responsibility of practitioners, relying on their own experience and knowledge of their patients, to make diagnoses, to determine dosages and the best treatment for each individual patient, and to take all appropriate safety precautions.

To the fullest extent of the law, neither the publisher nor the authors, contributors, or editors, assume any liability for any injury and/or damage to persons or property as a matter of products liability, negligence or otherwise, or from any use or operation of any methods, products, instructions, or ideas contained in the material herein.

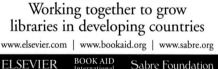

The publisher's policy is to use paper manufactured from sustainable forests

Last digit is the print number: 9 8 7 6 5 4

Printed in China

Contents

Preface

The disciplines of neuroanatomy and neurophysiology have the unique ability to fill veterinary students with fear; consequently, when those students then become veterinarians they remain uncomfortable with localising neurological lesions; they may be anxious or flummoxed when confronted with a neurological case. Lesion localisation is the foundation stone on which diagnostic neurology is built: without accurate lesion localisation, diagnosing and treating neurological cases becomes a stab-in-the-dark.

We are committed to sharing our enthusiasm about this fabulous field and so this book was written to help veterinarians and vets-in-training appreciate the neuroanatomical concepts that underlie the function and dysfunction of the nervous system.

The information provided in this book is based on that which we have found to be essential to understanding clinical neurology. It starts with the fundamentals of the gross structure and functional anatomy of the nervous system, and is followed by discussions of the different neural systems. It culminates in a chapter on the neurological examination and lesion localisation. We have tried our best to present the key concepts in simple, user-friendly language. We've also tried to cater for those readers with a deeper interest by supplying detail, but in such a way that it compliments rather than overwhelms the key concepts. We have exemplified the key concepts with images that illustrate how you can see the normal function of the nervous system in every animal that you watch. But as neural function is often graphically illustrated by dysfunction, we have also included many clinical case scenarios. Crucially, these clinical examples will also familiarise the practitioner, or student, with the clinical signs caused by specific lesions in the nervous system. The appendix contains 31 high-resolution, anatomical and histological images depicting detailed anatomy, and a comprehensive glossary that gives a brief summary of each structure and its function. In conjunction with the detail in the text, the Appendix should also make this book a useful reference text for anyone with a deeper interest in clinical neurology and neuropathology.

We very much hope that this book will help veterinarians and other neurophiles to better understand what is happening in the nervous system of the patients under their care: if we can achieve this goal then we will have repaid our mentors for all they have given us and, perhaps, help to inspire the next generation of veterinary neurologists.

May neuroanatomy 'live long and prosper'!

CH and CT
March 2012

Acknowledgements

The authors are board-certified, clinical neurologists who started their career with similarly limited neuroscience backgrounds, but had the great fortune of meeting four of the most inspirational people in this field: Alexander deLahunta, Ian Griffiths, Joe Kornegay and Joe Mayhew. Under their patient tutelage we came to understand how elegant and supremely logical the nervous system is, and what a thrill it is to make the correct neuroanatomical diagnosis on the basis of a neurological examination. My thanks also to Lola Hudson (NCSU-CVM) for giving me (CT) a great grounding in neuroanatomy.

The text is illustrated with clear, simple neuroanatomical diagrams drawn by the inimitable Quentin Roper, and anatomical specimens exquisitely prepared by Allan Nutman (Massey University).

The sheep brain used for gross specimens in the Appendix were prepared by Associate Professor Craig Johnson and Mr Neil Ward (Massey University).

Our thanks to Jaime Macdonald and Aaron Gilmour (Massey University), for their photography of Barney. Thanks also to the owners of Barney, the labrador retriever, and Timmy the whippet, for letting us use their canine models.

Our sincere thanks to the wise and experienced Dr. Tony Palmer of Cambridge University for providing the sheep brainstem histological sections and reviewing all of the Appendix images and their annotation.

Figs. 3.9B&C are reproduced from Thomson *et al*, Myelinated, synapsing cultures of murine spinal cord – validation as an in vitro model of the central nervous system, European Journal of Neuroscience, 2008, John Wiley and Sons.

Key references used in the writing of this book,

- Crosby EC, Humphrey T, Lauer EW. Correlative Anatomy of the Nervous system, Macmillan Co. New York, 1963
- deLahunta A and Glass E. Veterinary Neuroanatomy and Clinical Neurology, 3rd edition, Saunders, 2009
- Dyce KM, Sack WO, Wensing CJG. Textbook of Veterinary Anatomy, 4th Edition, Saunders, Philadelphia, 2010
- Evans HE. Miller's Anatomy of the Dog, 3rd Edition, Saunders, Philadelphia, 1993
- Gilbert SF. Developmental Biology. 8th edition, Sunderland, Mass. Sinauer Assoc, USA, 2006
- Gray's Anatomy. The Anatomical Basis of Clinical Practice, Ed Standring S. 39th Edition, Elsevier, Edinburgh, 2005
- Jenkins TW. Functional Mammalian Neuroanatomy. 2nd Edition, Lea&Febiger, Philadelphia, 1978
- King AS. Physiological and clinical anatomy of the domestic animals; v. 1. Central nervous system. Oxford; New York: Oxford University Press, 1987
- Mayhew IG. Large Animal Neurology. Wiley-Blackwell, Oxford, 2009
- Patten. Foundations of Embryology. 6th edition, McGraw-Hill, USA, 2002
- Roberts TDM, Understanding Balance, The Mechanics of Posture and Locomotion. Chapman & Hall, London, 1995
- Singer M. The brain of the dog in section. W.B. Saunders, Philadelphia, 1962
- Young B, Lowe JS, Stevens A, Heath JW. Wheater's Functional Histology. A text and colour atlas. Churchill Livingstone, Elsevier, 2006

Terminology, glossary and abbreviations

L = Latin, Gk = Greek.

Nomina Anatomia Veterinaria http://www.wava-amav.org/Downloads/nav_2005.pdf from the World Association of Veterinary Anatomists, has been used as a source of terminology throughout this book.

An extensive glossary of structures, their location and function is given in the Appendix.

Glossary of terms and abbreviations

Body – the entire physical structure including the head, neck, trunk, limbs and tail

CN; CNN – cranial nerves singular and plural

CNS – central nervous system

Decussation – to cross in the form of the letter 'X'; crossing the midline (*decussis* – L = intersection)

Dysmetria – altered rate, range or force of movement

Epaxial – above the axis of the spinal column

Ganglia – collections of nerve cell bodies, with similar functions, located outside the CNS

Hypaxial – below the axis of the vertebral column

LMN – lower motor neuron – neurons associated with motor function that have their cell body in the CNS and their axon leaves the CNS in a cranial or spinal nerve to synapse via a neuromuscular junction with striated, smooth or cardiac muscle. They could be considered to be peripheral motor neurons.

Neuraxis – brain and spinal cord

Neurocranium – the portion of the skull that houses the brain

Nuclei – collections of nerve cell bodies, with similar functions, located in the CNS

Paralysis – complete loss of strength in a limb or muscle group (*paralusis* – Gk = to disable, or *para* – Gk = beyond + *lysis* – Gk = loosening)

Paresis – reduction in motor function (*paralyein* – Greek = to be palsied)

Pathway – sequential tracts separated by synapses that are all involved in one neural function. For example, the visual pathway comprises the retinal ganglion neurons, optic nerve, optic chiasm, optic tract, a synapse in the lateral geniculate nucleus, optic radiation to the visual cortex

PNS – peripheral nervous system

Soma – Gk = body, pl = somata

Somatotopic organisation – the organisation of fibres within a tract, or region of the CNS in a precise pattern reflecting the anatomical arrangement of the body region being innervated (*soma* – Gk = body, *topos* – Gk = place)

Spinal cord segment – a section of spinal cord to which is attached a pair of dorsal and a pair of ventral nerve roots

UMN – upper motor neuron – neurons confined to the CNS that are associated with motor function. They could be considered to be central motor neurons.

Tract – a collection of neurons with the same function, that originate together and terminate together and do not synapse en route. Tract names often indicate their origin and destination. For example, the spinothalamic tract travels from the spinal cord to the thalamus

Anatomical terminology

Directional terms used for quadrupeds are different to those used in bipedal animals, which have an upright posture.

In regions located behind (caudal) to head–neck junction

- **Cranial**, caudal, dorsal, ventral

In regions located in front of (cranial) to the head–neck junction:

- **Rostral**, caudal, dorsal, ventral (*cranium* – L = skull, *cauda* – L = tail, *dorsum* – L = back, *venter* – L = belly, *rostrum* – L = beak)
- Use of the terms **anterior, posterior, superior, inferior:**
  Used in conjunction with the eye and the inner ear
  Otherwise ventral, dorsal, cranial/rostral and caudal (*ante* – L = before, *post* – L = behind/afterward)

Median plane – longitudinal midline of the animal, divides the animal into two symmetrical halves (*medius* – L = in the middle)

Sagittal plane – parallel to the median plane but off the midline; planes close the midline may be called paramedian (*sagitta* – L = arrow, as if it had pierced the body from front to back or back to front)

Dorsal/horizontal plane – parallel to the dorsal aspect of the animal

Lateral – towards the side; (*latus* – L = flank)

Medial – towards the midline; (*medius* – L = in the middle)

Transverse plane – transects the trunk, head, limb or appendage perpendicular to its long axis (*trans* – L = across or over, *versus* – L = turned so as to face)

Limbs:

- Cranial and caudal, if proximal to the carpus or tarsus
- Dorsal and palmar, if distal to, or involving the carpus; *palma* – L = palm of hand
- Dorsal and plantar, if distal to, or involving the tarsus; *planta* – L = sole of foot
- Proximal lies towards the junction with the body; *proximus* – L = near
- Distal lies further away from the junction with the body; *distare* – L = distance
- Axial – towards the axis/midline of the limb; *axle* – L = axle or pole around which rotation occurs
- Abaxial – away from the axis/midline of the limb; *ab* – L = from

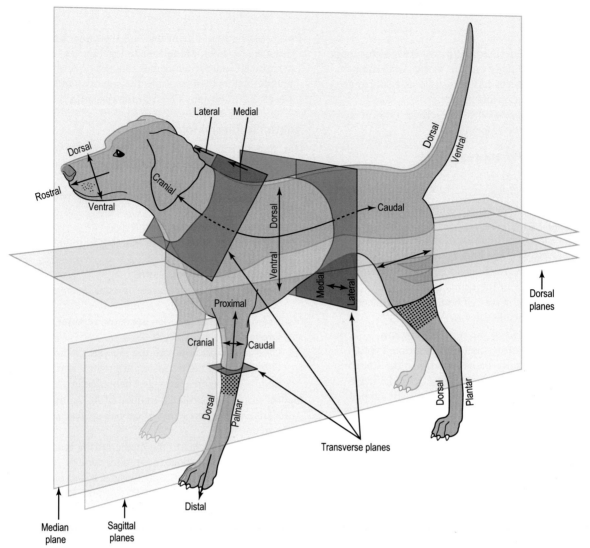

Reprinted with permission Dyce KM, Sack WO, Wensing CJG. *Textbook of Veterinary Anatomy*, 4th Edition, Saunders, Philadelphia, 2010.

Chapter 1
Regional neuroanatomy

Key points

- The peripheral nervous system consists of the nerves and ganglia located outside the brain and spinal cord.
- The myelin sheath surrounding the peripheral axons is formed by Schwann cells, whereas CNS axons are myelinated by oligodendrocytes.
- Dorsal and ventral nerve roots attach on each side of the spinal cord and carry sensory and motor axons, respectively. Lateral to the cord, the dorsal and ventral roots fuse to form mixed, spinal nerves. Adjacent spinal nerves may fuse, in a plexus, to form named nerves in the periphery.
- There are 12 pairs of cranial nerves that innervate the head and extend into the body.
- Areas of sensory innervation of the skin are categorised as dermatomes, cutaneous zones and autonomous zones.
- Somatic lower motor neurons innervating striated muscle of the body have their cell bodies sited in the CNS; their axons travel in the PNS to connect to the muscle at the neuromuscular junction. A motor unit comprises a single lower motor neuron (LMN) and the group of muscle fibres it innervates.

Basic systems arrangement of the nervous system

Neurons comprise a cell body, or soma (plural = somata), and cell processes/neurites. Dendrites are the processes that receive information, whereas axons/nerve fibres convey efferent information as action potentials/nerve impulses. The axons may be unmyelinated or myelinated with a lipid-rich, insulating myelin sheath that both speeds up nerve conduction and protects the axon. Ganglia are collections of nerve cell bodies outside the CNS. Nuclei are collections of neuronal cell bodies with a similar function, inside the CNS.

Nerve fibres are of three basic types:

1. Afferent/sensory fibres bring information into the central nervous system (CNS) from the periphery and convey that information to higher centres for processing.
2. Efferent/motor fibres take information from motor planning centres through the CNS to connect with other motor fibres that take information into the periphery.
3. Integrating fibres that may connect afferent fibres with storage centres, other processing centres or efferent fibres. They process, organise and/or store information.

Introduction to regions

The anatomical descriptions are based primarily on canine anatomy but they are also relevant to most domestic animals.

Anatomically there are two components: central and peripheral nervous systems. Functionally, there are the somatic and autonomic nervous systems.

Peripheral nervous system

The PNS consists of the nerves and ganglia located outside the brain and the spinal cord and principally functions to connect the central nervous system (CNS) to the head, body, limbs and viscera. With respect to nomenclature, a 'nerve(s)' is by definition, in the PNS, making the word 'peripheral' (as in 'peripheral nerve') redundant; it is myelinated by Schwann cells. Unlike the CNS, the PNS is not protected by bone, leaving it more vulnerable to mechanical injury. Schwann cells form the insulating myelin sheaths surrounding peripheral axons, whereas in the CNS that task is performed by oligodendrocytes. Afferent and efferent axons of the PNS form the spinal and cranial nerves (CNN).

Spinal nerves

Spinal nerves arise as roots from the spinal cord. A dorsal and a ventral root attach on each side of the spinal cord, and define each spinal cord segment. For example, the third cervical spinal cord segment has two dorsal roots and two ventral roots attaching to it. The dorsal roots convey primarily sensory nerve fibres into the spinal cord. Each dorsal root contains a spinal ganglion (old name 'dorsal root ganglion'), housing neuronal cell bodies of these sensory fibres (Fig. 1.1). The ventral roots convey motor nerve fibres away from the spinal cord. Motor fibres may be somatic and innervate striated muscle, or autonomic and innervate smooth or cardiac muscle. The dorsal and ventral roots fuse at the level of the intervertebral foramen to form a spinal nerve. Distal to the intervertebral foramen, the mixed sensory and motor spinal nerve usually splits into a dorsal and ventral branch. The dorsal branch supplies the

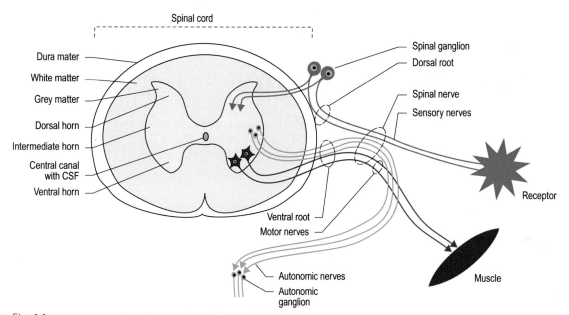

Fig. 1.1 **Transverse section of thoracic spinal cord showing the spinal nerve and its components. Note: arrows indicate direction in which action potentials travel, circles indicate neuronal cell bodies.**

epaxial muscles and skin, while the ventral branch supplies the hypaxial muscles and skin. A third branch, carrying autonomic fibres, may also arise and pass ventrally towards the midline to supply the viscera (Fig. 1.1).

Spinal nerves may remain as single, discrete nerves all the way out into the periphery, in which case they are named for the number of the spinal cord segment from which they arise, e.g. 'C3, ventral branch' is the ventral division of cervical spinal nerve 3; it supplies sensory and motor innervation to the hypaxial tissue of the neck. Alternatively, in a nerve plexus, the ventral branches of two or three adjacent spinal nerves may fuse, giving rise to nerves with specific names, such as radial nerve and femoral nerve (Fig. 1.2).

A cranial nerve arises from the brain; it is known by both the number of the nerve and a specific name, e.g. trigeminal nerve or cranial nerve, CN V (Fig. 1.6A).

The PNS comprises afferent (sensory) fibres and their receptors, and efferent (motor) fibres that link to effectors, such as striated, cardiac and smooth muscle.

Afferent nerve fibres originate at different types of sensory receptors and most of their fibres only synapse once they reach the CNS. The sensory nerve cell bodies of spinal nerves are located in spinal ganglia sited at the level of the intervertebral foramen. Cranial nerve ganglia are located just near, or inside, the neurocranium. The area of skin innervated by a spinal nerve is called a dermatome, while the area of skin innervated by a specific named nerve, which originates from two or more spinal nerves (for example, the radial nerve) is called a cutaneous zone. Adjacent dermatomes and cutaneous zones usually overlap. The area of skin innervated purely by one nerve is called an autonomous zone (Fig. 1.3). Autonomous zones are found on the head (Figure 10.13) as well as the body and limbs (Table 1.1).

Knowing the position of dermatomes and autonomous zones is useful for assessing sensory function of the PNS. However, there are species differences, for example, the horse does not have an autonomous zone specific to the radial nerve.

Motor neurons can be defined as upper motor neurons (UMNs) or lower motor neurons (LMNs). The UMN is confined to the CNS and its axon influences activity

Table 1.1 **Autonomous zones in the canine limb**			
Thoracic limb nerves	**Site for testing autonomous zone**	**Pelvic limb nerves**	**Site for testing autonomous zone**
Musculocutaneous nerve	Medial aspect of antebrachium	Saphenous nerve	Medial aspect of crus (stifle to hock)
Radial nerve	Dorsal aspect digits 2, 3, 4	Fibular (peroneal) nerve	Dorsal aspect digits 2, 3, 4
Ulnar nerve	Lateral aspect digit 5	Tibial nerve	Plantar aspect digits 3 and 4

of LMNs. They are the 'managers' of the motor system (see Chapter 4). The LMNs are found in cranial nerves, originating from the brainstem, and spinal nerves from the spinal cord. They form synapses at the neuromuscular junction and innervate striated muscle, smooth or cardiac muscle. They are the 'workers' of the motor system. The neurochemical that connects the electrical activity of the motor nerve to the striated muscle is acetylcholine (ACh). A nerve impulse arriving at the nerve termination triggers release of ACh (Fig. 1.4). The ACh crosses the synaptic cleft, binds to the receptors on the post-synaptic membrane and may stimulate muscle membrane depolarisation and muscle contraction, depending on stimulus strength and amount of ACh released. The ACh is broken down by acetylcholine esterase and recycled back into the distal end of the LMN. For striated muscle, the motor unit is defined as an axon and the muscle fibres it innervates. Motor units range in size from 3–150 muscle fibres per axon for muscles with fine versus coarse control, respectively. Small motor units are found in extraocular muscles, whereas large motor units are found in the large, postural muscles, e.g. the quadriceps femoris muscle.

Cranial nerves
In domestic mammals, there are 12 pairs of cranial nerves. Like the spinal nerves, these may convey sensory, motor and autonomic fibres of the parasympathetic nervous system (see p4). Cranial nerves are abbreviated to CN (singular) or CNN (plural).

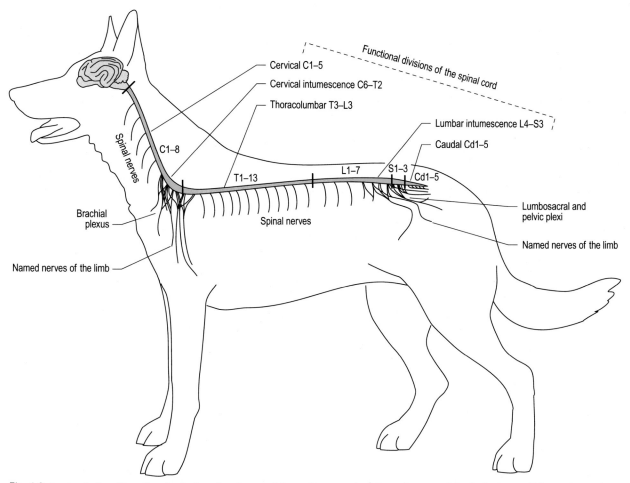

Fig. 1.2 **Anatomical and functional spinal cord regions and the main nerve plexi. Named nerves of the limbs (e.g. radial n. or femoral n.) are formed by the fusion of the ventral branches of 2+ spinal nerves, in the limb's neural plexus.**

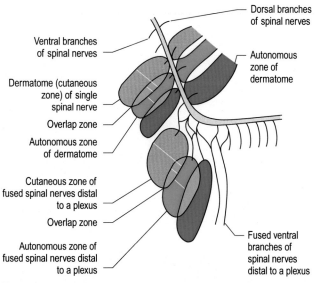

Fig. 1.3 **Sensory innervation of the skin depicting the basis of dermatomes, cutaneous zones and autonomous zones. The zones in this diagram are conceptual and not anatomically accurate to the thoracic limb.**

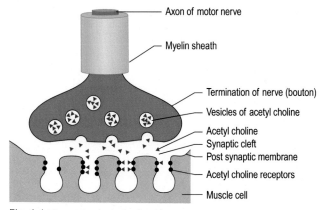

Fig. 1.4 **The neuromuscular junction.**

fibres generally remain distinct from other cranial nerves, but occasionally they may intermingle. For example, CN XI fibres travel in the vagus nerve to contribute to the recurrent laryngeal nerve. The nerves and their branches have specific names, e.g. auriculopalpebral branch of the facial nerve, CN VII.

Using Roman numerals, the nerves are numbered in rostro-caudal sequence based on their attachment to the brain. Assessing the function of the cranial nerves is an integral part of the clinical examination. They are covered in more detail in Chapter 10.

Sensory ganglia are located near, or just inside, the neurocranium whereas the somata of motor nerves are located primarily in the brainstem. The exception is the external branch of the accessory nerve (CN XI); these fibres originate in the cervical spinal cord. The cranial nerve

Autonomic nervous system

Key points

- The ANS consists of efferent and afferent fibres that innervate smooth and cardiac muscle of viscera. It has both central and peripheral components and its fibres travel in the PNS via cranial and spinal nerves.
- Functionally, the efferent side is divided into sympathetic ('fight or flight') and parasympathetic ('rest and digest') components.
- Anatomically, these divisions are also referred to as the thoracolumbar and craniosacral systems based on the origin of fibres from the CNS.

The ANS is variably defined depending on the source, but consists of efferent fibres that innervate smooth and cardiac muscle of viscera. In this book, afferent nerves from the viscera are considered to be part of the ANS. The ANS has both central and peripheral components; the latter are found in cranial and spinal nerves.

The ANS functions largely without conscious input to maintain homeostasis in the body at rest and during times of stress. It is divided on the basis of function into two components, the parasympathetic and sympathetic nervous systems. The parasympathetic system is known as the 'rest and digest' system and controls day-to-day activities such as digestion, elimination of wastes and activity that contributes to homeostasis. The sympathetic system is called the 'fight or flight' system and prepares the body for these activities by increasing heart and respiratory rate, dilating the pupils, redirecting blood flow to major limb muscles and away from activities such as digestion.

Anatomically, the two systems arise from different areas of the CNS. The parasympathetic system arises from the brainstem and sacral spinal cord, hence it is called the craniosacral system. The sympathetic system arises from the thoracolumbar spinal cord and is called the thoracolumbar system. For both parasympathetic and sympathetic systems, the nerve fibres leaving the CNS will synapse in a ganglion once en route to their target organ.

Central nervous system

Key points

- The CNS consists of the spinal cord and the brain.
- The spinal cord is divided into five clinically important, functional regions: cervical, cervical intumescence, thoracolumbar, lumbar intumescence and caudal regions.
- Anatomically, the divisions of the brain are the forebrain, the midbrain and the hindbrain. Functionally, the divisions of the brain are the forebrain, brainstem and cerebellum and each portion is associated with distinctive functions.
- Grey matter houses neuronal somata. White matter is formed by axons, many of which have lipid-rich myelin sheaths, causing the white appearance.
- In the spinal cord, neurons forming the sensory, autonomic or motor regions of grey matter are centrally located; they form longitudinal columns extending the length of the cord. In the brainstem, the grey matter columns are fragmented into clusters of cells called nuclei. In the forebrain, there are both superficial and deeply located grey matter.

The CNS comprises the spinal cord and brain. Externally, it is covered by three layers of fibrous, supporting tissue, the meninges (see Chapter 3). Internally, the ventricular system forms a series of fluid-filled spaces that connect to the externally located, subarachnoid space. The ventricular system contains cerebrospinal fluid (CSF) (see Chapter 3).

Spinal cord

The spinal cord is protected by the vertebral column. It is divided into five anatomical regions based on the vertebral column, and five functional regions based on the innervation of the limbs. Table 1.2 refers to canine neuroanatomy.

The number of vertebrae varies for different types of animals; consequently the number of spinal cord segments will also vary (Table 1.3).

In transverse section the spinal cord is tubular in shape, with a small central canal filled with CSF. It is divided anatomically into peripheral white matter and central grey matter. The butterfly-shaped grey matter is where somata are located; this is divided functionally into two or three main regions called horns. The horns form continuous columns of nerve cells that extend along the spinal cord. The white matter comprises tracts travelling cranially (ascending/sensory), caudally (descending/motor) and between segments (intersegmental). It is divided into anatomical regions called funiculi (Fig. 1.5). The spinal cord is covered in more detail in Chapter 4.

Table 1.2 Anatomical and functional regions of the canine spinal cord (see also Fig. 1.2)

Anatomical region	Spinal cord segments	Functional region and area supplied	Spinal cord segments
Cervical	C1–C8	Cervical: neck	C1–C5
Thoracic	T1–T13	Cervical intumescence: thoracic limb	C6–T2
Lumbar	L1–L7	Thoracolumbar: thorax and abdomen	T3–L3
Sacral	S1–S3	Lumbar intumescence: pelvic cavity, pelvic limb, perineum	L4–S3
Caudal	Cd1–Cd5	Caudal: tail	Cd1–Cd5

Table 1.3 Numbers of vertebrae in different types of animals

Animal	Cervical	Thoracic	Lumbar	Sacral	Caudal
Dog and cat	7	13	7 (occasionally 6)	3	20+
Horse	7	18	6	5	20
Ox	7	13	6	5	18–20
Sheep	7	13	6 (7)	4	16–18
Goat	7	13	6 (7)	5	16–18
Swine	7	14–15	6–7	4	20–23
Camelid	7	12	7	4	13–15
Bird	8–25	7 – four fuse to form notarium	Synsacrum – last 1–2 thoracic, plus the lumbar, sacral and first caudal vertebrae		5–6 free vertebrae, then pygostyle

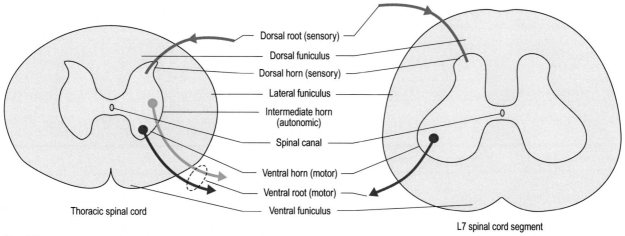

Fig. 1.5 **Thoracic and lumbar spinal cords in transverse section depicting the basic arrangement of white and grey matter.**

Table 1.4 **Functions of the different regions of grey and white matter in the spinal cord**

Grey matter	Function	White matter	Function
Dorsal horn	Sensory	Dorsal funiculus	Cranially projecting sensory (proprioceptive, tactile and nociceptive) Bidirectional, intraspinal connections
Intermediate horn (thoracolumbar and sacral segments only)	Autonomic	Lateral funiculus	Cranially projecting sensory (proprioceptive, tactile, nociception, thermal) Caudally projecting motor facilitating flexor muscle activity Bidirectional, intraspinal connections
Ventral horn	Motor	Ventral funiculus	Caudally projecting motor facilitating extensor muscle activity Some cranially projecting sensory (nociceptive) Bidirectional, intraspinal connections

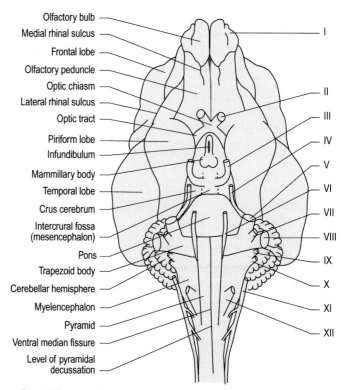

Fig. 1.6A **Canine brain, ventral aspect (see Fig. A3).**

The basic anatomy and associated function of the different components of the spinal cord are outlined in Table 1.4.

The sulcus limitans is a small transverse fissure located laterally in the walls of the central canal of the spinal cord; it extends rostrally into the brainstem. This fissure arose during embryological development. It demarcates the dorsal, sensory component (alar plate) from the ventral, motor component (basal plate) (see Chapter 2).

Brain – forebrain, brainstem, cerebellum

The brain is housed in the protective neurocranium comprising frontal, parietal, occipital, temporal, ethmoid and sphenoid bones.

It can be divided anatomically and functionally. Anatomically there are three major divisions called the forebrain or prosencephalon, the midbrain or mesencephalon, and the hindbrain or rhombencephalon. These anatomical divisions may be subdivided further.

The three major functional divisions of the brain are the forebrain, brainstem and cerebellum. For functional reasons, we define the brainstem to include the midbrain, pons and medulla oblongata; however, some authors include the diencephalon in the brainstem as it is the stem on which the telencephalon and cerebellum sit (Table 1.5).

Anatomically, on the dorsal and lateral aspects, the brain is dominated by two large, ovoid cerebral hemispheres that are elongated in the longitudinal direction. Caudal to the hemispheres, on the midline and extending for a variable distance laterally, (species specific) is the cerebellum. The longitudinal fissure separates the hemispheres from each other, whilst the transverse fissure separates the hemispheres from the cerebellum (see Fig. A1 in the appendix).

Ventrally, the rostral aspect of domestic animals is dominated by the paired olfactory bulbs (Fig. 1.6A). These are small in humans (Fig. 10.3) and miniscule, or totally absent, in many cetaceans. Caudally, the olfactory bulbs are connected via the olfactory tract to the more laterally placed, piriform lobes. On the midline is the diencephalon with the optic chiasm, hypophysis (pituitary gland), and mamillary

Table 1.5 **Regions of the brain, their general function and associated cranial nerves UMN = upper motor neuron**

Anatomical division and components	Functional division	Main functions	Cranial nerves
Telencephalon Part of the prosencephalon Paired cerebral hemispheres	Forebrain	Reception and processing of sensory input, information integration, voluntary motor control, memory, behaviour	I
Diencephalon Part of the prosencephalon, includes the thalamus, hypothalamus, subthalamus, epithalamus and metathalamus	Forebrain	Gateway to the forebrain Relay centre for information entering the cerebrum Alertness (arousal) and awareness Autonomic and homeostatic regulatory control including salt/water balance and the pineal gland (circadian and seasonal reproductive activity) Part of UMN system	II
Mesencephalon Dorsal aspect = tectum Ventral aspect = the cerebral peduncle (tegmentum, substantia nigra and crus cerebri)	Midbrain – rostral brainstem	UMN nuclei Passing through it are cranially projecting sensory input from the limbs, body and head, caudally projecting motor output from forebrain Arousal Reflex function for hearing and vision	III IV
Metencephalon part of the rhombencephalon Ventral = pons Dorsal = cerebellum	Pons (part of the brainstem) and the cerebellum	Pons: UMN nuclei Passing through it are cranially projecting sensory input from the limbs, body and head, caudally projecting motor output from forebrain Arousal/awareness Cerebellum: coordination of motor function. Originates from the metencephalon, but is functionally distinct from the brainstem	V
Myelencephalon Part of the rhombencephalon Also called medulla oblongata	Medulla oblongata (caudal brainstem)	UMN nuclei Passing through it are cranially projecting sensory input from the limbs, body and head, caudally projecting motor output from forebrain Arousal Main cardiovascular and respiratory control centres	VI VII VIII IX X XI XII

UMN = upper motor neuron.

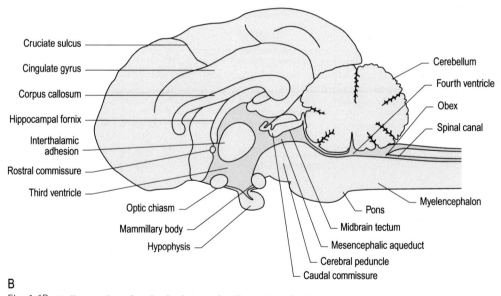

B

Fig. 1.6B **Median section of canine brain (see also Figs. 3.11 and A4).**

bodies (Fig 1.6B). Caudal to this is the midbrain with the crus cerebri (cerebral peduncles) conveying efferent information from the forebrain to the brainstem; the intercrural fossa is sited between the paired crura. Caudal to the midbrain is the pons of the ventral metencephalon, and then the medulla oblongata with the trapezoid body and the pyramids extending to the spinal cord junction.

Brainstem
The brainstem forms a stalk connecting between the spinal cord and the cerebral hemispheres. The brainstem has a similar cross-sectional arrangement to that of the tubular

spinal cord except that in the medulla oblongata, the dorsal aspect of the tube has been opened up and the roof plate expanded (Fig. 1.7). The fluid-filled ventricular system is enlarged in this region, forming the fourth ventricle; this ventricle connects to the subarachnoid space via the lateral apertures (see Chapter 3). Rostral to the fourth ventricle is the mesencephalic aqueduct and caudally, the roof plate tapers and fuses on the midline at the site of the obex, reducing the ventricular system to the tube that continues caudally as the central canal.

The white matter is superficial and the grey matter is located deeper within the brainstem. The sulcus limitans

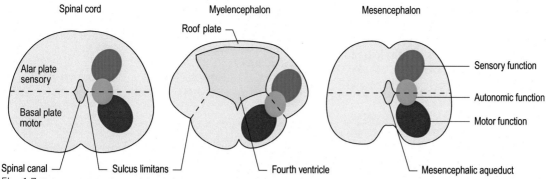

Fig. 1.7 **Transverse sections of the spinal cord, medulla oblongata and midbrain and the function of the nuclei in the different dorsoventral regions.**

is more visible in parts of the brainstem than it is in the spinal cord. It still separates dorsal, sensory areas from the ventral, motor areas; however, in the fourth ventricle region it is displaced to a ventrolateral position. Autonomic (parasympathetic) grey matter is located at the level of the sulcus limitans at the intermediate position.

In the spinal cord, the grey matter forms continuous longitudinal columns, such that the sensory dorsal horn observed in cross-section is continuous along the length of the spinal cord. The same applies to the motor ventral horn. The autonomic nerve cells of the intermediate horn are present in the thoracolumbar area (sympathetic function) and the sacral area (parasympathetic function). The grey matter of the brainstem is similar to that of the cord in that it is longitudinally arranged, but the columns have become fragmented to form clusters of cell bodies with the same function. These clusters are called nuclei and many nuclei are associated with the cranial nerves (Fig. 10.2).

Nuclei are collections of neuronal cell bodies, with similar functions, located *within* the CNS (Fig. 1.7). Ganglia are collections of nerve cell bodies, with similar functions, located *outwith* the CNS. Thus, it is inaccurate to refer to the 'basal ganglia' of the forebrain. The correct term is basal nuclei.

The dorsal aspect of the midbrain is associated with four bulges that together form the paired rostral and caudal colliculi (*colliculus* – L = hill) (Figs. A5, A7). The two pairs of colliculi form the corpora quadrigemina (L = four bodies). The caudal colliculi are more widely separated from each other than are the rostral colliculi.

The reticular formation (*rete* – L = net) is a diffuse network of neurons extending from the medulla oblongata to the thalamus. It has a variety of functions including arousal/awareness, UMN function, cardiac and respiratory control centres.

Cerebellum

Prenatally, the cerebellum develops as a dorsal outgrowth of the metencephalon and adopts a complex structure. It has a highly convoluted surface with sulci (grooves) and folia (ridges). Grossly, it has a longitudinal, median ridge, the vermis, and two lateral hemispheres. The vermis is divided into approximately ten lobules (Fig. 7.1) that are associated with coordinating different aspects of motor function. For example, the caudoventral lobule, the nodulus and its adjacent hemispheres, the flocculus, together form the flocculonodular lobe. This lobe is also called the vestibulocerebellum as it connects to the vestibular nuclei

Table 1.6 **Regions of the diencephalon and their major functions**		
Region of diencephalon	**Anatomical location**	**Main functions**
Thalamus	Midline: paired thalamic nuclei connected via the interthalamic adhesion, which passes through centre of third ventricle	Relay centre for incoming information, except olfaction Integration between cerebral areas Cerebral arousal
Hypothalamus	Ventral to the thalamus, forming the walls and floor of third ventricle Includes rostral (supraoptic) intermediate (tuberal) and caudal (mammillary) areas	Brain centre regulating autonomic motor activity
Subthalamus	Caudolateral to hypothalamus; ventral to the thalamus	Part of UMN motor control system
Metathalamus	Caudodorsal to thalamus; between the thalamus and the midbrain Includes the geniculate bodies	Relay centre for visual or auditory stimuli
Epithalamus	Dorso-medial to thalamus Includes the pineal gland and habenular nuclei. The latter has connections with the limbic system and olfactory regions	Circadian rhythms Autonomic responses to olfactory and emotional stimuli

of the brainstem. It is responsible for coordinating motor function to maintain the animal's balance (see Chapter 7).

Forebrain

The forebrain comprises the two cerebral hemispheres (cerebrum/telencephalon) and the thalamus (diencephalon). The thalamus acts like a gateway between the brainstem and the cerebrum such that all incoming information (except olfaction) approaches the cerebrum via the thalamus of the diencephalon. Thus the thalamus acts like a post office, receiving incoming mail from the brainstem, sorting it and sending it on to specific addresses within the cerebrum. It also receives local mail from the cerebrum and posts it back to other telencephalic areas. The diencephalon has five major subdivisions each associated with different functions, as outlined in Table 1.6.

The cerebrum comprises two hemispheres (Figs. 1.8, A1). The surface of the hemispheres may be smooth (lissencephalic) or convoluted (gyrencephalic), forming gyri (ridges) and sulci (troughs) (Figs. 1.9, A2). The convolutions permit more cortical surface area to be contained in the same volume of cranial vault. The convoluted cortex is usual in most species of veterinary interest; however, rodents, lagomorphs, birds and most marsupials are naturally lissencephalic (Fig. 1.8). Developing carnivores and primates are lissencephalic until relatively late in gestation.

Most of the grey matter is located superficially forming the cerebral cortex (Fig. 1.12). Grey matter is also located deep within the hemispheres in the hippocampus, the basal nuclei and septal nuclei. The hemispheres are divided into lobes named mainly for the overlying bone (Figs. 1.10 and 1.11 and Table 1.7). These lobes are loosely associated with different functions.

In vertebrate animals, brain weight is closely correlated with body weight, thus an adult sperm whale has a brain that weighs five times more than that of a human. However, the white matter increases as a cubic function while the surface area and grey matter content only increase as a square function: thus brains from larger animals have a higher white matter to grey matter ratio. In an evolutionary

Table 1.7 **Lobes of the cerebrum and their major functions. Cognition is the ability to integrate a sensory input with other information such as memory. Thus an object that has been sensed can be recognised**		
Region of cerebral hemisphere	**Anatomical location**	**Main functions**
Frontal lobe	Deep to the frontal bone, forming rostral third of the hemisphere	Motor cortex, association areas involved in planning actions and movement
Parietal lobe	Deep to the parietal bone. Dorsal midline strip caudal to frontal lobe, extending one-third of the way down lateral aspect	Somatosensory (somesthetic) cortex and association areas Cognitive association areas involved in perceiving sensory input
Temporal lobe	Deep to the temporal bone Ventrolateral mid portion of cerebral hemispheres	Audition, limbic system, learning and memory
Occipital lobe	Deep to the occipital bone, caudal third of hemispheres	Vision Cognitive association areas
Rhinencephalon	Ventro-lateral aspect of each hemisphere, ventral to lateral rhinal sulcus, dorsal to the sphenoid bones and caudal to ethmoid bone. Includes the olfactory bulbs, piriform lobe and hippocampus	Olfaction, limbic system, learning and memory

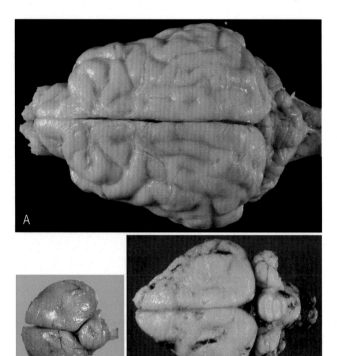

Fig. 1.8 **Comparative anatomy of dog (A), bird (B) and rabbit brains (C) (dorsal aspects). Note the convoluted, gyrencephalic hemispheres in the dog brain, but lissencephalic hemispheres of the bird and rabbit brains. (Brains not to scale.)**

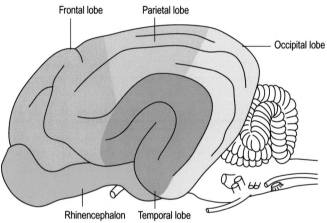

Fig. 1.10 **Mammalian brain, lateral aspect, depicting lobes of brain.**

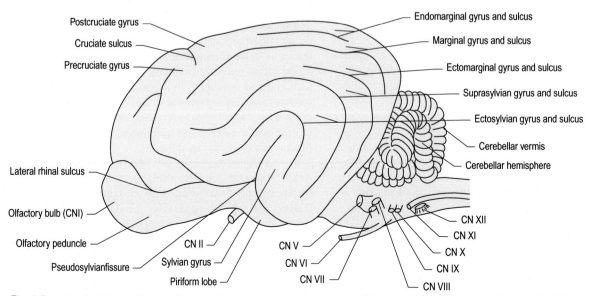

Fig. 1.9 **Canine brain from the lateral aspect. Roman numerals refer to the cranial nerves. Note: the pattern of gyri and sulci is species specific.**

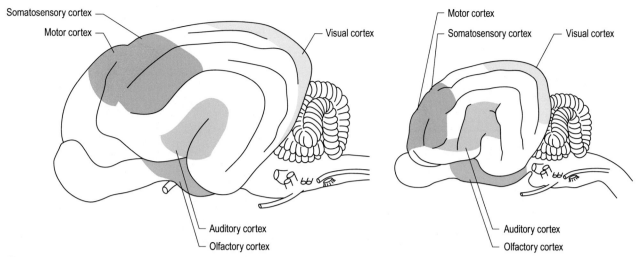

Fig. 1.11 **Lateral aspect of the brains of the dog (left) and cat (right) depicting the main functional areas of the brain.**

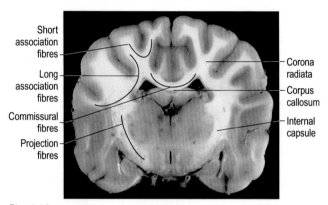

Fig. 1.12 **Dog brain, transverse section, at the level of the thalamus, illustrating white matter connections.**

Fig. 1.13 **Sheep brain, paramedian section, depicting white matter connections of the cerebrum to the brainstem via the internal capsule (courtesy of the Veterinary Virtual Museum, IVABS, Massey University).**

sense, the cortex is divided into primitive, old and new regions. These are the paleopallium (*paleo*, derived from the Greek for ancient; *pallium* – L = cloak), archipallium (*archi* – Gk = primitive) and the neopallium (*neo* – Gk = new). The paleopallium is ventral to the lateral rhinal sulcus and is largely associated with olfaction. It is relatively large in domestic animals compared with primates. The archipallium, which includes the hippocampus, is a region of the brain that originally functioned to correlate olfactory input with other sensory information, but evolved to acquire other functions such as behaviour (see Chapter 11). It is medially located. The neopallium is the largest part of the cerebrum, separated from the archipallium by the splenial sulcus medially and from the paleopallium by the lateral rhinal sulcus, ventrally (see Figs. A2, A4). It includes the primary receiving areas for vision, audition and sensory inputs, as well as integration areas.

White matter tracts form connections within the forebrain (association and commissural fibres) and to other parts of the CNS (projection fibres) (Fig. 1.12). Association fibres connect within a hemisphere. Short association fibres connect within a lobe between adjacent gyri, while long association fibres connect between lobes within the same hemisphere. Commissural fibres connect across the midline between hemispheres. The main commissural fibres are bundled together as the corpus callosum. This forms an elongated, transverse band of white matter at the base of the longitudinal fissure. Projection fibres connect between the hemispheres and the brainstem (Fig. 1.13). Corticopetal and corticofugal projection fibres enter and leave the cerebrum, respectively; they do so via the internal capsule.

Functional systems: introduction to the neurological examination

The nervous system is organised into functional systems. Most diseases principally affect one, or more, functional systems due to their proximity, so the nervous system needs to be considered functionally and not just anatomically (Table 1.8, see specific chapters).

Neuroanatomy and lesion localisation

Key point

■ The primary goal of the neurological examination is to anatomically localise the lesion(s). As diseases are often region specific, neuroanatomical localisation is critical for constructing a sensible list of diagnostic possibilities.

Table 1.8 **Motor and sensory classification of the nervous system**

Motor or sensory	Functional system	Functions and locations of the neural system
Motor	Somatic efferent	UMNs and LMNs influencing striated muscle, all spinal nerves to body, limbs and head CNN III, IV, V, VI, VII, IX, X, XI, XII
	Autonomic efferent	Autonomic UMNs and LMNs. To smooth and cardiac muscle of the viscera and vasculature, and to glandular myoepithelium
		Sympathetic: thoracolumbar spinal nerves
		Parasympathetic: sacral spinal nerves and CNN III, VII, IX, X, XI
Sensory	Somatic afferent	Touch, temperature, mechanoreception from body, limbs and head. All spinal nerves, CN V, VII, IX and X
	Special senses	Olfaction: CN I
		Vision: CN II
		Taste: CN VII, IX, X
		Hearing: CN VIII
	Autonomic afferent	Sensory impulses from viscera and blood vessels (distension, chemical changes, e.g. pH) CNN VII, IX, X, spinal nerves
	General proprioception (conscious and subconscious)	Muscle and joint position and movement, tactile input from body, limbs and head. All spinal nerves, CN V
	Vestibular proprioception	Vestibular input from inner ears and spinal cord, CN VIII, spinal nerves
	Nociception	From body, limbs and head CNN VII, IX, X and all spinal nerves

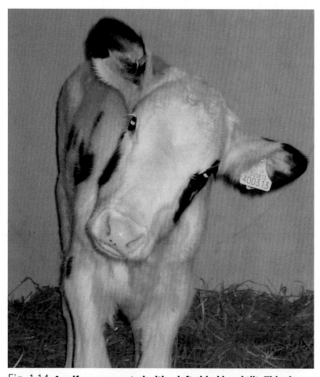

Fig. 1.14 **A calf was presented with a left-sided head tilt. This sign combined with the loss of extensor tone on the left side strongly suggested a deficit in the vestibular system on the left side. But the head tilt did not indicate if the lesion was in the brain (vestibular nuclei in the brainstem) or inner ear (semicircular ducts). However, on neurological examination, no other cranial nerve deficits, general proprioceptive deficits or upper motor neuron paresis were identified: this indicated that the lesion did not affect the motor tracts arising in the brainstem, the sensory tracts going through the brainstem, or the cranial nerve nuclei in that region of the brainstem. Thus both normal and abnormal clinical signs were used to localise the lesion. As there were no brainstem signs, the lesion was localised to the inner ear. A presumptive inner ear infection was successfully treated with antibiotics.**

The primary goal of the neurological examination, and a good reason to study neuroanatomy, is to localise the lesion. The location of a lesion, or lesions, is fundamental to making a diagnosis in a case with neurological signs and cannot be replaced by other diagnostic tests such as advanced imaging. Not all abnormalities noted by imaging are clinically significant. The location of the abnormality must be able to explain the clinical signs.

Localising a neurological lesion relies on identifying both those neural systems that are dysfunctional AND those systems that are functioning normally (Fig. 1.14).

It matters little where a lesion is located on a pathway (origin, midway along the pathway, or termination), it will still produce similar signs of dysfunction. Most regions of the nervous system are associated with a number of functions either because a neural pathway begins or ends in that region, or is passing through it. The key to localising the lesion is based on having knowledge about which functional pathways are associated with that region, and conversely, which pathways are not.

If a lesion is in a particular region, then it could cause signs of dysfunction due to damage to pathways in that region. However if a pathway does not pass through that region, then it will not be affected. Thus knowledge of those neural systems that are functioning normally indicates to the examiner that the lesion is not located in the region that those systems occupy (Fig. 13.1). For example, if the lesion is in the thoracolumbar spinal cord, then pathways passing through that part of the cord may be damaged; these include proprioception and UMN tracts to the pelvic limbs. But the lesion will not affect the cranial nerves or the function of the thoracic limbs, as the neural systems do not pass through that region. Therefore, noting the normal CNN and normal thoracic limb function is just as important as noting the UMN signs and proprioceptive deficits in the pelvic limbs.

Chapter 2
Neuroembryology

Key points

- During early embryonic development, the neuroectoderm forms the neural tube and neural crest; these structures give rise to the central nervous system (CNS) and cells of the peripheral nervous system (PNS), respectively.
- The neural tube forms the spinal cord and brain, and the neural canal forms the inner ventricular system. The brain divides into prosencephalon, mesencephalon and rhombencephalon.
- Dorsal outgrowths of the neural tube give rise to the cerebrum and cerebellum. The degree of cerebellar development at birth determines the mobility of a neonatal animal.
- Germinal cells surrounding the neural canal give rise to neurons and glial cells; these cells migrate to form grey and white matter. The germinal layer becomes the ependyma in the postnatal animal.
- Neuronal differentiation is determined by extracellular morphogens. Sonic Hedgehog protein triggers motor neuron development in the ventral spinal cord, while Bone Morphogenetic Protein induces sensory neuron differentiation in the dorsal spinal cord. Different homeobox proteins signal the longitudinal differentiation of the spinal cord.
- Neuronal precursors migrate in response to molecular signals. Axonal growth is directed by chemoattractants or chemorepellants in the extracellular environment.

Development of the CNS

Formation of the neural tube

The notochord is derived from the mesoderm and establishes the cranial–caudal axis of the embryo. It induces the overlying ectoderm to become neurectoderm. The neurectoderm thickens to form the neural plate along the dorsal, longitudinal axis of the embryo. A longitudinal trough appears in the midline of the neural plate, forming the neural groove. The sides of the plate rise up and seal over the top of the groove to form the neural tube, which surrounds a fluid-filled, neural canal. Closure of the neural tube is called primary neurulation; it occurs at about 20 days in the canine fetus (canine gestation is approximately 60 days). Closure starts in the cervical region and extends rostrally and caudally from that point. The ends of the tube may remain open for a period as the rostral and caudal neuropores. Just prior to neural tube formation, neural crest cells develop, located dorsolaterally at the junction between the neurectoderm and the ectoderm. The neural crest cells separate from the neurectoderm and the ectoderm as the tube develops. Columns of neural crest cells form along the dorsolateral aspects of the neural tube, while the ectoderm separates and fuses dorsal to the neural tube creating the overlying skin (Fig. 2.1). The neural tube extends the length of the embryo including into the head region and forms the basis of the spinal cord and the brain. The neural canal will develop into the inner ventricular system (see Chapter 3). Inside the head, the neural tube develops into three regions, the prosencephalon (forebrain = telencephalon and diencephalon), the mesencephalon (midbrain) and the rhombencephalon (hindbrain = metencephalon and myelencephalon). The sulcus limitans is a groove that forms in the lateral walls of the neural canal. It demarcates the tube into dorsal/alar and ventral/basal plates that are associated with sensory and motor functions, respectively (Fig. 2.2).

During differentiation of the neural tube, three cell layers develop from the original pseudostratified, single cell layer. Innermost, sited around the neural canal, is the germinal layer, in which cellular proliferation occurs giving rise to both neurons and the supporting glial cells, oligodendrocytes and astrocytes. The post-mitotic cells migrate so that the neurons are located in the middle or mantle layer, while their axons extend into the marginal layer (Fig. 2.2). Astrocytes are found in both the mantle and marginal layer, while oligodendrocytes settle in the marginal layer to myelinate the axons. After development has finished the germinal layer becomes the ependymal layer surrounding the ventricular system of the brain and the spinal cord. The mantle layer becomes the grey matter and the marginal layer becomes the white matter (except in the telencephalon, see later). The grey and white matter form continuous columns; these extend the length of the spinal cord and into the brainstem. Overall, the brainstem develops from the neural tube in a similar way to the spinal cord (see Figs. 1.7, 10.2). However, the columns of grey and white matter become fragmented with the grey matter forming nuclei. Additionally, in the rhombencephalon, the dorsal aspect of the tube opens back up forming a groove-like structure, but with a thin cover called the

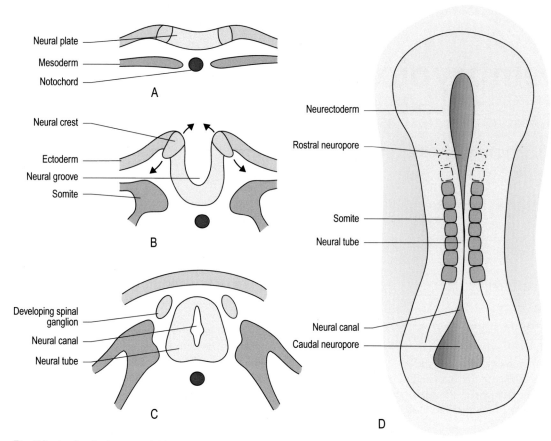

Fig. 2.1 **The developing neural tube. (A–C) Transverse sections at sequential developmental stages. (D) Dorsal aspect, without overlying ectoderm, after neurulation.**

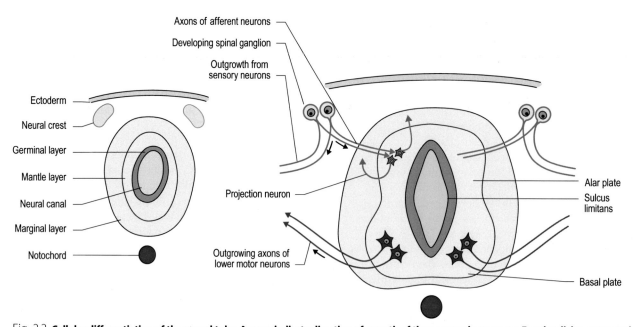

Fig. 2.2 **Cellular differentiation of the neural tube. Arrows indicate direction of growth of the neuronal processes. For simplicity, autonomic motor neurons have been left off this diagram. See figure 1.1 for further information.**

medullary velum (*velum* – L = awning). The neural canal is expanded to become the fourth ventricle. The tube reforms in the midbrain, with a small-diameter neural canal, the mesencephalic aqueduct (see Fig. 1.7).

Development of the brain

The cerebellum and the cerebral hemispheres develop as dorsal outgrowths of the neural tube. The cerebellum forms from the dorsal aspect of the metencephalon (part of the rhombencephalon) arising as bilateral, rhombic lips that grow dorsally and fuse. Neurons arising from the germinal layer surrounding the future fourth ventricle migrate dorsally into the developing cerebellum to form the Purkinje cells and the neurons of the cerebellar nuclei. The external germinal layer is a second proliferative zone for the cerebellum. It develops on the dorsal, superficial aspect of the cerebellum and is the source of the remaining neurons for the cerebellum. The timing of cell proliferation in the external germinal layer is species specific. It may be complete before birth as in precocial animals such as many prey species. Or it continues postnatally, as in altricial animals, such as carnivores, and some prey species, such as rabbits and mice. An animal's ability to ambulate in the perinatal period is directly related to the degree of cerebellar development. Prey species born in the open environment need to be able to get up and run with the herd immediately. Altricial species are usually born into a protective environment, such as a den or burrow and brain development can continue after birth (see Fig. 7.5).

The forebrain (prosencephalon) develops as two regions, the diencephalon and the telencephalon (cerebrum). The thalamus of the diencephalon represents the rostral end of the neural tube and hence, the neural canal. Proliferation of tissue across the midline joins the walls of the neural tube and forms the interthalamic adhesion that splits the neural canal into dorsal and ventral components. These canals reunite rostral to the interthalamic adhesion, thus forming a vertically oriented, ring-like structure, the third ventricle. Bilateral outgrowths from the ventral prosencephalon form the optic cups and give rise to the neurons of the retina and the optic nerve. An outgrowth from the ventral midline joins a dorsal outgrowth from the future nasopharynx, to form the hypophysis, comprising the neuro- and adenohypophysis, respectively.

The cerebral hemispheres arise from the dorsal aspect of the prosencephalon as massive, bilateral outgrowths. Each one is associated with a dorsolateral recess of the neural canal forming the lateral ventricles. These ventricles retain a connection to the third ventricle of the thalamus via the interventricular foramens. The germinal layer, which is still sited adjacent to the ventricles, is called the ventricular zone. It may continue to be a source of new neurons well into the postnatal period. Neurons migrate from the ventricular zone to the periphery of the developing cerebrum and their axons grow centrally from the surface. Thus much of the grey matter in the hemispheres is located superficially in the cerebral cortex with the white matter being located deep to that; this is the opposite of the spinal cord arrangement. However, some grey matter, such as the septal and basal nuclei and the hippocampus, end up being deeply located within the cerebral hemispheres, adjacent to the lateral ventricles. In many species, the migration of so many neurons to the surface results in the cortical surface becoming convoluted and thrown into folds comprising gyri (ridges) and sulci (troughs). Some animals, such as rodents, lagomorphs and birds retain a smooth cerebral cortex; these species are called lissencephalic (see Fig. 1.8).

Molecular basis of differentiation

Differentiation of the neural tube is based on the expression of different genes and occurs in all three planes – ventrodorsal, mediolateral and craniocaudal (Fig. 2.3A–C). Ventrodorsally, two major morphogens affect differentiation of the neural tube. Sonic Hedgehog (SHH) protein arising from the notochord and subsequently the floor plate, causes nerve cells in the ventral aspect of the cord to differentiate into motor neurons. Bone Morphogenetic Protein (BMP) from the overlying ectoderm, and then the roof plate, causes cells in the dorsal aspect to differentiate into sensory neurons. Diffusion of these morphogens sets up dorsoventral and mediolateral concentration gradients. Thus cells at different locations on the x–y grid will be exposed to

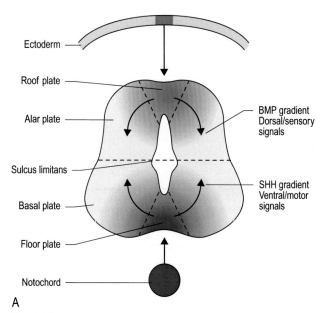

A

Fig. 2.3A **Dorsoventral differentiation of the neural tube.**

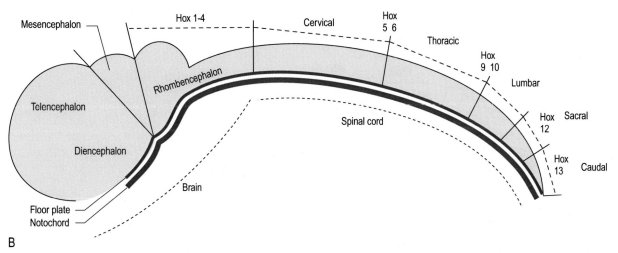

B

Fig. 2.3B **Craniocaudal differentiation of the neural tube is determined by homeobox genes.**

different concentrations of morphogen, thereby determining their differentiation. In the craniocaudal direction the homeobox genes determine the regional specification along the neural tube that forms the spinal cord. There are many other genes involved in differentiation of the brain. It is also recognised now that astrocyte differentiation is regionally specified in a similar manner.

Glial cells lay down cellular scaffolds that assist migration of neuronal precursor cells to their final position in the developing cerebellum and the cerebrum. The process by which the neurons travel along the glial fibres involves signalling and recognition of specific proteins, such as astrotactin or reelin, which are expressed by glial or neuronal cells.

Neurons must connect to their appropriate target. The tips of axons arising from differentiating neurons navigate

through the developing CNS by responding to molecular signals that may either attract or repel the tip (Fig. 2.4).

Formation of the PNS

Initially, the neural crest cells form continuous, longitudinal columns of cells on the dorsolateral aspects of the neural tube. Cells migrate from the neural crest giving rise to melanocytes, noradrenaline-secreting cells of the adrenal medulla, Schwann cells and postsynaptic nerve cell bodies of the autonomic ganglia. The neural crest columns then fragment to form cell clusters. A cluster of cells is located bilaterally at each developing spinal cord segment. The clusters become spinal ganglia, comprising nerve cell bodies associated with sensory nerves of the PNS (Figs. 2.1, 2.2). Motor nerve cell bodies of the somatic and autonomic systems are located in the ventral and intermediate horns of the spinal cord grey matter, respectively.

As in the CNS, axonal growth in the PNS also uses molecular tracking systems. The growing axonal tip responds to chemoattractants or chemorepellants present in the extracellular environment.

Malformations of the nervous system

When development does not proceed according to plan, then a variety of malformations can occur. Several examples of malformations are given. If cerebrospinal fluid (CSF) flow in the neural canal is blocked then the CSF accumulates, resulting in hydrocephalus. This causes dilation of the ventricular system and pressure on the surrounding brain tissue, which atrophies or fails to develop. The pressure may cause bulging of the skull (Fig. 2.5A). Failure of closure of the caudal neuropore can result in spina bifida (failure of vertebral arch fusion), abnormal spinal cord formation and cystic dilation of the meninges, forming meningoceles. Similarly, if the rostral neuropore fails to close, forebrain development is

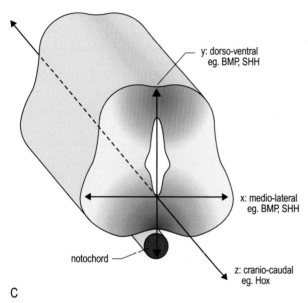

C

Fig. 2.3C **Three-dimensional gradient of differentiation of the neural tube.**

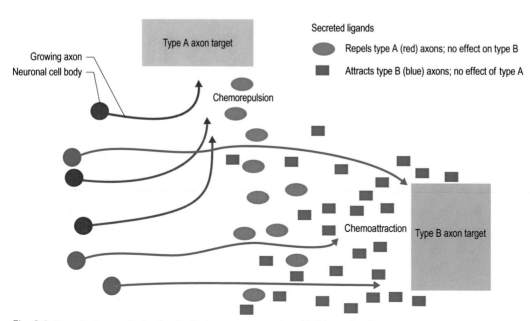

Fig. 2.4 **Growth of axons in the developing nervous system is guided by molecular cues that attract or repel them.**

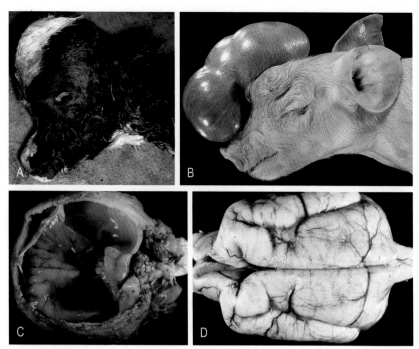

Fig. 2.5 **Malformations of the nervous system resulting in (A) hydrocephalus, (B) menigocele, (C) hydranencephaly and cerebellar hypoplasia and (D) lissencephaly. Note, (C) and (D) depict the dorsal aspect of the brains. Images courtesy of the Pathobiology Group, IVABS, Massey University.**

compromised. The meninges may protrude through the defect forming meningoceles (Fig. 2.5B) or the forebrain may fail to develop (anencephaly). Teratogens (e.g. viruses or drugs) can cause abnormal development by destroying proliferating cells, resulting in hypoplasia, e.g. of the cerebellum causing cerebellar signs. Similarly teratogens may block proliferation in the developing forebrain resulting in compensatory ventricular distension, called hydranencephaly (Fig. 2.5C). Disturbed neuronal migration or axonal growth can result from mutations in genes encoding signalling proteins that are used by migrating cells or for directing axons. Failure of neuronal migration results in underpopulated cerebral cortices and lissencephaly (Fig. 2.5D).

Chapter 3
Neurohistology, physiology and supporting structures

Neurophysiology • Assoc. Prof Craig Johnson, IVABS, Massey University
Supporting structures • Assoc. Prof Craig Johnson, IVABS, Massey University

Neurohistology

Key points

- Neurons are excitable cells that receive and integrate afferent information from receptors and other neurons, and transmit information to other neurons or effector organs.
- Nissl substance (rough endoplasmic reticulum) is a prominent feature of many healthy, neurons. The majority of neurons lack centrioles and cannot divide.
- Dendrites receive and integrate multiple synaptic inputs. Dendritic spines are specifically involved in learning and memory; they serve to increase the number of possible contacts between neurons.
- Axons are long, non-tapering cytoplasmic processes that transmit impulses; they contain organelles and a cytoskeletal transport system.
- Neuroglia provide support and nutrition, maintain homeostasis, form myelin, and participate in signal transmission in the nervous system. They include astrocytes, oligodendrocytes and microglia in the CNS. Schwann cells form myelin in the PNS.
- Synapses are the junction between the axon terminals of a neuron and a receiving cell. The majority are categorised as chemical synapses, however electrical synapses also occur.

Cells of the nervous system

The principal functional unit of the nervous system is the neuron (*neuron* – Gk = cord, nerve). This is a highly specialised and polarised cell that receives, integrates and transmits information.

In the human brain it is estimated that there are 100 billion neurons. In contrast, the well-studied nematode, *Caenorhabditis elegans*, manages to go through life with a grand total of 302 neurons. Neuroglia are 5-10 fold more numerous than neurons and function to support them. Neuroglia do not transmit action potentials (although some have synapses) but are vital for the normal function of the nervous system.

Neurons

Neurons are the core components of the vertebrate brain, spinal cord and nerves. Neurons are excitable cells that receive and integrate incoming information from sensory receptors and other neurons, and transmit information to other neurons or effector organs. A typical neuron consists of a cell body or soma. It has a series of branching processes called dendrites that receive information from surrounding excitable cells or receptors. The output of the neuron is through a single process, the axon, although this may then split into a number of collateral branches.

The soma (plural = somata) contains a relatively large, round nucleus with a prominent nucleolus (Fig. 3.1A). The size of the cell body ranges from 5 μm to more than 100 μm, for interneurons and motor neurons innervating striated muscle, respectively. The soma contains a cytoskeleton made up of neurofilaments and neurotubules. The cytoskeleton extends into the dendrites and axon, setting the diameter of, and providing internal support for, these slender processes.

The soma contains most of the synthetic machinery of the cell, such as the Golgi apparatus and endoplasmic reticulum, while mitochondria are located in both the soma and axons. Nissl substance is granular material that stains with basophilic dyes; it is composed of rough endoplasmic reticulum. Nissl substance is the site of protein synthesis and its prominence in neurons indicates that they are highly metabolically active. In neurons that are damaged, especially after axonal injury, the Nissl granules disperse; this reaction is called chromatolysis (Fig. 3.1B).

Most neurons lack centrioles, organelles involved in the organization of the cytoskeleton and the movement of chromosomes during mitosis. Consequently, most neurons cannot divide. One exception is the neurons of the olfactory mucosa. These cells can divide and replace cells destroyed by pathogens contacting the olfactory mucosa. Olfactory mucosa neurons could provide stem cells for repairing

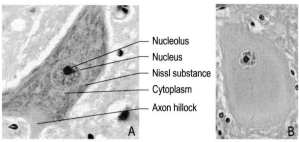

Fig. 3.1 **(A) Normal neuron with prominent Nissl granules. (B) Damaged, chromatolytic neuron.**

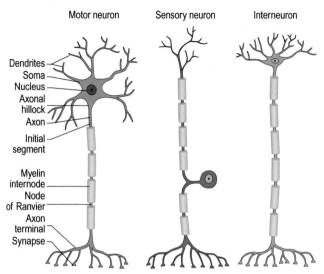

Fig. 3.2 **Basic structure of the three main classes of neurons – motorneurons, sensory neurons and interneurons. Neurons are not drawn to scale with each other.**

injured CNS tissue; this is an area of active research. Neural stem cells exist in some areas of the brain, too, such as the subventricular zone of the forebrain. They may be the source of new neurons after birth.

Dendrites (*déndron* – Gk = tree) are the branched projections of a neuron that receive input from many other neurons and conduct it to the soma. For example, the average mouse neuron receives input from 500 other neurons and has 8000 synapses. The input may be excitatory or inhibitory. The dendrites integrate the incoming information, and the balance of input determines whether action potentials will be produced by the neuron. The dendrites of some neurons are covered with small membranous protrusions called dendritic spines. Each dendritic spine may synapse with multiple axons; thus one dendrite could communicate with hundreds of axons. Abnormal spines have been shown in the brains of humans with cognitive impairments. The dendritic branching pattern of a neuron can change: it may increase or decrease. An enriched or stimulatory environment, such as when the animal is learning, is associated with dendritic growth.

Axons are cytoplasmic processes that can propagate electrical impulses. Axons may be only a few micrometres long, as in interneurons, whilst axons in blue whales may be over 10 metres long. Neurites is a term that encompasses both axons and dendrites. Efferent neurites (axons) may be differentiated from afferent neurites (dendrites) in two ways: (a) efferent neurites usually maintain a constant radius, while afferent neurites often taper; (b) efferent neurites are often much longer than afferent neurites, although this may not be the case for sensory neurons. For example a sensory neuron from the distal limb has a long afferent neurite, a cell body in the spinal ganglion and an efferent neurite that synapses in the adjacent spinal cord dorsal horn.

Owing to their length, axons usually contain the majority of the cell cytoplasm, and organelles such as neurofibrils, neurotubules, small vesicles, lysosomes, mitochondria and various enzymes. However, the majority of axonal proteins are synthesised in the soma, which may be located some distance from the distal portion of an axon (for example, consider the distance between the spinal cord and a distal limb muscle) in a horse. The axonal transport system is essential to carry material between the soma and the axonal tip. Microtubules (made of tubulin) run along the length of the axon and provide the main cytoskeletal tracks for axonal transport. The motor proteins, kinesin and dynein, move cellular cargoes in the anterograde (towards the axon tip) and retrograde (towards the cell body) directions, respectively. Motor proteins bind and transport several different cargoes including organelles such as mitochondria, cytoskeletal elements and vesicles containing neurotransmitters. Fast axonal transport is used to move

organelles, structural proteins and neurotransmitters from their sites of synthesis in the cell body to the distant reaches of the axon at rates of hundreds of centimetres per day. Slow axonal transport moves components of the cytoskeleton at speeds of up to 2.5 mm/day. A retrograde transport system runs in the opposite direction, moving organelles from the distal axon back to the cell body at rates of up to 200 mm per day.

There are many types of neurons and they differ in the size of the soma, the length of the axon and the dendritic arborisation. Neurons are the most diverse kind of cell in the body with hundreds of different types, each with specific, message-carrying abilities. Neuronal types can be divided into three main groups:

1. Sensory neurons (of the PNS) carry information from the sense organs to the neuraxis. They interface with many different types of receptor cells.
2. Motor neurons (of the PNS) carry information from the neuraxis to somatic and visceral muscles.
3. Interneurons (most common in the CNS) connect between neurons (Fig. 3.2). They may be long conveying afferent or efferent information, or shorter and used for integrating information.

Neuroglia

Neuroglia (*glia* – Gk = glue), are non-neuronal cells that provide support and nutrition, maintain homeostasis, form myelin, and participate in signal transmission in the nervous system. A number of types of neuroglia are recognised, principally astrocytes, oligodendrocytes, Schwann cells (collectively called macroglia) and microglia.

Astrocytes (*astro* – Gk = star shaped) are a heterogeneous population of cells. Morphologically distinct examples of astrocytes include the protoplasmic astrocytes of the grey matter, fibrous astrocytes of the white matter and radial astrocytes of the retina and cerebellum. Most astrocytes express glial fibrillary acidic protein (GFAP) that is used histologically as a cell-specific marker (Fig. 3.3). Astrocytes perform many functions, including contributing to the blood–brain barrier, regulation of blood flow, provision of nutrients to the nervous tissue, insulating synapses intercellular communication and maintenance of extracellular ion balance. Astrocytes have important roles

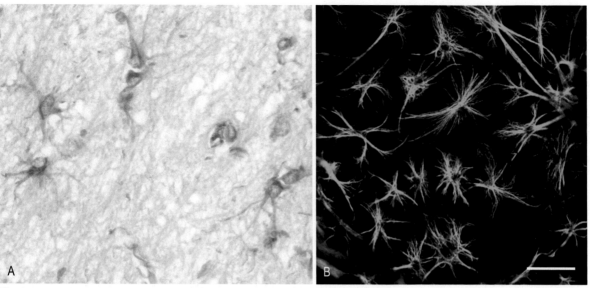

Fig. 3.3 **Astrocytes immunostained with glial fibrillary acidic protein (GFAP). (A) Reactive astrocytes in dog brain (courtesy of Prof Brian Summers, University of London). (B) Astrocytes grown in cell culture; size bar = 50 μm.**

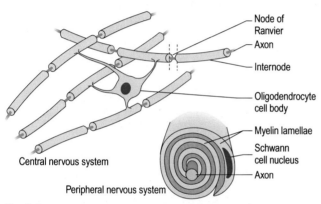

Fig. 3.4 **Oligodendrocytes myelinate one to many segments of CNS axons, whereas Schwann cells in the PNS myelinate only one axonal segment.**

in the repair and scarring process of the neuraxis following traumatic injuries or inflammatory disease. Bidirectional communication between astrocytes and neurons occurs, and their role in disease processes is increasingly being recognised.

Oligodendrocytes (*oligo* – Gk = few branches) produce the myelin sheaths that surround many axons in the CNS. Schwann cells myelinate axons in the PNS (Fig. 3.4). A single oligodendrocyte can myelinate one large diameter axon or up to 100 small diameter axons, whereas Schwann cells only myelinate single axons. Myelin is essential for rapid, targeted conduction of nerve impulses and axonal protection. The myelin sheath is formed by outgrowth of cell processes from the myelinating cell, spiralling around the axon to form the numerous layers of membrances; most of the cytoplasm is extruded and the membranes compacted, forming myelin. Adjacent segments of myelin are called internodes. Internodes are separated by 1 μm gaps called the node of Ranvier. Ion channels clustered in the axonal membrane at the node are used to propagate action potentials along the axon. The myelin sheath is lipid-rich, providing effective insulation and blocking the exchange of ions across the axonal membrane in the internodal regions. Thus the action potential skips over the internodal areas as it jumps between nodes. This is called saltatory conduction (*saltus* – L = to leap or bound).

The myelin sheath also physically protects the axon. Its loss renders the axon vulnerable to chemical and mechanical damage.

Microglia are the resident macrophages of the CNS, and thus act as the first and main form of active immunity. Microglia comprise 20% of the total glial cell population within the brain and are constantly surveying the neuraxis for damaged neurons, plaques, and infectious agents. The brain and spinal cord are considered immune-privileged organs in that they are separated from the rest of the body by the blood–brain barrier (BBB) (see Fig. 3.19). This barrier prevents many pathogens from reaching the nervous tissue, but it also blocks most antibodies from accessing the neuraxis, due to their large size. Hence, microglia must be able to recognize foreign bodies, phagocytose them and act as antigen-presenting cells to activate other immune cells.

Synapses
The term synapse designates the point where the axon of one neuron makes a functional connection with another excitable cell such as a neuron, astrocyte or effector cell. (*sunapsis* – Gk = point of contact) (see Neurophysiology section).

Neurophysiology

Key points

- Myelination increases the speed at which impulses are propagated along the myelinated fibre by enabling saltatory conduction.
- Action potentials trigger the release of neurotransmitter at a chemical synapse or neuromuscular junction. The neurotransmitter crosses the synaptic cleft and binds to receptors on the postsynaptic membrane causing chemically-gated ion channels to open. Ion transfer causes change in the postsynaptic membrane potential.
- Neurotransmitters are classed as excitatory or inhibitory depending on whether they depolarise or hyperpolarise the postsynaptic membrane potential.

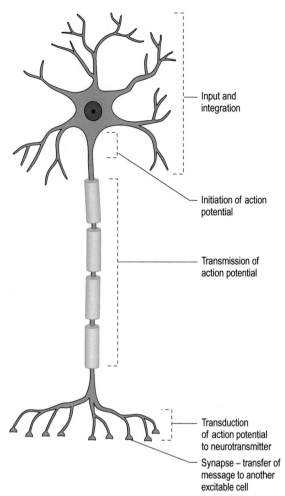

Fig. 3.5 **Functional regions of a neuron.**

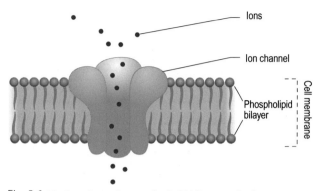

Fig. 3.6 **The ion channel spans the lipid bilayer and, when open, permits ions to flow between the inside and the outside of the cell.**

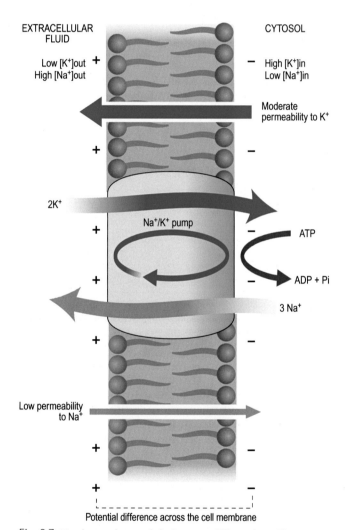

Fig. 3.7 **Membranes have a default permeability to ions. The sodium–potassium ATPase pump establishes ion concentration gradients across the plasma membrane; this is the basis of the resting membrane potential.**

There are many different types of neurons, all of which are designed to perform different functions, yet all types work using the same principles and components. Information processing occurs within the components of the neuron (Fig. 3.5) as well as at the connections between neurons. The functional capacity of the central nervous system to process information is due to both the complexity of individual neurons and their connections. Most types of neuron only connect with other neurons and glia. Some types connect with sensory receptors, while others connect with effector tissues such as muscle of the body, viscera, blood vessels and glands.

Membrane potential of excitable cells

The cell membrane is composed of a lipid bilayer that has a hydrophilic surface and a hydrophobic interior. Embedded in the cell membrane are proteins such as molecular pumps and ion channels; these are important for electrical activity. The cell membrane is responsible for the generation and maintenance of the membrane potential. In addition, the membrane of excitable cells can propagate an action potential. The membrane potential is formed by concentration gradients of ions across the plasma membrane. The gradient is formed by the high resistance of the lipid bilayer and the action of ion channels embedded in the cell membrane (Fig. 3.6).

The generator of the membrane potential is the molecular co-transporter sodium-potassium ATPase pump (Fig. 3.7). This molecule uses chemical energy in the form of ATP to transport sodium ions out of cells and potassium ions into cells. For every three positively charged sodium ions removed from the cell, two positively charged potassium ions replace them. Thus, the inside of the cell is negative with respect to the outside as the ionic gradients generate an electrical potential difference across the membrane, called membrane potential. The size of a cell's membrane potential depends on how permeable that cell's membrane is to particular ions. Permeability is a consequence of the number and type of ion channels. Ion channels allow ions to diffuse across the plasma membrane, down their concentration gradient. For example, a smooth muscle cell typically has a membrane potential of –50 mV whereas that of striated muscle will be about –95 mV. The membrane potential for a particular cell can be calculated using the Goldman equation. This equation takes into account the concentrations of ions inside and outside the cell, and the permeability of that cell membrane to those ions.

Cell membranes have an inherent permeability to ions such as sodium and potassium. The ATPase pump establishes a concentration gradient of ions, such that the ions diffuse down their concentration gradient until the charge thus generated, balances the osmotic force of the concentration gradient.

Action potential

An action potential is generated when the membrane potential of the axon hillock (see Fig. 3.2) depolarises (becomes less negative) sufficiently such that it reaches threshold potential. When threshold potential is reached, voltage-gated sodium and potassium channels open allowing massive ion diffusion across the membrane. Sodium ions move more rapidly than potassium ions and so for a brief period the membrane potential becomes much less negative as positively charged sodium ions flow into the cell. The further reduction in membrane potential allows even more voltage-gated channels to open. The change in membrane potential spreads to adjacent areas of the plasma membrane and they, too, pass threshold and become highly permeable to sodium and potassium ions. Eventually the neuron reaches a point where the membrane potential is reversed and the voltage-gated channels begin to close. The closure of the voltage-gated ion channels brings the movement of ions to an end and the membrane potential equilibrates to normal values. This change in membrane potential continues to spread along the length of the axon and is the basis for the electrical conduction of information along nerves (Fig. 3.8).

Myelination and nerve conduction

The rate at which an action potential travels along an axon is influenced by many factors including the diameter of the axon and the number of ion channels in the plasma membrane. Many axons are wrapped in a layer of lipid-rich myelin. Myelin prevents ion exchange in the internodal areas and consequently these sections of axon have few ion channels and molecular pumps. Thus action potentials are generated only at the nodes of Ranvier. In myelinated axons, action potentials travel by jumping from one node of Ranvier to the next in a process called saltatory conduction.

This makes action potential conduction both much faster (nerve impulses are conducted at speeds of up to 120 m/s) and more energy efficient. In non-myelinated axons, ion channels and molecular pumps are spread along the length of the axon. This reduces the speed of action potential conduction as well as increasing the energy expenditure.

Synapses

Neurons can be connected to each other in two distinct ways:

1. Chemical synapses in which a chemical neurotransmitter bridges the 30–50 nm space between the pre- and postsynaptic membrane (Fig. 3.9).
2. Electrical synapses in which gap junctions (protein pores) form physical contact between cells. They allow faster conduction of membrane potential changes between neurons. Unlike chemical synapses they cannot amplify signals and are usually bidirectional. They are common in invertebrates and are found in the retina and cerebral cortices of vertebrates.

The vast majority of the synapses in the mammalian brain are chemical synapses; the neuromuscular junction is also a chemical synapse.

When an action potential arrives at a chemical synapse, it stimulates release of a chemical neurotransmitter from the axonal terminus into the synaptic cleft. This neurotransmitter binds to receptors on the postsynaptic membrane, stimulating chemically gated ion channels. These channels open and induce ion fluxes changing the postsynaptic membrane potential. Depending on its location in the nervous system, the recipient neuron can receive tens or even hundreds of thousands of inputs from other neurons; each one can induce changes in the local membrane potential. The numerous changes are collated and the recipient cell processes all the incoming information. The collated input may stimulate the recipient cell to depolarise or not. If it depolarises, then information continues to be spread through the nervous system.

Under normal circumstances, information processing does not occur at the neuromuscular junction. Thus the arrival of an action potential at the axonal terminus activates calcium channels resulting in the release of neurotransmitter into the synaptic cleft and an action potential in the postsynaptic muscle fibre and muscle contraction. The number of action potentials arriving at the axonal terminus determines the strength of the muscle contraction.

Excitatory and inhibitory neurotransmitters

Neurotransmitters are chemicals that transmit nerve impulses across a synapse. They can be either inhibitory or excitatory. Excitatory neurotransmitters open ion channels allowing extracellular positive ions, such as sodium, to diffuse into the cell. This makes the inside of the cell less negative, thereby decreasing the potential difference across the membrane. An example of an excitatory neurotransmitter is glutamate. Inhibitory neurotransmitters open ion channels permitting extracellular negative ions, such as chloride, to diffuse into the cell, or intracellular positive ions such as potassium to diffuse out. The inside of the cell becomes more negative and increases the potential difference existing across the membrane. In the brain the major inhibitory neurotransmitter is GABA, while in the spinal cord it is glycine. An individual neuron will generally

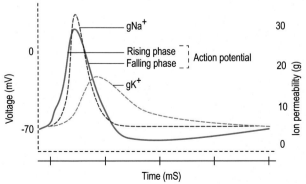

Fig. 3.8 **Schematic diagram illustrating the generation of an action potential owing to the changing permeability of the cell membrane to Na⁺ and K⁺.**

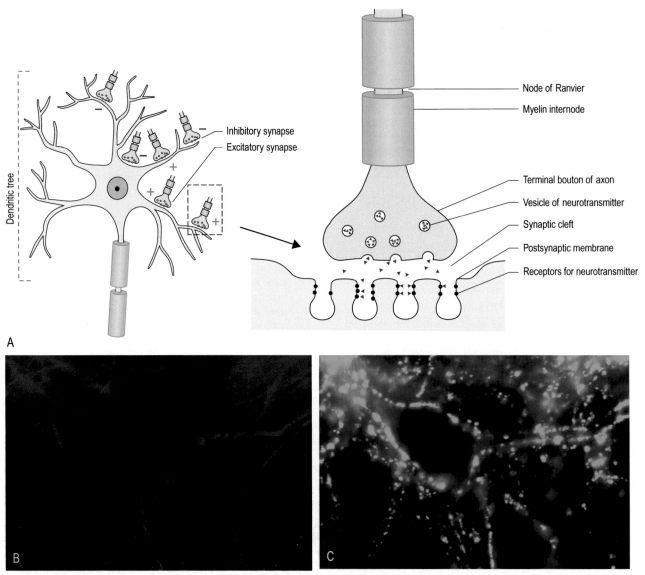

Fig. 3.9 **Chemical synapse. (A) The electrical energy of the action potential is transmitted between adjacent neurons, or from neurons to muscle cells, by the release of chemical neurotransmitters. (B,C) Cultured murine spinal cord neurons colabelled for tubulin (red) a neuronal cytoskeletal protein and synaptophysin (green) to identify synapses. The neuronal nucleus can be seen as a negatively stained shadow in the centre of the neuronal cell bodies in figure 9B; it is approximately 7-8 μm in diameter (reproduced with permission from Thomson et al, 2008).**

release only one type of neurotransmitter molecule, thus neurons can be termed excitatory or inhibitory.

The generalised neuron
Even though there is a huge variety in the shape and degree of connectivity of different neurons, the concept of the generalised neuron covers most of the variations and is a useful way to describe the concepts of neuronal function. Neurons process incoming information and may generate and propagate electrical charges as follows. The neuron receives information from many other neurons via chemical or electrical synapses. These inputs cause local fluctuations in membrane potential at the postsynaptic membrane. The changes in the membrane potential spread over the surface of the neuron. The dendritic processes of the neuron together with the cell body integrate all of the changes in membrane potential from all regions of the neuron's sensory field. The summated changes affect the membrane potential at the axonal hillock. This is the critical area for the propagation of information. If this area reaches the threshold potential

for the neuron, then an action potential will develop, spread along the axon to its synaptic termination where it will stimulate, or inhibit, the next neuron in the chain.

Information processing within and between neurons
The primary function of the nervous system is to receive inputs, process information and produce the appropriate output. The processing of information is carried out at several levels. Individual neurons process information from their receptive field to produce changes in the rate at which they generate action potentials. Neurons are interconnected into groups that work together to carry out specific processing tasks. Groups of neurons are interconnected into systems that deal with specific functions and systems interconnect at progressively higher levels to produce an animal's nervous system. This multi-level, modular design allows powerful and rapid information processing that enables the organism to sense its environment and behave in a manner appropriate to its perception. This modular concept is explained further in Chapter 4.

Supporting structures

Meninges

The brain and spinal cord are surrounded by three layers of connective tissue called meninges (Fig. 3.10). From superficial to deep, these are the dura mater, the arachnoid mater and the pia mater (*meninx* – Gk = membrane; *dura* – L = tough; *mater* – L = mother; *arachnoid* – Gk = cobweb like; *pia* – L = tender).

Key points

- The brain and spinal cord are surrounded by three layers of meninges – the dura mater, arachnoid mater and pia mater.
- Cerebrospinal fluid is produced by choroid plexi in the ventricular system of the brain. Its flow is largely rostral to caudal in the ventricular system and subarachnoid space from which it is drained.
- The CNS receives 20% of the total cardiac output, with the metabolically active grey matter receiving more than the white matter.
- The arterial blood supply to the brain is based around four pairs of arteries arising from the cerebral arterial circle, and one pair originating from the basilar artery. There are major, clinically important, species differences in the pattern of this arterial supply.
- The blood–brain barrier surrounding blood vessels is selectively permeable to bloodborne components. This protects the CNS from microorganisms but also limits drug permeability. However, CNS disease can compromise the function of blood–brain barrier.

The dura mater is composed of a thick layer of fibrous tissue and is also known as the pachymeninx (*pachys* – Gk = thick). The arachnoid mater is a thin membrane that encloses the cerebrospinal fluid (CSF) in the subarachnoid space. The arachnoid mater has numerous, fine filaments that traverse the subarachnoid space connecting with the pia mater (see Figs. 3.11B and 7.1). The pia mater is fused to the surface of the neuraxis. The arachnoid and pia mater comprise the leptomeninges (*lepto* – Gk = thin). The epidural space exists in the spinal canal and contains epidural fat and blood vessels. Inside the neurocranium, the dura is fused to the periosteum and the epidural space is a potential space only. The dura and arachnoid mater are fused in both regions; the subdural space is also a potential space. Potential spaces may be opened forming an actual space by pathological processes such as haemorrhage.

In two places, the dura mater folds inwardly to form double-layered curtains that hang from the roof of the cranial vault. The falx cerebri runs longitudinally separating the two cerebral hemispheres. The tentorium cerebelli runs transversely separating the caudal poles of the hemispheres from the rostral aspect of the cerebellum (Fig. 3.11A).

The meninges extend around the spinal nerve roots as sleeves and may reach as far peripherally as the intervertebral foramina (Fig. 1.1). At this level, the meninges fuse with the epineurium to form distinct cuff zones. At the cuff zones, drugs can diffuse more easily into the CNS. This characteristic is utilised in epidural anaesthesia to block nerve conduction in the spinal roots.

The ventricular system

The ventricular system is derived from the fluid-filled centre of the embryonic neural tube. In the brain, it comprises four expanded regions forming ventricles, interconnecting foramens and tubes (see Figs. A4, A5, A9-27). There is a curved lateral ventricle oriented longitudinally in each cerebral hemisphere that is connected to the third ventricle via an interventricular foramen. The third ventricle is a dorsoventrally oriented ring, surrounding the interthalamic adhesion. It connects via the mesencephalic aqueduct to the fourth ventricle located ventral to the cerebellum. Caudally, the dorsal aspect of this ventricle closes over at the obex to form the spinal canal. Laterally, the fourth ventricle is connected via two lateral apertures to the subarachnoid space. The ventricular system and the subarachnoid space contain cerebrospinal fluid (CSF) (Fig. 3.12).

Cerebrospinal fluid: production and circulation

Cerebrospinal fluid (CSF) is produced by small arteries and arterioles in the leptomeninges and the choroid plexuses. A choroid plexus is a collection of capillaries interposed in

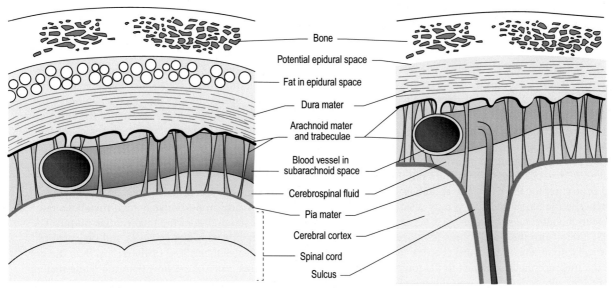

Bone
Potential epidural space
Fat in epidural space
Dura mater
Arachnoid mater and trabeculae
Blood vessel in subarachnoid space
Cerebrospinal fluid
Pia mater
Cerebral cortex
Spinal cord
Sulcus

Fig. 3.10 **Sections through meninges surrounding the spinal cord (left) and brain (right).**

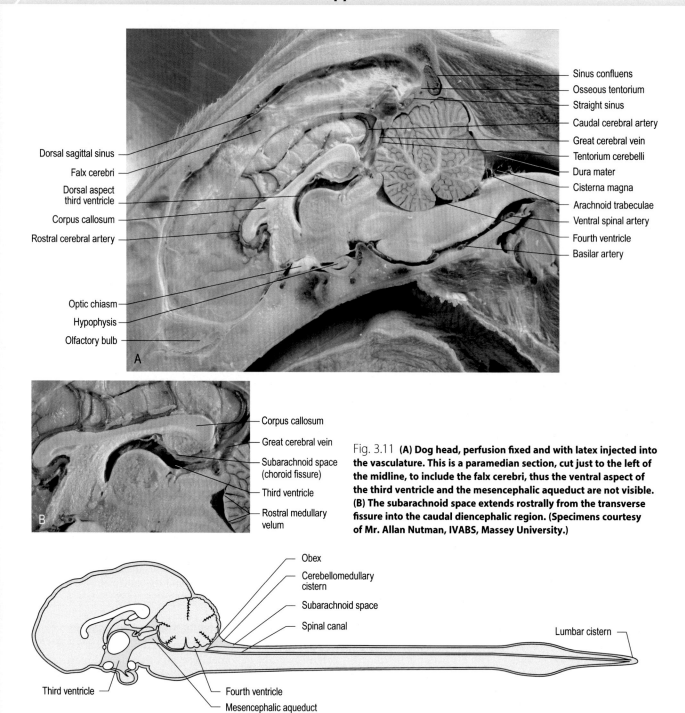

Dorsal sagittal sinus
Falx cerebri
Dorsal aspect third ventricle
Corpus callosum
Rostral cerebral artery

Optic chiasm
Hypophysis
Olfactory bulb

A

Sinus confluens
Osseous tentorium
Straight sinus
Caudal cerebral artery
Great cerebral vein
Tentorium cerebelli
Dura mater
Cisterna magna
Arachnoid trabeculae
Ventral spinal artery
Fourth ventricle
Basilar artery

Corpus callosum
Great cerebral vein
Subarachnoid space (choroid fissure)
Third ventricle
Rostral medullary velum

B

Fig. 3.11 **(A) Dog head, perfusion fixed and with latex injected into the vasculature. This is a paramedian section, cut just to the left of the midline, to include the falx cerebri, thus the ventral aspect of the third ventricle and the mesencephalic aqueduct are not visible. (B) The subarachnoid space extends rostrally from the transverse fissure into the caudal diencephalic region. (Specimens courtesy of Mr. Allan Nutman, IVABS, Massey University.)**

Obex
Cerebellomedullary cistern
Subarachnoid space
Spinal canal
Lumbar cistern

Third ventricle
Fourth ventricle
Mesencephalic aqueduct

Fig. 3.12 **Median section of the canine brain, ventricular system and subarachnoid space of the CNS. The lateral ventricles are lateral to the plane of this image.**

the choroid membrane (tela choroidea). The tela choroidea comprises pia mater fused directly to the ependyma (which is lining epithelium of the ventricular system) with no intervening neural tissue. There is a choroid plexus in each of the four ventricles of the brain. Cerebrospinal fluid is produced by ultrafiltration of blood plasma through the choroid plexus and modified by secretions from the epithelial secretory cells. The CSF provides physical and chemical protection for the CNS. The endothelial–epithelial barrier between the blood and CSF is only selectively permeable to bloodborne substances.

The CSF flows from the lateral ventricles, through the interventricular foramens to the third ventricle, caudally through the mesencephalic aqueduct to the fourth ventricle. From here some flows down the central canal of the spinal cord. The majority of CSF leaves the central space through lateral apertures of the fourth ventricle and enters the

sub-arachnoid space. The CSF is drained from the sub-arachnoid via three main routes: (a) by the venules of the sub-arachnoid space; (b) into the venous sinuses of the brain through invaginations in the wall of the sinus called arachnoid villi; and (c) by the lymphatic vessels of the cranial and spinal nerve roots.

Blood supply
Although the CNS accounts for only 2% of the body weight, it has a disproportionately high metabolic rate and receives about 20% of the total cardiac output. The oxygen requirements of the synapses and neuronal cell bodies are greater than those of the axons, thus the grey matter receives more blood flow than the white matter. Additionally, association/integration areas have greater requirements than other areas and so the forebrain is more vascular than other CNS regions.

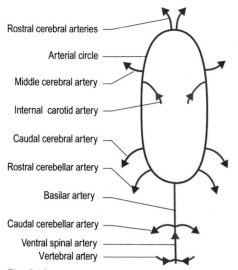

Rostral cerebral arteries

Arterial circle

Middle cerebral artery

Internal carotid artery

Caudal cerebral artery

Rostral cerebellar artery

Basilar artery

Caudal cerebellar artery

Ventral spinal artery

Vertebral artery

Fig. 3.13 **Schematic of the blood supply to the brain of the dog.**

Arterial blood supply of the brain is based around five pairs of arteries (Figs. 3.13–15, A3). Four of these arise from the cerebral arterial circle located on the ventral surface of the forebrain. These arteries include the rostral, middle and caudal cerebral arteries and the rostral cerebellar artery. The caudal cerebellar arteries originate from the basilar artery. The basilar artery is continuous with the ventral spinal artery at the foramen magnum. It runs longitudinally on the ventral aspect of the brainstem and connects with the caudal aspect of the arterial circle. The major brain arteries traverse the surface of the brain in the sulci, and send smaller branches to perfuse the deep tissues. Whilst there are anastomoses between the arteries on the surface of the CNS, the penetrating arteries do not communicate with each other and so blockages of individual end-arteries lead to ischaemia of defined parts of the CNS.

Although there are some species differences in the arteries of the brain, these are relatively minor. However, there are major differences in how blood gets to the brain; these differences are clinically important. Generally speaking there are four possible routes by which the blood may arrive at the arterial circle; the internal carotid artery, the basilar artery, the maxillary artery and the vertebral artery. The common domestic animals have various combinations of these routes. The maxillary artery may have a rete mirabile (*rete* – L = net, *mirabile* – L = marvellous) where the major vessel breaks into many convoluted small branches before re-anastomosing. The rete mirabile may act as a heat exchanger to protect the brain from major temperature changes and act to reduce pulsations in the blood perfusing the CNS. The cat, sheep (Fig. 3.15) and ox have one, or more, rete mirabile.

Patterns of arterial supply to the brain
1. General form (dog, human). The internal carotid artery and the basilar artery both carry blood to the cerebral arterial circle. Carotid blood reaches most of the cerebral hemispheres except the caudal portion. Vertebral blood supplies the rest of the brain (Fig. 3.16).
2. Sheep and cat. The proximal two-thirds of the internal carotid artery is absent in the adult and the direction of blood flow is caudad in the basilar artery. The only supply of blood to the cerebral arterial circle originates from the maxillary arteries via a rete mirabile. Maxillary blood supplies all the brain except the caudal part of the medulla.
3. Ox. As in the sheep and cat the proximal two-thirds of the internal carotid is absent in the adult and the direction of blood flow is caudad in the basilar artery. Unlike the sheep there are two anastomosing branches, one from the maxillary artery and one from the vertebral artery, both of which have rete mirabile. Maxillary and vertebral blood supplies the whole of the brain.

Blood supply and animal slaughter
Animal welfare legislation in many countries prohibits slaughter without prior stunning in order to ensure that animals do not suffer pain during throat cutting and exsanguination. Cutting the throat cuts the common carotid artery and jugular veins. The teaching of some religions does not allow for stunning to take place prior to slaughter and legislation in some countries provides them with an exemption from the general requirement for stunning. In these animals that are not stunned there will be a period of time after the throat cut and before the onset of insensibility. It has recently been shown that the animal may perceive pain during this period. The duration of sensibility following the throat cut will depend on whether the vertebral arteries can keep the brain supplied with oxygen. This period varies between species because of anatomical differences. It is thought that the period of sensibility is between 8 and 20 seconds in the sheep, but between 34 and 85 seconds in cattle.

Arterial supply to the spinal cord
The spinal cord is supplied segmentally by spinal branches arising from the vertebral artery and aorta, and entering the vertebral canal at the intervertebral foramens. Within the spinal canal, each branch divides into a smaller dorsal, and larger ventral branch. The dorsal branches enter the spinal cord with the dorsal root. The ventral branches unite to form the unpaired, median, ventral spinal artery.

Venous drainage of the CNS
The neuraxis and meninges are drained by veins and sinuses (see other texts for details of the veins). In sinuses, valves are absent or poorly developed, hence retrograde blood flow can occur. Sinuses in the brain form a dorsal and ventral set. The dorsal set is primarily midline with the dorsal sagittal sinus, sited in the falx cerebri draining caudally to meet the straight sinus at the confluences of the sinuses located at caudal end of the falx cerebri. The straight sinus drains the great cerebral vein from the deeper cerebrum. Drainage from the confluence is laterally into the ventrally directed, paired transverse sinuses, beginning in the dorsal part of the occipital bone. The transverse sinus terminates by dividing into the sigmoid and temporal sinuses in the ventrocaudal aspect of the skull. The ventral set of sinuses begins with the paired cavernous sinus lying subdurally on the floor of the middle cranial fossa, surrounding the hypophysis. The cavernous sinus receives venous drainage from the ophthalmic plexus, and may, depending on the species, interconnect across the midline by the intercavernous sinus. The cavernous sinuses drain caudally into the ventral petrosal sinus that connects to the sigmoid sinus. The dorsal petrosal sinus drains the basal vein of the cerebrum into the transverse sinus. The sinuses drain into the maxillary, vertebral, occipital and internal jugular veins (Fig. 3.17).

The spinal cord has an internal vertebral venous plexus lying on the floor of the vertebral canal, with paired vessels

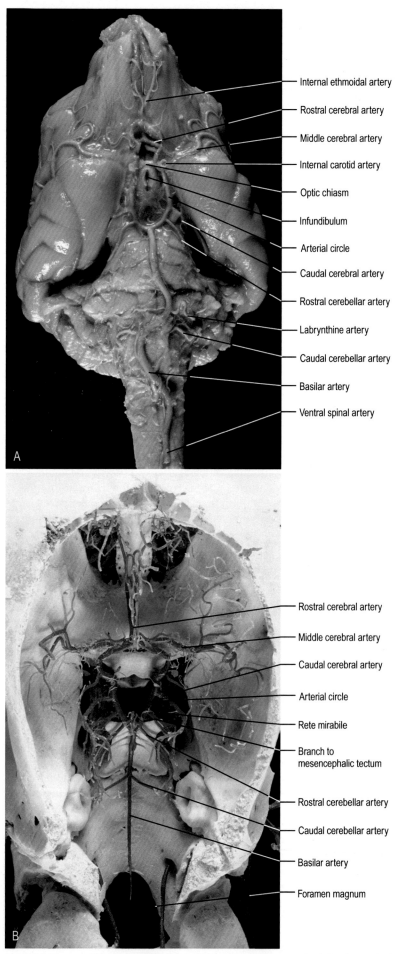

— Internal ethmoidal artery

— Rostral cerebral artery

— Middle cerebral artery

— Internal carotid artery

— Optic chiasm

— Infundibulum

— Arterial circle

— Caudal cerebral artery

— Rostral cerebellar artery

— Labrynthine artery

— Caudal cerebellar artery

— Basilar artery

— Ventral spinal artery

— Rostral cerebral artery

— Middle cerebral artery

— Caudal cerebral artery

— Arterial circle

— Rete mirabile

— Branch to mesencephalic tectum

— Rostral cerebellar artery

— Caudal cerebellar artery

— Basilar artery

— Foramen magnum

Fig. 3.14 **The arterial supply of the dog and sheep brain. The vessels of the dog brain have been infused with latex, while the sheep vasculature is a resin cast. (Specimens prepared by Mr. Allan Nutman, IVABS, Massey University.)**

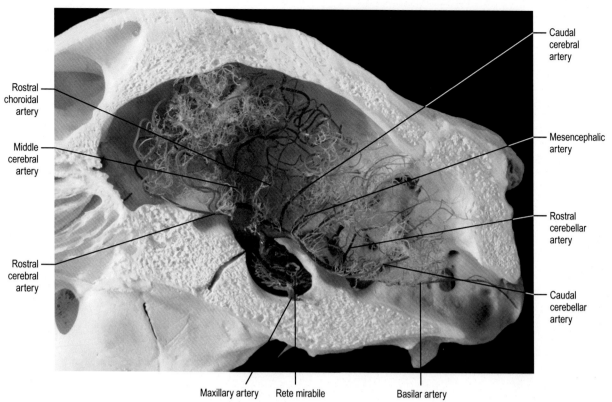

Rostral choroidal artery

Middle cerebral artery

Rostral cerebral artery

Caudal cerebral artery

Mesencephalic artery

Rostral cerebellar artery

Caudal cerebellar artery

Maxillary artery   Rete mirabile   Basilar artery

Fig. 3.15 **The rete mirabile of the sheep brain. (Vascular cast prepared by Mr. Allan Nutman, IVABS, Massey University.)**

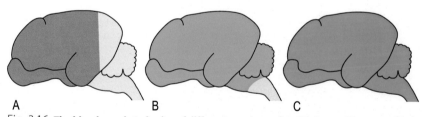

A   B   C

Fig. 3.16 **The blood supply to brains of different species varies; (A) dog and humans, (B) sheep and cat, (C) ox. Magenta represents supply from the internal carotid artery; yellow from the vertebral artery; blue from the maxillary artery and green is from both the vertebral and maxillary arteries.**

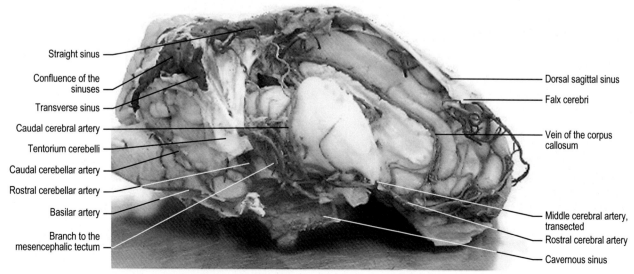

Straight sinus

Confluence of the sinuses

Transverse sinus

Caudal cerebral artery

Tentorium cerebelli

Caudal cerebellar artery

Rostral cerebellar artery

Basilar artery

Branch to the mesencephalic tectum

Dorsal sagittal sinus

Falx cerebri

Vein of the corpus callosum

Middle cerebral artery, transected

Rostral cerebral artery

Cavernous sinus

Fig. 3.17 **Sheep brain lateral aspect, vasculature filled with latex (red for arteries and blue for veins and sinuses). The right hemisphere has been removed to show deeper vessels. (Specimen prepared by Mr. Allan Nutman, IVABS, Massey University.)**

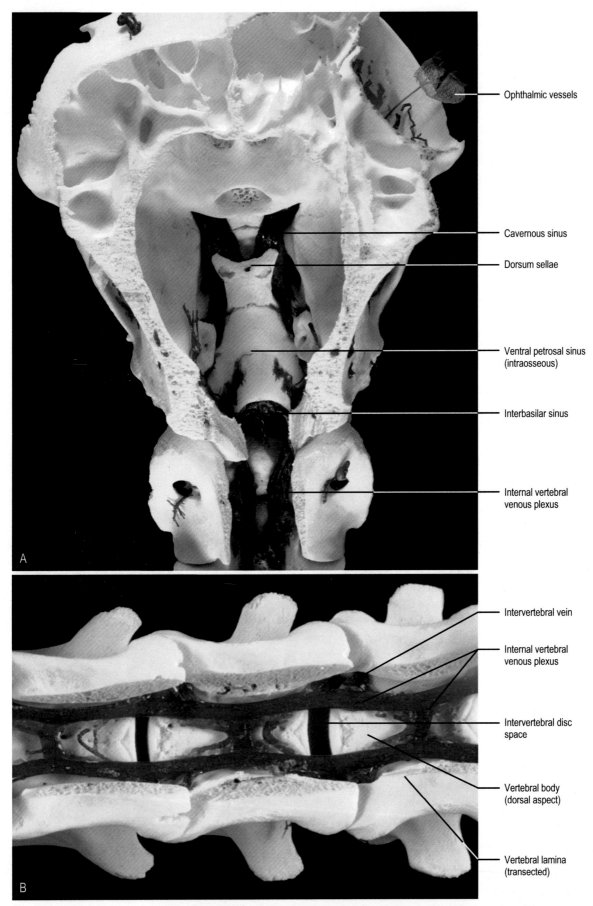

— Ophthalmic vessels

— Cavernous sinus

— Dorsum sellae

— Ventral petrosal sinus (intraosseous)

— Interbasilar sinus

— Internal vertebral venous plexus

A

— Intervertebral vein

— Internal vertebral venous plexus

— Intervertebral disc space

— Vertebral body (dorsal aspect)

— Vertebral lamina (transected)

B

Fig. 3.18 **Resin casts of the venous sinuses and veins on the ventral aspect of the neuraxis in the sheep. (A) Base of the neurocranium of sheep, dorsal aspect. (B) Base of the spinal canal of sheep, dorsal aspect. (Specimens prepared by Mr. Allan Nutman, IVABS, Massey University.)**

that diverge to drain into intervertebral veins at each intervertebral foramen (Fig 3.18).

Blood–brain barrier

The blood–brain barrier (together with the blood–CSF barrier) prevents some molecules that may be present in the blood from diffusing into the CNS parenchyma. This protective mechanism aims to limit the exposure of the CNS tissues to pathogens and molecules that could have a deleterious effect. Because of these barriers, the composition of the CSF and the extracellular fluid in the CNS is different to that in the rest of the body.

Structurally the blood–brain barrier has three components: (a) tight junctions between the capillary endothelia; (b) a thick basement membrane; and (c) a layer of astrocyte foot processes that surround the capillaries (Fig. 3.19). The barrier is highly permeable to water, carbon dioxide, oxygen and lipid-soluble substances, and less permeable to electrolytes. Carrier molecules mediate transport of glucose and some other small molecules. It is almost totally impermeable to proteins and larger molecules, especially those that bear an electrical charge. Some areas, such as the hypothalamus, the area postrema and pineal gland, lie outside of the blood–brain barrier. These areas contain sensors for osmolarity, glucose concentration and pH, and send information into regulatory areas of the CNS. The blood–brain and blood–CSF barriers function to maintain a highly controlled CNS environment,

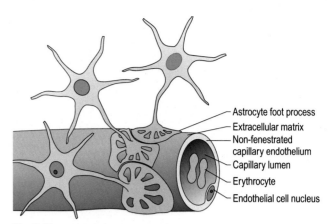

Fig. 3.19 **The blood–brain barrier.**

- Astrocyte foot process
- Extracellular matrix
- Non-fenestrated capillary endothelium
- Capillary lumen
- Erythrocyte
- Endothelial cell nucleus

but also have clinical significance with respect to medical treatment of the CNS as they will exclude many drugs. However, the blood–brain barrier in developing and senescent animals is more porous than that of mature adults.

Examples of drugs that cannot normally cross the blood–brain barrier include some antibiotics and neuromuscular blocking agents. However, pathological processes, such as inflammation, can compromise the function of these barriers allowing entry of compounds that are normally excluded.

Chapter 4
Hierarchical organisation in the nervous system

Key points

- Functionally, the nervous system is organised hierarchically; this is analogous to a business corporation with workers and managers.
- The hierarchy consists of effectors (sensory and motor) and different levels of information processing and integration in the spinal cord, brainstem and forebrain.

The functional arrangement of the nervous system is hierarchical and can be likened, in some ways, to corporate structure (Fig. 4.1, Table 4.1). There are workers and management systems. The workers are those nerves that interact directly with the sensory receptors in the body and with the effectors (muscle). Thus the majority of the 'worker' nerves are found in the PNS. Conversely, management is confined to the CNS. It receives and processes sensory inputs, integrates information, and directs the worker outputs. There are a number of levels of management: junior, senior and executive. These levels are located to different extents in the spinal cord, brainstem and forebrain. There are also maintenance systems that keep the basal level of activity going in the body. These are represented largely by the autonomic nervous system and include visceral reflexes. For example, stimulation of baroreceptors results in cardiovascular changes to maintain appropriate blood pressure.

Overview of motor and sensory systems

Key points

- The motor system maintains static and dynamic posture, controls voluntary movement, gait and visceral motor function. It can be divided into two components, upper motor neurons (UMN) and lower motor neurons (LMN).
- The neuromuscular junction connects the electrical activity of the LMN to the depolarisation of the muscle via chemical messengers.
- Planning and direction of voluntary movement is centred in the forebrain. The forebrain and the cerebellum communicate with UMNs in the motor cortex and brainstem. The UMNs interact with LMNs in the brainstem and spinal cord.
- Sensory receptors can be classified based on morphological criteria, the type of sensory modality to which they are receptive and by the type of the animal's environment they are sensing.
- Sensory receptors are distributed throughout the body and head. Their axons project into the CNS, making local connections with LMNs for reflex function. They also project to centres in the brainstem and forebrain for integration.

Overview of motor (output) systems

The functions of the motor system are (a) to maintain posture and provide a stable platform for movement, (b) voluntary movement and locomotion, and (c) visceral motor function (see Chapter 5).

Upper motor neurons, lower motor neurons and the neuromuscular junction

The motor system can be divided into two main components – upper motor neurons (UMNs) and lower motor neurons (LMNs). The UMNs are completely contained within the CNS, thus an alternative name for them could be 'central motor neurons'. The UMN cell body is located in a motor nucleus of the brainstem or the motor cortex of the forebrain. Their axons connect to LMNs either by synapsing on them directly or indirectly, via interneurons. The LMNs have their cell body in the CNS (brainstem or spinal cord). Their axons project into the PNS, via cranial or spinal nerves, to connect with striated or smooth muscle at the neuromuscular junction; thus an alternative name for them could be 'peripheral motor neurons'. Note that while

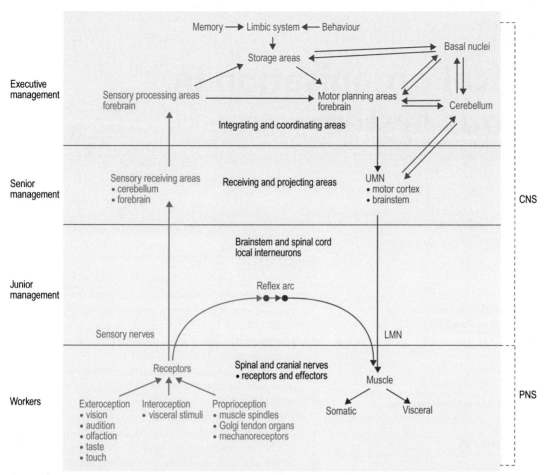

Fig. 4.1 **Schematic of hierarchical structure of the nervous system. Green = sensory systems; purple = interneurons, red = motor systems.**

Table 4.1 **Hierarchical arrangement of the nervous system**

Hierarchical position	Location of sensory system	Location of motor system
Workers Link between the PNS target organs and the CNS Involved in reflex functions	Sensory receptors and sensory nerves, with input via spinal and cranial nerves	LMNs connecting via NMJ to muscle
Junior management Interneuronal circuitry which links between input from sensory fibres, or UMNs, to LMN Involved in reflex functions	Spinal cord for afferent spinal nerves Brainstem for sensory input from CNN V, VIII, IX, X Forebrain for sensory input from CNN I, II	Spinal cord for connecting to LMNs of spinal nerves Brainstem for connecting to LMNs of CNN III–VII, IX–XII
Senior management Primary receiving areas or UMN centres	Primary sensory receiving areas Cerebellum – subconscious proprioception Forebrain – visual, auditory, somatosensory and olfactory cortices	UMN nuclei of the brainstem and the motor cortex of the forebrain
Executive management Processing and integrating areas	Diverse areas of the brain processing and interpreting sensory input. Interconnections between sensory association areas, storage (memory), behaviour and emotion centres and motor planning centres with links to the cerebellum and basal nuclei	

the cell body of the LMN connecting to striated muscle lies in the CNS, its long axon is located in the PNS. The ANS has two LMNs in series, with the cell body of the second LMN located in a peripheral ganglion (see Chapter 12). The UMNs, along with other management components of the motor system, organise and direct the activity of the LMN. When stimulated LMNs induce muscle contraction. Thus the UMNs are part of a motor management system, while the LMNs with their associated muscles are analogous to the workers.

The neuromuscular junction (NMJ) (see Fig. 1.4) connects the electrical activity of the LMN to the depolarisation of the muscle, using chemical messengers, such as acetylcholine (ACh). Even in the absence of action potentials, acetylcholine is continually being released at the

NMJ causing miniature depolarisations of the muscle end plate. These miniature end plate potentials result in end plate noise that can be detected electromyographically using needle electrodes. Release of ACh also contributes trophic support to the muscle fibres, which when lost, as occurs when the LMN is destroyed, is associated with rapid, severe, neurogenic atrophy of the muscle fibres (see Chapter 5). When a volley of action potentials arrives at the motor end plate, large amounts of ACh are released and the muscle is stimulated to contract proportionally.

There are two main activities of striated muscles in the body and limbs, extension and flexion of joints. Extensor muscles are antigravity muscles as they permit the animal to resist the effects of gravity. Extensor muscles increase the joint angle. For the thoracolumbar vertebral column,

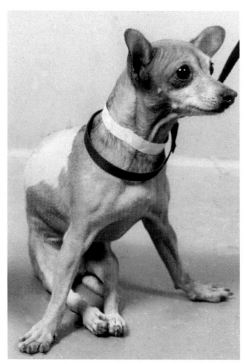

Fig. 4.2 **Extensor dominance in the pelvic limbs of a dog due to a lesion disrupting UMN tracts in the caudal thoracic spinal cord. The thoracic limbs are also in increased extension (braced) to carry the weight that is no longer being borne by the pelvic limbs and extensor muscles of the caudal half of the trunk.**

flexor (hypaxial) muscles work in conjunction with extensor (epaxial) muscles to resist the effects of gravity on the trunk. Antigravity muscle activity has to dominate flexor muscle activity, otherwise the animal would be recumbent. However, in the normal animal, extensor dominance is modulated by the action of inhibitory UMNs synapsing on the LMN supplying extensor muscles. Thus the overall descending UMN activity in the normal animal is inhibitory to antigravity extensor muscles. Damage to these inhibitory UMN pathways results in extensor dominance and spasticity (Fig. 4.2; see also Chapter 5 – UMN signs).

Overview of sensory (input) systems

Sensory receptors can be classified in several ways, based on morphological criteria (e.g. encapsulated or non-encapsulated) or the type of sensory modality type to which they are receptive, e.g. touch, sound. They can also be classified based on what part of the animal's environment they are sensing. This could be the external environment (exteroceptors), or the internal environment (interoceptors) or receptors that specialise in stimuli used in spatial orientation of the animal (proprioceptors). Examples of exteroception include vision, audition, olfaction, gustation and touch. Examples of interoceptors include receptors in the viscera sensitive to stretch, pH, and chemical changes such as CO_2. Proprioceptors are located throughout the body and head, and in the vestibular apparatus of inner ears. They include muscle spindles (stretch receptors), Golgi tendon organs, joint receptors, tactile/pressure receptors, especially of the feet, and hair cells of the inner ear.

Worker and management systems
Motor systems
The workers comprise the LMNs in which the motor neuron connects directly with the muscle. Superimposed on the workers are the various levels of management. Sitting in a role analogous to junior management is interneuronal circuitry that connects sensory and motor nerves and different groups of LMNs so they can function as integrated, coordinated worker systems: it has a key role in polysynaptic reflexes. Junior management is located near the LMN cell bodies in the spinal cord or brainstem and connects to the LMNs of the spinal or cranial nerves, respectively. It receives direction from senior management.

Senior management comprises the traditional UMN tracts that, in domestic mammals, originate primarily in the brainstem and in the motor cortex of the cerebral hemispheres.

Executive management has its head office mainly in the cerebral cortex, but it also has diverse connections and feedback loops throughout the brain including with the cerebellum and basal nuclei.

Functionally, executive management holds primary responsibility for planning and directing voluntary and complex movement. It talks to senior management. Senior management receives instructions from the executive, has feedback loops with some areas of the brain, especially the cerebellum, and directs junior management (interneurons) in the brainstem and spinal cord. Senior management can also interact with workers (LMN) directly. When the UMNs fire, they can stimulate, or inhibit, the activity of the LMN. Junior management is like the foreman on the workshop floor, listening to input from both the workers and the managers, and coordinating the outputs of worker groups to produce the specific patterns of movements that are required for actions like locomotion.

Sensory systems
For the sensory systems, the workers are the receptors distributed throughout the body (extero-, intero- and proprioceptors) with their axons projecting via cranial and spinal nerves into the CNS.

Once inside the CNS, the fibres make connections with local circuitry (junior management) for reflex function. For spinal nerves, these connections are made primarily with interneurons in the dorsal horn, which then ultimately connect with LMNs in the ventral horn. For example, a noxious stimulus applied to the foot travels via the spinal nerves to the dorsal horn. From there it connects via interneurons to LMNs in the ventral horn of several spinal cord segments stimulating LMNs supplying limb flexor muscles and the foot is withdrawn from the stimulus. Many of the cranial nerves convey sensory input to brainstem cranial nerve nuclei. This input connects via interneurons to LMN in other brainstem nuclei. For example, in the palpebral reflex, input to the sensory nucleus of CN V nucleus connects via interneurons (junior management) to the facial nucleus so that touch around the palpebrum triggers reflex blinking.

Connections from sensory spinal nerves can also travel cranially in the cord to synapse in brainstem nuclei and make connections with UMNs (senior management of the motor system). Sensory information is also projected directly to primary sensory receiving areas in the cerebellum (for subconscious proprioception) and the somatosensory cortex of the cerebrum (senior management). Input from cranial nerves is projected to the forebrain where it is received in auditory, somatosensory, olfactory and visual cortices of the cerebrum. Input from the vestibular system (head proprioception) is also projected to the cerebellum via CN VIII. These primary receiving areas are like the senior management for the sensory system.

Sensory input that is received in the primary sensory cortices is projected to nearby association areas where it is processed, ranked in terms of importance and, from there, integrated with other information. The association and integration areas are the equivalent of the executive management for the sensory systems. For example, visual input via cranial nerve II is received in the visual cortex in the occipital lobes. The executive system for visual input will process that information in the nearby visual association area and link it with other processed sensory inputs (e.g. touch, audition), stored information (memory), emotion-generating areas of the brain (limbic system) and information from other integrating and coordinating centres such as the cerebellum and basal nuclei.

The locations of the main functional regions of the cortex are comparable in all mammals, but their extent varies: for example in the carnivore the primary sensory and motor areas and olfactory cortex comprise 80% of the cortical surface whereas in primates the same zones make up less than 20%. The relationship is reversed for the associative cortex in these two groups of animals, while rodents and lagomorphs have almost no associative functions at all (see Fig. 4.16).

The sensory executive areas will also link with the executive motor areas for planning of voluntary movement. Thus sensory systems can modify motor output directly at the local level via reflexes utilising junior management, or indirectly via connections to the motor system hierarchy at senior and executive management levels.

The workers and maintenance crew: The reflex arc

A large amount of motor activity used for basic functions such as postural support, locomotion or visceral function

Key point

■ The simplest reflex arc has a receptor in the PNS, a sensory axon projecting to the CNS where it connects with LMNs that project to a muscle. Via reflex arc wiring a stimulus results in a stereotypical motor output. Reflex arcs occur in somatic and visceral systems.

involves reflex activity. The reflex activity can then be modulated by input from higher centres.

A reflex arc involves both the PNS and the CNS. It has a sensory/afferent nerve in the PNS that brings information into the CNS where the input is linked to a motor/efferent nerve that connects back to a muscle (Fig. 4.3). Via that linkage, the stimulus of the sensory nerve elicits a stereotypical motor output and muscle activation. The neural wiring of a reflex arc is laid down during embryological development. Thus, unlike a learned motor response, its function does not depend on experience. An example of a learned motor activity is the menace response in which the animal blinks in response to a menacing gesture made to the eye. By comparison, the palpebral reflex, in which the animal blinks in response to tactile stimulation of the palpebrum, is present from birth.

A typical reflex is the patellar, or 'knee jerk' reflex, in which tapping the patellar ligament with a plexor (patellar hammer), causes reflex contraction of the quadriceps muscle and stifle extension (Fig. 4.4). Simultaneously, the antagonistic semitendinosus and semimembranosus muscles are reflexively inhibited from contracting. Sensory input is via the femoral nerve. In dogs, this nerve synapses directly onto the LMNs in the ventral horns of L4–L6 spinal cord segments, which supply the quadriceps muscle, also via the femoral nerve. Note: a monosynaptic reflex like this is unusual but may include stretch/myotatic reflexes (see Chapter 5); interneurons are usually interspersed between afferent and efferent neurons, resulting in a polysynaptic reflex. Simultaneously, the sensory input also travels

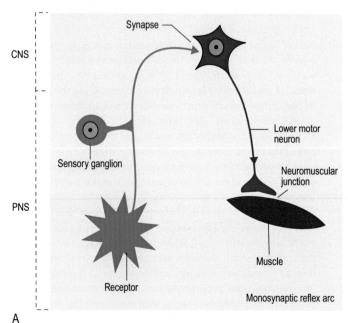

A

B

Fig. 4.3 **Basic reflex arcs: (A) monosynaptic arc; (B) polysynaptic arc.**

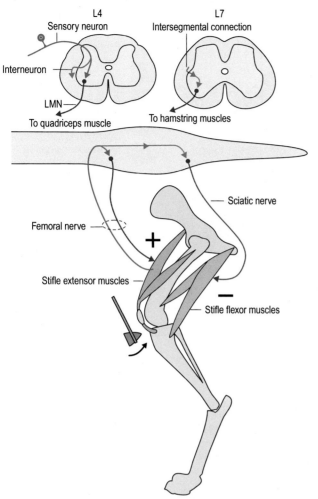

Fig. 4.4 **Basic wiring involved in the patellar reflex. Reflexes utilise input from exteroceptors, interoceptors or proprioceptors. They use spinal nerves and cranial nerves and may affect striated or smooth muscles. For example, gut activity is stimulated by the sight and/or smell of food.**

caudally, via interneurons, to spinal cord segments L6–S1 to synapse on interneurons that inhibit LMN-induced contraction of the hamstring muscles. Thus, contraction of the quadriceps muscle is unopposed.

Junior management: Spinal cord and brainstem

Key points

- Interneurons in the spinal cord and brainstem enable local connections between sensory and motor neurons for reflex activity.
- Both the grey and white matter can be divided functionally into distinct regions.
- The dorsal funiculus carries cranially projecting sensory tracts. The lateral funiculus carries cranially projecting sensory tracts and caudally projecting motor tracts facilitating flexor muscle activity. The ventral funiculus carries mainly caudally projecting motor tracts facilitating extensor muscle activity. Each funiculus also transmits fibres connecting between spinal cord segments.

- Some tracts remain ipsilateral whilst others decussate. Knowing whether a tract influences the ipsi- or contralateral side of the body, is clinically significant.
- LMNs innervating the limbs are confined to the cervical and lumbar intumescences. The cranial part of the intumescence innervates cranial and proximal muscles of the limb. The caudal intumescence innervates the distal and caudal muscles of the limb.
- UMN tracts in the spinal cord originate in the brain and mainly influence γ-LMN, via interneurons.
- Nerve fibre diameter varies between tracts. Larger diameter fibres are more vulnerable to injury. Thus spinal cord compression sequentially results in proprioceptive dysfunction, paresis, autonomic dysfunction, loss of tactile sensation, paralysis and finally, loss of all nociception caudal to the lesion.

Overview of the spinal cord

The spinal cord has a variety of functions that can be summarised as the following:

1. Receiving and distributing information to the PNS;
2. Local integration (junior management) of sensory and motor functions for reflex activity, both within a limb and between limbs;
3. Relaying afferent/sensory information to the brain centres (senior management);
4. Relaying efferent/motor information from senior motor management centres (UMN nuclei and motor cortex), via UMN tracts to connect with LMN;
5. Forming connections between caudally directed tracts from the brain and cranially directed tracts, such that the former can regulate transmission of impulses in sensory systems. This is part of the mechanism by which nociceptive stimuli are modified.

The spinal cord has central grey matter and peripheral white matter. The grey and white matter can be divided functionally (Fig. 4.5). Each grey matter horn, or white matter funiculus, can be divided into distinct regions. There are ten different zones of the grey matter and more than a dozen specific tracts in the white matter. The details of those divisions are summarised in Fig. 4.5 and Table 4.2.

Spinal cord grey matter

The function of different areas of grey matter is outlined in Table 4.2.

The motor neurons of the lateral aspect of the ventral horn supplying the limbs are somatotopically arranged. Longitudinally, this arrangement means that cranial segments of the intumescence supply the cranial and proximal muscles of the limb and the caudal segments supply the caudal and distal muscles. This is clinically relevant. For example, a lesion in the cranial cervical intumescence (C6–C7) will damage the innervation to the shoulder muscles resulting in a shortened stride due to loss of shoulder movement. Damage to the caudal cervical intumescence (C8–T2) will compromise the radial, median and ulnar nerves resulting in failure to extend the elbow and bear weight on the limb, decreased movement of the carpus and digits and a shortened stride.

Species differences include an additional nucleus (retrodorsal n.) located at C8–T1 and S1–S3 provides fine digital control in certain species, such as humans.

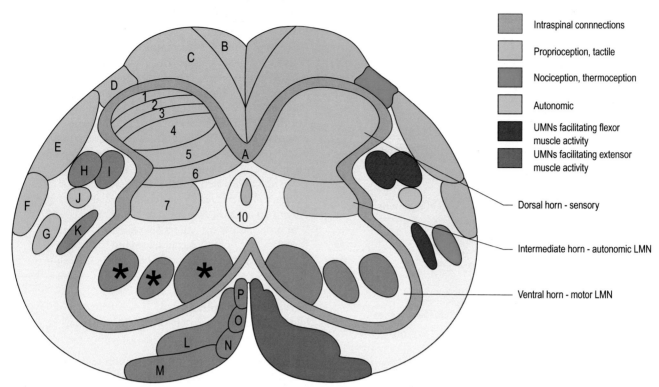

Fig. 4.5 **Transverse section of spinal cord identifying grey matter zones and white matter tracts on one side and their general functions on the other. This is a hybrid diagram and the specific white matter tracts do not appear in all regions of the spinal cord. In the cervical region there are additional tracts, which are not depicted and there is no intermediate horn of grey matter (GM). Cranially and caudally directed tracts intermingle and are not as discrete as the diagram would imply. Grey matter is divided into ten zones (Rexed's laminae) based on cellular architecture; this histological division has some correlation with function. The arrangement of all zones are variable throughout the cord, especially for zones 8 and 9; these are indicated by an asterisk (*). Details of tracts and laminae are given in Tables 4.2 and 4.3. Note that nociception is also conveyed in the dorsal and ventral funiculi as well as other parts of the lateral funiculi (see Chapter 6). Green colours = sensory, turquoise = autonomic, red colours = motor.**

Table 4.2 **The location and function of different regions of grey matter of the spinal cord; approximate correlations with the laminae are noted**

Location	Grey matter column	Function
Top of dorsal horn (1,2,3)	Marginal nucleus and substantia gelatinosa	Nociception
DH deep to substantia gelatinosa (3,4)	Nucleus proprius	Interneurons and projection neurons
Base of DH, T1–L2 (5)	Visceral nuclei	Projection of visceral afferent stimuli to brain
Base of DH, T1–L4, medial aspect (5,6)	Nucleus thoracicus (also called nucleus of the dorsal spinocerebellar tract)	Projection of proprioceptive input from caudal half of body to cerebellum and nucleus Z
IH T1–L3 (7)	Intermediomedial and intermediolateral nuclei	Efferent, sympathetic presynaptic neurons
IH S1–S3 (7)	Sacral parasympathetic nuclei	Efferent, parasympathetic presynaptic neurons
Medial VH all segments excluding L7 and S1 (8,9)	Medial motor neurons	LMNs supplying truncal/axial muscles
Central VH C1–C6 (8,9)	LMNs of spinal accessory nerve (CN XI) and phrenic nucleus	Innervation of shoulder and neck muscles, and the diaphragm
Lateral aspect especially at the intumescences (9)	Lateral motor neurons	Innervation of the appendicular muscles
Surrounding the central canal (10)	Central intermediate substance	Nociception

DH = dorsal horn, IH = intermediate horn, VH = ventral horn.

origin and termination. For example, the vestibulospinal tract originates in the vestibular nuclei and ends in the spinal cord.

The white matter of the spinal cord is summarised in Table 4.3.

There is a general pattern to the functions conveyed by spinal cord white matter. Each funiculus has the propriospinal tract making intersegmental connections between cranial and caudal spinal cord segments. The dorsal funiculus carries cranially projecting sensory tracts; the lateral funiculus carries both cranially projecting sensory tracts and caudally projecting motor tracts facilitating flexors and the ventral funiculus carries mainly caudally projecting motor tracts facilitating extensors. However, it should be noted that there are some exceptions to this general pattern. For example, the following cranially directed tracts are found in the ventral funiculus.

1. Spinoreticular tracts – sensory and nociceptive input to the reticular formation and then to the thalamus and cerebrum, for alerting and motivational purposes.
2. Spinovestibular tracts – proprioceptive input from the cervical region to the caudal vestibular nuclei (head proprioception).
3. Spinomesencephalic tract to midbrain and the thalamus. This tract may be involved in the activation of a caudally directed analgesia system.
4. Spino-olivary fibres – convey sensory feedback to the olivary nucleus and hence cerebellum. Spino-olivary fibres are found in the spinoreticular tract (VF) the ventral spinocerebellar tract (LF) and the fasciculus cuneatus (DF).

Spinal cord white matter

Within the CNS, nerve bundles form functional tracts that have common origins and destinations. Such tracts may also be called fasciculi (*fasciculus* – L = little bundle). The specific name of a tract, or fasciculus, usually indicates its

Table 4.3 **The function of the white matter tracts indicated in** Fig. 4.5

Label	Tract name	Function: S = sensory, M = motor
A	Propriospinal (spino-spinal)	Connections between spinal cord segments; used in reflex activity
B	Fasciculus gracilis	S: Proprioception and tactile input from caudal ½ of body, projecting to the nucleus gracilis in the medulla oblongata. Post-synaptic tract intermingled conveying pinprick pain*
C	Fasciculus cuneatus	S: Proprioception and tactile input from cranial ½ of body, projecting to the medial nucleus cuneatus in the medulla oblongata. Post-synaptic tract intermingled conveying pinprick pain*. Cuneocerebellar tract fibres at base of FC, conveying proprioception from cranial half of the body
D	Dorsolateral fasciculus	S: Nociception, thermal, multisynaptic. Most fibres terminate in the substantia gelatinosa
E	Dorsal spinocerebellar	S: Proprioception from body caudal to thoracic limb
F	Ventral spinocerebellar	S: Proprioception from caudal half of the body. The cranial spinocerebellar tract is found on the medial aspect and conveys proprioceptive input from the cranial half of the body
G	Spinothalamic	S: Nociception, touch and temperature, multisynaptic. These modalities are also conveyed by other tracts in lateral and ventral funiculi*
H	Rubrospinal	M: Flexor activity of body and limbs, limb protraction during locomotion
I	Lateral Corticospinal	M: Flexor and extensor activity especially of the distal limbs (voluntary, skilled movement leading to dexterity), also urinary bladder function
J	Lateral tectotegmentospinal	M: UMN sympathetic supply to the body (head, neck, trunk and limbs); function best observed by pupillary dilation
K	Medullary (lateral) reticulospinal tract	M: Strongly inhibitory to extensor activity such as standing; it has a key role in flexor phase of gait. This tract arises from the medial medullary motor nucleus
L	Pontine (ventral) reticulospinal	M: Facilitates extensor activity, e.g. standing and antigravity muscles; key role in extensor phase of gait
M	Lateral vestibulospinal	M: Vestibulospinal: Ipsilateral extension, inhibition of ipsilateral flexion and contralateral extension; key role in extensor phase of gait
	Spinovestibular	S: Spinovestibular: proprioception of head–neck junction to vestibular nuclei
N	Tectospinal	M: Contraction of neck muscles for reflex turning of head in response to auditory and visual stimuli
O	Ventral corticospinal	M: Facilitation of voluntary movement in the neck and trunk
P	Medial vestibulospinal and medial longitudinal fasciculus	M: Ipsilateral extension of neck muscles and inhibition of contralateral extension

*See tables 5.1 and 6.1 for more details

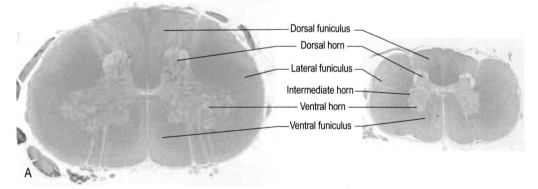

A

Fig. 4.6A **Dog spinal cord, transverse sections, at the levels of the cervical intumescence (left) and cranial lumbar spinal cord (right). Note the increased size of the dorsal and ventral horns in the cervical intumescence compared with the lumbar cord and the presence of an obvious intermediate horn supplying autonomic efferent fibres to the viscera, in the latter. Spinal cord sizes are in proportion with each other; this illustrates that the cord diameter is larger at the intumescence. Spinal cord sections stained with luxol fast blue and cresyl violet.**

There are also other caudally directed tracts in the lateral funiculus, such as fibres from the locus ceruleus, which is a collection of adrenergic neurons in the pons, and the raphe nuclei of the rostral medulla oblongata. Both tracts are involved in modulating the response to noxious stimulation, the first by releasing noradrenaline and the second by releasing serotonin.

Note that tracts and pathways are not the same. A tract, or fasciculus, is a specific bundle of axons in the CNS extending from dendrites to synapse. Tracts are usually named for their origin and termination, e.g. the vestibulospinal tract. A pathway is a route through the nervous system that may involve several tracts in sequence, synapsing successively with each other. For example, the proprioceptive pathway from the thoracic limbs is as follows: afferent impulses from the PNS travel cranially in the spinal cord via the fasciculus cuneatus, synapse in the cuneate nucleus of the medulla oblongata, travel via the medial lemniscus to the thalamus, synapse and then go via thalamo-cortical fibres to the somatosensory cortex.

Many tracts decussate (e.g. corticospinal, rubrospinal tracts) meaning they cross the midline in the CNS, thus the origin and termination of the tract are on opposite sides.

Spinal cord functions: Links with the PNS

During embryonic development the neural tube has a relatively uniform diameter along its length. However, if a neuron fails to connect to a target, the neuron degenerates. There are more peripheral targets in limb regions, hence in the postnatal animal the spinal cord diameter is larger in regions supplying the limbs as it houses more nerve cell bodies and nerve fibres. These areas of increased diameter are called the cervical and lumbar intumescences (*tumere* – L = to swell up). In a transverse section of the spinal cord at an intumescence, the dorsal and ventral horns are enlarged (more neuronal cell bodies and processes) and the nerve roots are more prominent (Fig 4.6A, B).

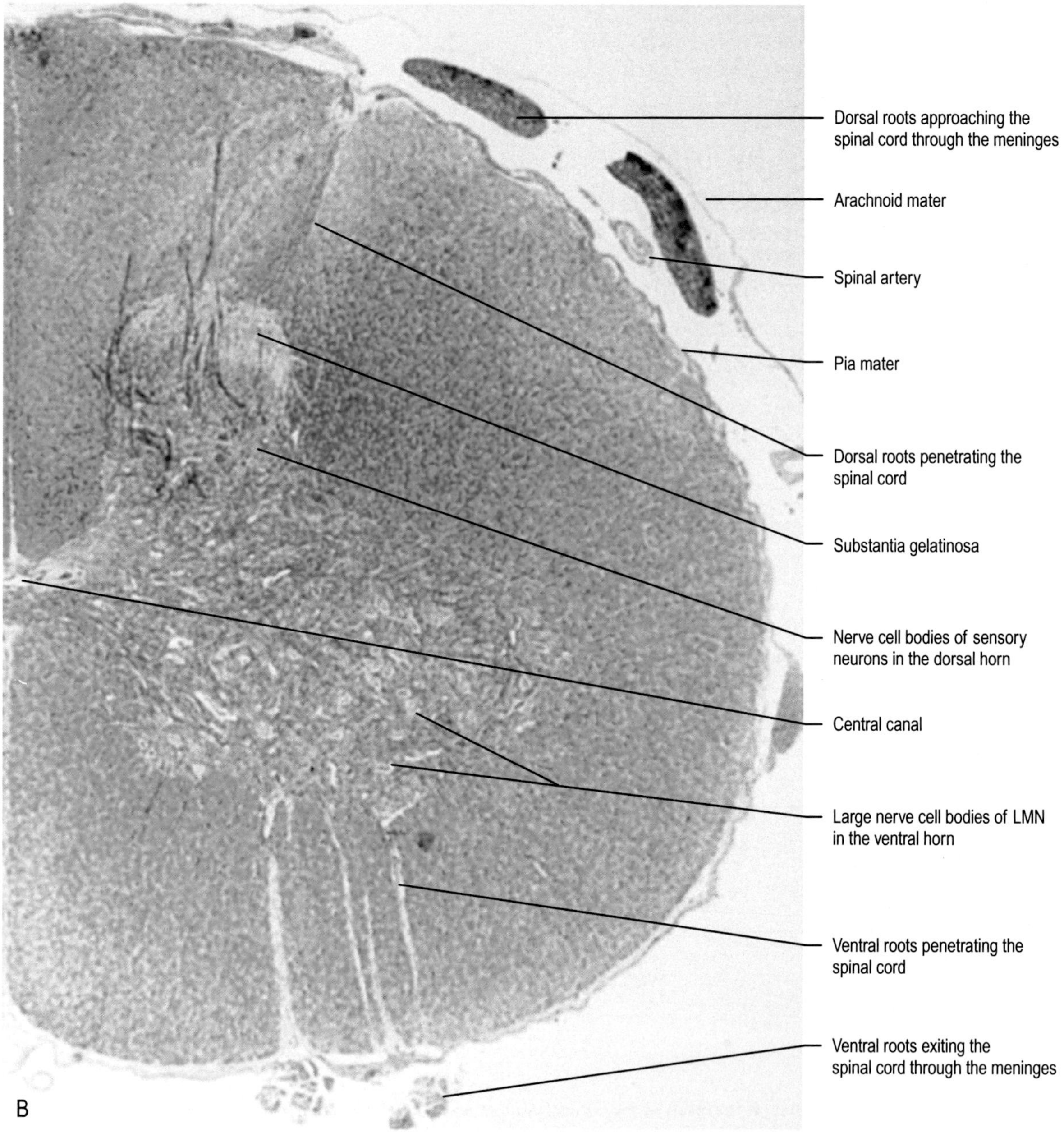
Dorsal roots approaching the spinal cord through the meninges
Arachnoid mater
Spinal artery
Pia mater
Dorsal roots penetrating the spinal cord
Substantia gelatinosa
Nerve cell bodies of sensory neurons in the dorsal horn
Central canal
Large nerve cell bodies of LMN in the ventral horn
Ventral roots penetrating the spinal cord
Ventral roots exiting the spinal cord through the meninges
B

Fig. 4.6B **Higher magnification of the C7 cord segment.**

Longitudinally, the different regions of the intumescences innervate different aspects of the limbs, via the brachial or lumbsosacral plexi (see Fig. 1.2). The pelvic plexus innervates pelvic viscera. Spinal nerves attached to the cranial part of the intumescence will mingle in the cranial part of the associated plexus and then innervate the proximal and cranial muscles of the limb. Spinal nerves attached to the caudal part of the intumescence will mingle in the caudal part of the associated plexus, and then innervate the distal and caudal muscles of the limb. This leads to a general rule that the cranial intumescence and plexus innervate cranial and proximal muscles of the limb, whilst the caudal intumescence and plexus innervate the caudal and distal muscles of the limb. Knowing which spinal cord segments contribute to the intumescence allows the clinician to localise the lesion based on observed signs. For example, observing that the supraspinatus muscle is atrophied and the animal cannot extend the shoulder would indicate a lesion in the cranial part of the brachial plexus or the cervical intumescence (Fig. 4.7).

Clinically, the spinal cord can be divided into functional areas, based around which cord segments supply the limbs, into the C1–C5, C6–T2, T3–L3, L4–S3 and Cd1–5 regions for the dog (see Fig. 1.2). Knowing these divisions is key to interpreting the clinical neurological examination of the spinal cord (see Chapter 13).

A lesion in any region of the cord can affect both the grey matter and white matter. Damage to grey matter causes loss of neurons and their axons will degenerate. Clinically, this is particularly important if the lesion affects the nerve cell bodies of the LMNs in an intumescence. Their LMN fibres connecting to the NMJ in the limb muscles will degenerate and the muscles will atrophy. Damage to other neurons in the grey matter, or their axons in the white matter, will lead to loss of axons distal to the lesion. If sensory somata, or their cranially-projecting neuronal processes are damaged, axons cranial to the lesion will be lost. Conversely damage

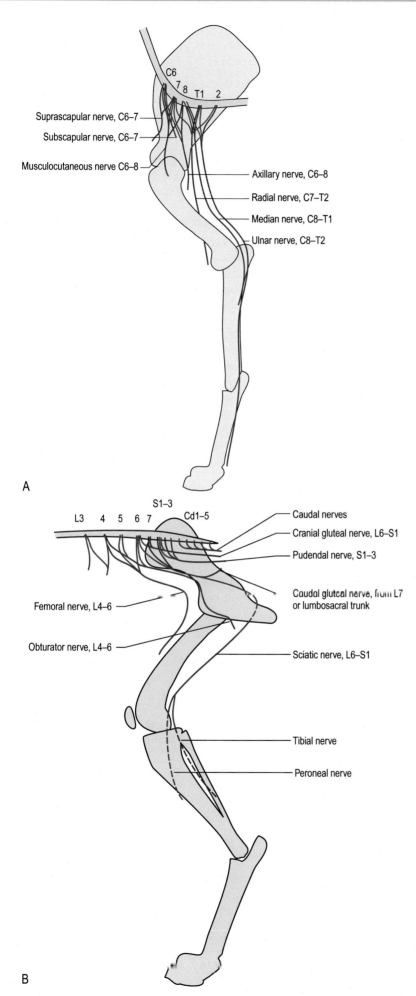

C6
7 8 T1 2

Suprascapular nerve, C6–7

Subscapular nerve, C6–7

Musculocutaneous nerve C6–8

Axillary nerve, C6–8

Radial nerve, C7–T2

Median nerve, C8–T1

Ulnar nerve, C8–T2

A

S1–3

L3 4 5 6 7   Cd1–5

Caudal nerves

Cranial gluteal nerve, L6–S1

Pudendal nerve, S1–3

Caudal gluteal nerve, from L7
or lumbosacral trunk

Femoral nerve, L4–6

Obturator nerve, L4–6

Sciatic nerve, L6–S1

Tibial nerve

Peroneal nerve

B

Fig. 4.7 **Innervation of the thoracic and pelvic limbs
from the intumescences via the plexi, viewed from the
medial aspects. The cranial intumescence and plexus
innervates the proximal, cranial muscles of the limb.
The caudal intumescence and plexus innervates the
distal and caudal muscles of the limb.**

to neurons whose axons connect to caudal segments (e.g. for reflex function) or damage to UMN fibres, will cause loss of axons caudal to the lesion. These patterns of damage can be recognised histopathologically. Damage to white matter can cause loss of sensation or motor function, resulting in anaesthesia and paresis/paralysis caudal to the site of the lesion.

Localising lesions in the spinal cord revolves around evaluating spinal **R**eflexes, muscle **A**trophy and **T**one – or the 'Neuro RAT' (see Fig. 5.6 and Table 5.2). Incoming sensory fibres from the thoracic and pelvic limbs enter the cervical or lumbosacral intumescences, respectively. Those fibres can synapse with the LMNs supplying that limb, which then connect via the NMJ to striated muscles in that limb. Thus, as long as those spinal cord segments of the intumescence are functioning normally, reflex arcs will be intact and the limb muscles will have tone. If the spinal cord segments supplying the limbs are damaged, this can cause loss of reflex function, loss of tone and marked wasting of the muscles (neurogenic atrophy) due to loss of the LMN ('LMN lesion') and degeneration of the neuromuscular junction. In contrast, damage to the segments cranial to the intumescence can result in deficits in the body and limbs caudal to the lesion. The animal may have sensory deficits and, due to damage to UMN ('UMN lesion'), paresis/paralysis. However, the reflexes and limb muscle tone will still be intact in the limbs caudal to the lesion and any atrophy will be mild and due to disuse of the muscle. Note that reflexes and tone may actually be increased with such lesions due to damage to UMNs that are inhibitory to LMN.

Spinal cord functions: Links within the spinal cord

Sensory input from the periphery enters the cord via the dorsal root and may synapse on interneurons in the dorsal horn or pass through the dorsal horn into the white matter or ventral horn without synapsing (Fig. 4.8). Output from the dorsal horn may:

   I. Link to LMNs in the ipsilateral ventral horn of the same spinal cord segment for reflex function;
  II. Decussate in the white commissure to the contralateral ventral horn of the same spinal cord segment for reflex function;
 III. Enter the white matter to travel cranially or caudally to another spinal cord segment, ipsilateral or contralateral to the original side, and synapse with LMNs for reflex function;
  IV. Enter the white matter to travel cranially to the brain.

Interneurons are involved in all of these connections, excluding the monosynaptic relay found in some myotatic/stretch reflexes. Axons that connect between spinal cord segments form the propriospinal tract; this is also known as the spino-spinal tract as it starts and finishes within the spinal cord.

By virtue of links described in I–III above, input from one limb can result in reflex activity within that limb, utilising just one, or many, of the spinal cord segments involved in that intumescence. It can also affect the contralateral limb and the limbs of the other girdle. For example, stepping on a sharp object with the left pelvic limb will cause reflex withdrawal of that limb and simultaneous extension of the contralateral pelvic limb and potentially, the thoracic limbs too to accommodate the change in weight distribution.

Locomotion involves synchronised flexion and extension of the limbs, much of which is coordinated through wiring that forms reflexes (see Chapter 9), thus, it also utilises links described in 1–3. Events in each limb are linked temporally and spatially, to events in the other limbs. The basic

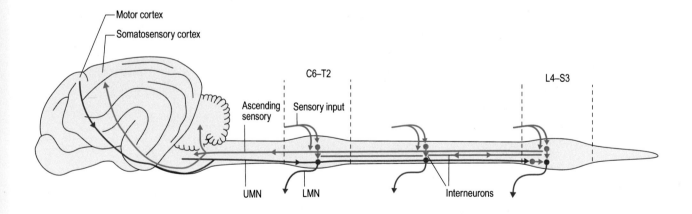

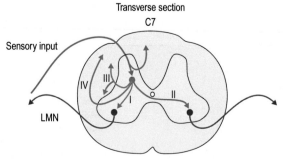

Fig. 4.8 **Links within the spinal cord. See text for explanation of Roman numerals.**

circuitry for coordinated, rhythmical flexion and extension of the limbs is located in the spinal cord. But the spinal cord circuitry alone is insufficient for gait; input from brain centres is also required.

Spinal cord functions: Links to the brain

Most incoming sensory fibres from the PNS synapse in the dorsal horn. Fibres make local connections for reflex function or enter the white matter to travel cranially to the brain in specific, defined tracts within the dorsal, lateral or ventral funiculi. Such cranially directed fibres may or may not synapse in the dorsal horn first. Once they reach the brain they may: (a) terminate by synapsing in the brainstem on specific nuclei; (b) travel to the cerebellum without synapsing en route; (c) synapse in relay nuclei in the brainstem, from which they continue to the somatosensory cortex of the forebrain (Fig. 4.8).

The UMN tracts in the spinal cord link the UMN motor centres of the brain with the LMNs of the spinal cord. The majority of UMN nuclei important for quadrupedal movement are located in the brainstem. The UMN input from the motor cortex of the forebrain directs voluntary, learned movements. The UMN systems initiate, modulate and terminate LMN activity and reflex function for posture and locomotion, voluntary movement and visceral function.

Most UMN axons in the spinal cord synapse on interneurons, which then synapse onto the LMN. There are some exceptions to this rule, depending on the species. The corticospinal tract and vestibulospinal tracts may synapse directly onto the LMN. Whether a UMN synapses directly or indirectly on LMNs is relevant clinically as indirect synapses onto diverse interneurons allow for divergence and convergence of information (Fig. 4.9). If there are several synapses, loss of a component of the pathway may be compensated for by rerouting the information through other neurons. The nervous system is relatively plastic and co-opting of alternative routes may assist in recovery after spinal cord injury. Conversely, if the synapse of the UMN is directly onto the LMN, then there are no alternative routes, using interneurons, by which information can get to the LMN. Humans have a much greater dependence on direct connections; this is one reason why a cerebrovascular

accident ('stroke') affecting blood supply to the motor cortex or its efferent pathways, can cause significant motor deficits.

Many tracts decussate, such that their axons cross the midline, either near their origin, e.g. rubrospinal tract, or near their termination, e.g. ventral corticospinal tract, thus tract input and termination are on the opposite sides of the body. Decussation of the nervous system may have evolved from the development of the coiling reflex in primitive chordates. A noxious stimulus on one side results in contraction of contralateral muscles, thus moving the animal away from the stimulus. A few tracts may cross the midline more than once, e.g. ventral spinocerebellar tract. Other tracts mainly influence the ipsilateral side, e.g. vestibulospinal tract. Sensory tracts travelling to the cerebellum ultimately terminate in the ipsilateral cerebellum. Sensory tracts travelling to the cerebrum, remain ipsilateral in the spinal cord, but after synapsing in the brainstem, their rostral continuation crosses to the opposite side. The exceptions to this rule are tracts like the spinothalamic tract that conveys nociception in quadrupeds. The spinothalamic tract travels cranially on both sides of the spinal cord in lateral funiculi, and in and out of the grey matter synapsing multiple times.

Decussation is clinically relevant as indicated by the example of an animal with a lesion that affects the pathway conveying touch and proprioception. Consider the cat in Fig. 4.10 that is bearing weight on the dorsal aspect of the right forepaw indicating abnormal paw position sense. The proprioceptive pathway originates in tactile and joint receptors of the forepaw, travels via the nerves (e.g. the radial nerve) into the dorsal horn of the C7–T1 spinal cord segments, into the dorsal funiculus (fasciculus cuneatus) cranially to the medulla oblongata where it synapses (nucleus cuneatus). From there the pathway decussates (deep arcuate fibres) and continues rostrally (medial lemniscus), synapsing in the thalamus and hence to the somatosensory cortex on the left side of the brain. This cat's signs could be due to a lesion anywhere along that pathway from origin to termination. If the lesion were in the spinal cord, it would have to compromise the right dorsal funiculus, but if it were in the forebrain or rostral brainstem, it would have to be on the left side. Localising the lesion depends on the results of the rest of the neurological examination. For example, if the lesion was in the spinal cord, there may be signs of ipsilateral limb paresis, while if it was in the forebrain there may be signs of contralateral visual deficit (see Fig. 13.1).

The function of spinal cord tracts, and their vulnerability to compressive lesions, is related to their microanatomy; this vulnerability explains the sequence of neurological signs observed in compressive spinal cord lesions. Factors determining vulnerability are axonal diameter, thickness of the myelin sheath and fibre location in the cord. The conduction velocity of a nerve fibre is proportional to both the diameter of the fibre and the degree of myelination. Thus large-diameter, heavily myelinated fibres are fast conducting (e.g. myelinated, 20 μm diameter fibres conduct at velocity of up to 120 m/s), while small, lightly or non-myelinated fibres are slow conducting (e.g. 1 μm diameter conducting at 1 m/s). Examples of such fibres are proprioceptive and nociceptive fibres, respectively.

In compressive lesions of the spinal cord, the first fibres to be compromised are the proprioceptive fibres, as they

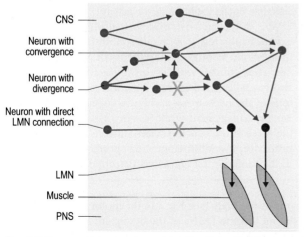

Fig. 4.9 **Upper motor neurons connect directly or via interneurons to LMNs. Lesions as depicted by the green 'X' will result in complete loss of LMN control if UMNs make a direct link from the motor centre in the brain. However, those that connect via interneurons may be able to reroute information and thereby still control the LMN.**

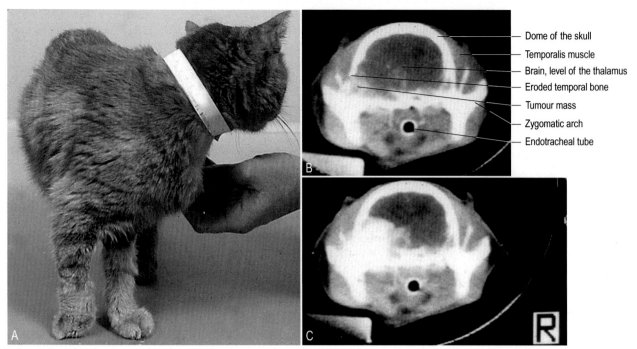

Labels on image B:
- Dome of the skull
- Temporalis muscle
- Brain, level of the thalamus
- Eroded temporal bone
- Tumour mass
- Zygomatic arch
- Endotracheal tube

Fig. 4.10 **(A) Cat with abnormal paw position due to a lesion affecting termination of the proprioceptive tract; specifically the cat had a tumour in the left forebrain. The cat was not paretic, but it did have a visual deficit in the right eye. The majority of the visual pathway from the right eye decussates in the optic chiasm ventral to the diencephalon (forebrain) to the left visual cortex. Hence clinical signs in the right side of the body were due to a left forebrain lesion. This contralateral location of the lesion relative to the clinical signs reflects decussation of the involved sensory pathways. Precontrast (B) and post-contrast enhanced (C) CT scans depicting a large extradural mass on the left side of the cranial vault.**

are large diameter and heavily myelinated. The last fibres to be compromised are those conveying nociception. That it takes a severe, extensive lesion to cause loss of nociception reflects the fact that nociceptive fibres are small diameter and lightly myelinated and, also, that there are several tracts that convey nociception; these tracts are located in different areas of the spinal cord (see Chapter 6). Other sensory fibres and motor fibres have axonal diameters and myelin sheath thickness that is between these two extremes.

For compressive spinal cord lesions of increasing severity, the signs will begin with spinal hyperpathia/sensitivity (due to meningeal irritation), proprioceptive dysfunction, then paresis, loss of superficial (pinprick) pain, paralysis, and finally loss of all nociception even from an intense crushing stimulus such as applied across a digit by a pair of large haemostats. Loss of urinary and faecal continence occurs when the spinal cord damage is severe enough to cause marked paresis or paralysis.

Senior management: Brainstem and motor cortex

UMNs and the brain

Senior management of the motor system comprises UMN nuclei located primarily in the brainstem and the motor cortex of the cerebrum (Figs. 4.11, 4.12). It makes feedback loops with the cerebellum. It talks with junior management (interneurons) in the brainstem and spinal cord and may communicate directly with the worker LMNs. The UMN system is managed by the executive officers located mainly in the forebrain.

The senior management UMN system located in the forebrain is the motor cortex. It is organised somatopically such that specific regions of the cortex relate to specific

Key points

- The majority of UMN nuclei in quadrupeds are located in the brainstem; however skilled movements are controlled by UMNs mainly located in the forebrain.
- UMN originating in the motor cortex travel to the brainstem and synapse on LMNs in cranial nerve nuclei (corticonuclear tract). Or they continue caudally via the pyramids of the medulla oblongata to synapse on LMNs in the spinal cord (corticospinal or pyramidal tract).
- Nuclei associated with maintaining posture (antigravity support) are the vestibular and pontine reticular formation. The red nucleus and medullary reticular nuclei facilitate flexor activity.
- UMNs in the caudal brainstem that ultimately inhibit extensor muscle activity require input from midbrain or forebrain to function: facilitators of extension do not. Thus animals with lesions in the mid brainstem and rostral cerebellum can show increased extensor tone of the neck, trunk and limbs (opisthotonus).
- Senior management of the sensory system includes the cerebellum, which receives subconscious proprioceptive information, and specific receiving areas in the forebrain for conscious perception.

regions of the body (see Fig. 4.14 for motor homunculi). Its output links to LMNs of the brainstem and the spinal cord via the corticonuclear (old name = corticobulbar) and corticospinal tracts, respectively.

The output from the motor cortex travels via the internal capsule in the forebrain and the crus cerebri into brainstem forming the longitudinal fibres of the pons. The

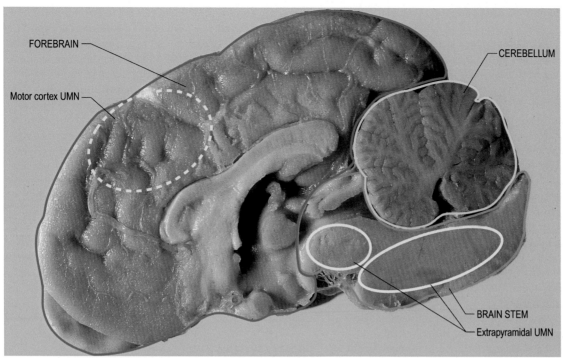

Fig. 4.11 **Dog brain median section depicting location of UMN centres and nuclei in yellow outline. Note the motor cortex (dotted outline) in the forebrain is located primarily on the lateral aspect of the hemisphere with some extension over the medial edge into the brain bordering longitudinal fissure.**

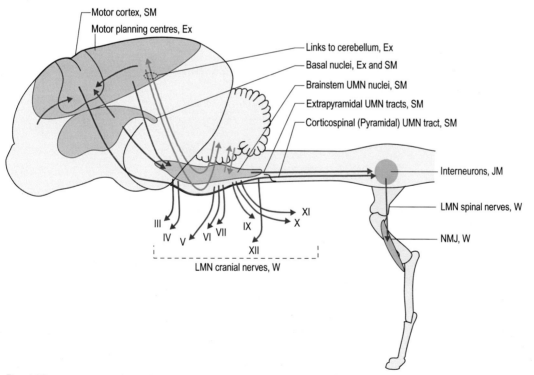

Fig. 4.12 **Motor system hierarchy in the quadrupedal mammalian brain, including the motor planning centres of the executive management (see next section). Ex = motor executive, SM = senior management, JM = junior management, W = worker.**

corticonuclear fibres terminate on the cranial nerve nuclei in the brainstem. (Termination is primarily ipsilateral (CN IV) bilateral (CNN III, V, VII, IX–XI) or contralateral (CNN VI, XII).) The remaining tracts, which are corticospinal, project caudally in the superficially located pyramids on the ventral aspect of the medulla oblongata forming the pyramidal system (see Chapter 5). In the spinal cord, the corticospinal tract divides into the lateral and ventral tracts, travelling caudally in the relevant funiculi. These tracts

decussate, thus the motor cortex influences the contralateral side of the body. Decussation is either at C1 level (lateral corticospinal tract) or just prior to terminating (ventral corticospinal tract). The motor cortex and its outputs are much more important in primates, and especially in humans, than in domestic mammals. For example, in equids the corticospinal tract only extends as far as the second cervical spinal cord segment. An animal's ability to perform skilled, dextrous movements is directly related to the development of the motor cortex and the pyramidal system (see Fig. 5.4).

In quadrupeds, the main UMN nuclei are found throughout the brain, but particularly in the brainstem. The UMN tracts arising from brainstem nuclei do not travel through the medullary pyramids and are thus known as the extrapyramidal system.

In the midbrain, UMN nuclei include the red nucleus (in the ventral midbrain, tegmentum) and tracts arising from the tectum (dorsal midbrain). The pons is associated with the pontine reticular formation and the medulla oblongata with the medial and lateral medullary reticular formation and the vestibular nuclei. The locations and functions of the tracts arising from these UMN centres are given in Fig. 4.5 and Table 4.3. In summary, brainstem nuclei associated with maintaining posture (antigravity support) are in the vestibular and pontine reticular formation, while UMN centres associated with facilitating flexor activity/protraction are the red nucleus, medullary reticular formation and the motor cortex of the forebrain.

Executive management centres located throughout the cerebral cortex activate the UMN system (Fig. 4.12).

Many of the UMN pathways facilitate movement, but some, especially the medial medullary reticulospinal tract, are major inhibitors of movement. However, the inhibitory UMNs, particularly those in the pons and medulla

oblongata, require input from centres in the midbrain or forebrain to function – facilitators of extension do not. Thus an animal with a caudal cranial fossa lesion, i.e. a lesion in the caudal part of the cranial vault, disrupting connections between the forebrain and caudal brainstem can show greatly exaggerated, generalised, extensor tone called 'opisthotonus' (see Fig. 9.6). Extensor (antigravity) muscle activity is stronger than flexor muscle activity. Therefore, in spinal cord lesions that damage UMN tracts, loss of LMN inhibition by the medial medullary reticulospinal tract, and loss of input from other tracts that facilitate flexor activity (e.g. corticospinal and rubrospinal), can result in significant spasticity, hypertonus and uninhibited reflexes (Fig. 4.2).

All of these UMN centres have bidirectional links with the cerebellum, forming feedback circuits. Thus the UMN centre informs the cerebellum of its intended activity and the cerebellum then can regulate the movement as it occurs. To do this the cerebellum uses continuous subconscious proprioceptive feedback from the parts of the body that are moving and those that are involved in postural support (see Chapters 6 and 7).

Sensory systems
Senior management of the sensory systems comprises the primary receiving areas for incoming information, which are located in the cerebellum and forebrain (Fig. 4.13). The

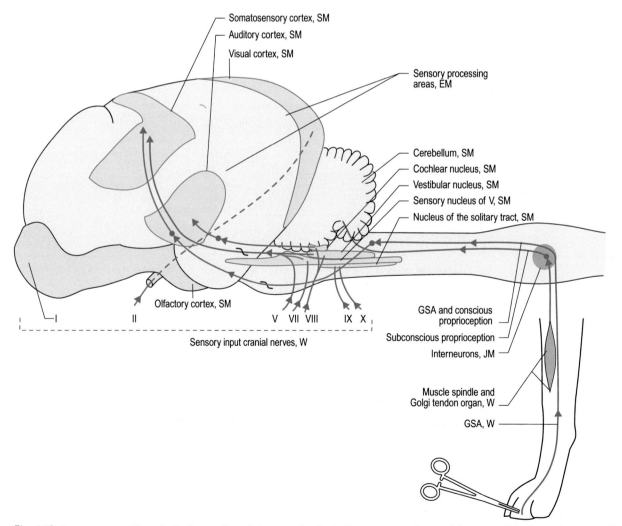

Fig. 4.13 **Sensory system hierarchy in the quadrupedal mammalian brain. Roman numerals = cranial nerves, GSA = general somatic afferent, which includes tactile, thermal and nociception. Note, not all the executive components (e.g. association and interpretation areas) are noted on this figure. See next section.**

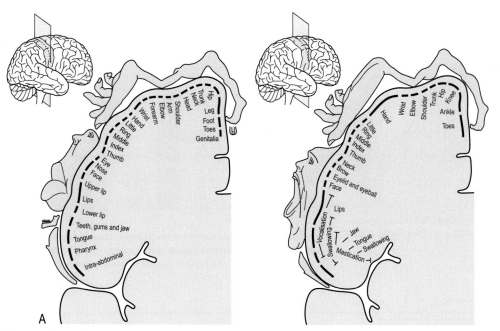

Fig. 4.14A **The human sensory (left) and motor (right) homunculus (redrawn with permission from _Gray's Anatomy_ 39th edition, fig 22-13).**

cerebellum receives subconscious proprioceptive information from muscle spindles and Golgi tendon organs of the body and limbs via the PNS and spinal cord. Subconscious proprioception for the head, originating in the vestibular apparatus of the inner ear, is sent to vestibular nuclei of the brainstem and hence to the cerebellum. Proprioceptive information from the head musculature is forwarded from the trigeminal nuclei in the brainstem. Conscious proprioceptive, tactile, nociceptive, thermal and gustatory information is received in the somatosensory cortex of the forebrain (see Fig. 4.14 for human and feline sensory homunculi). Auditory, visual and olfactory stimuli project to specific receiving areas in the forebrain, such as the auditory, visual and olfactory cortices (Fig. 4.13).

Both the motor cortex and somatosensory cortex are somatopically arranged, such that the body areas can be mapped to specific areas of each cortex. This mapping results in the homunculus image (L = little man) (Fig. 4.14A), or in the case of the cat, the felunculus (Fig. 4.14B).

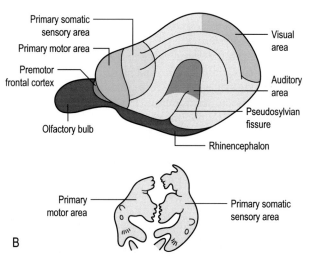

Fig. 4.14B **The feline sensory and motor homunculi (redrawn with permission from King A.S. Physiological and Clinical Anatomy of the Domestic Mammals. Volume 1, Central Nervous System. Oxford University Press, 1993, figure 8.2b, page 102). The two figures are drawn at the same scale. The lower image of the homunculi can be superimposed on the primary motor and sensory areas, by spreading them over both the medial and lateral aspects of the hemispheres.**

Executive management: Forebrain

Key points

- The executive management links inputs from sensory association areas, storage areas, behaviour and emotion-generating areas with motor planning areas.
- The output from the executive system can stimulate complex and varied patterns of motor activity and voluntary, learned tasks.
- The variability with which an animal can respond to stimuli is determined by the degree of cerebrocortical development. In non-primates only a minority of the cerebral cortex is dedicated to the association of information.

The executive management sits at the top of the hierarchical arrangement. It has its head office located mainly in the forebrain. It talks with senior management, but not with junior management, or the workers, directly.

The executive component of the motor system hierarchy is responsible for planning motor activity. It involves diffuse regions of the forebrain and subcortical connections. It draws on brain regions used for integrating sensory information (association areas), storage of information (memory), behaviour and emotion (limbic system) and motor coordinating/regulating areas, such as the basal nuclei and cerebellum. It is the site where an appropriate output is determined, based on integration of all inputs, experience and prediction of the outcomes. The executive motor planning centres also include areas involved in

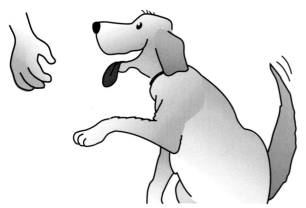

Fig. 4.15 **Dog using association areas to integrate sensory inputs, memory and behaviour centres, to produce a specific, learned motor output**

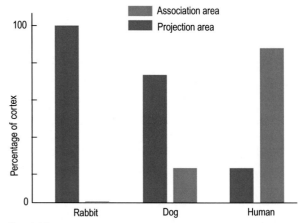

Fig. 4.16 **Percentage area of cerebral cortex used for receiving or projecting information (senior management – purple columns) versus integrating information (executive management – orange columns) in different species.**

abstract thought and problem-solving in animal types with those abilities. Thus the range of responses that an animal can display to a stimulus is determined by the degree of cerebrocortical development. Complex, varied responses require a high degree of neuronal connections to permit learning, memory, assessment of input, differential processing and conceptualisation. In many invertebrates, stimuli can only evoke outputs that are stereotypical or reflexive.

Outputs from the executive system are delegated to different UMN centres in the motor cortex and brainstem nuclei (senior management); these ultimately direct the worker LMNs and result in muscle activity. Through such hierarchical organisation the simplest motor components (individual LMN function or reflex arcs) can be recruited into complex patterns of activity. This is the basis of the diverse array of complex motor functions that animals use.

Thus the cerebral cortex draws on a wide range of storage, processing and integrating areas to produce an output that filters down through the hierarchical motor system and is finally expressed as a voluntary, complex, learned task, such as a dog learning to shake 'hands' (Fig. 4.15).

The executive components of the sensory system are the association areas. Association areas integrate input from their adjacent, primary receiving area. Primary receiving areas include auditory, sensory, visual and olfactory cortices. The association area rates that input in terms of importance and compares it with previous experience by drawing on storage/memory areas. Association areas connect with executive motor areas, and their input assists with planning a suitable response and predicting the outcome. Connections are via short interneurons, which form complex patterns of circuitry linking executive sensory and motor systems, memory, emotion and behaviour centres.

In primates and humans, association areas of the brain are well developed. In cats and dogs, the projections areas (primary receiving areas and motor cortex) account for the vast majority (approximately 80%) of the cerebral cortex. The remainder of the cortex is the association area. The situation is opposite in humans in which the majority of the cortex is used for association of information (Fig. 4.16).

Chapter 5
Reflexes and motor systems

Key points

- A reflex is a stereotypical somatic or autonomic activity triggered by a specific stimulus. The reflex arc involves sensory input, connection in the CNS to the UMN, the LMN, neuromuscular junction and muscle.
- Muscle tone and bulk depends on LMN function.
- UMNs initiate, regulate, modify and terminate the activity of the LMN. UMNs may inhibit or facilitate LMNs. Loss of inhibitory UMN function results in increased muscle tone and spinal reflexes, whereas loss of facilitatory UMNs results in paresis or paralysis.
- The UMN system originating from the motor cortex is responsible for voluntary and learned movement of the face, body and limbs using the corticonuclear and corticospinal/pyramidal tracts, respectively. It is more important in primates and humans than quadrupeds.
- The extrapyramidal system is responsible for maintaining posture and rhythmical/semiautomatic activities including locomotion. Extrapyramidal UMN tracts originate primarily in the brainstem and their fibres do not travel in the pyramids. In quadrupeds, this system is of primary importance.
- Specific UMN tracts are excitatory or inhibitory to LMNs. Movement is ultimately expressed through the LMNs stimulating muscles.

- Loss of UMN input typically results in paresis or paralysis with normal to increased muscle tone and spinal reflexes caudal to the lesion. Muscle atrophy is mild and due to disuse.
- Loss of the LMNs results in paresis/paralysis, with decreased to absent muscle tone and reflexes. Muscle atrophy can be severe and is neurogenic in origin.
- The 'Neuro RAT' helps differentiate between UMN and LMN signs – **R**eflexes, **A**trophy and **T**one.
- Planning of motor activity takes place in the forebrain and motor function is modulated by input from the cerebellum and basal nuclei.

General introduction

Normal posture, gait and voluntary movement require input from sensory systems, planning and coordination centres, storage (memory) areas, and output through motor systems using UMNs and LMNs. Upper motor neurons are the 'managers' and are confined to the CNS. Lower motor neurons are the 'workers' and have their neuronal cell body in the CNS, but the axon, which forms the majority of the cell, travels via spinal or cranial nerves in the PNS to synapse at the neuromuscular junction. Thus we suggest that motor neurons could be described as either UMNs / central motor neurons, which are managers; and LMNs / peripheral motor neurons, which are workers. In the case of the autonomic efferent fibres, there are a pre-synaptic and a post-synaptic LMN (peripheral motor neuron). The terms central and peripheral motor neurons are more descriptive than upper motor neuron and lower motor neuron, however UMN and LMN are widely used, despite their propensity to cause significant confusion.

The strength of muscle contraction is directly proportional to the frequency of action potentials in the nerve supplying the muscle. Conversely, the precision of muscle function is inversely proportional to the size of the motor unit, where a motor unit is defined as a single α-LMN axon and the muscle fibres with which it synapses. Muscles with large motor units, such as proximal limb muscles, are used for imprecise movements. Small motor units, such as found in the extraocular muscles, enable fine, specific movement of the target organ, such as the eye.

Muscle activity for maintaining posture (at rest or during motion) arises largely at a subconscious/subcortical level, whereas voluntary movement arises primarily from a conscious/cortical level. The subconscious level utilises reflex arcs linking function within, and between, limbs. Subcortical control results in postural changes (sitting, standing, etc.) and repetitive movement, such as breathing, basic locomotion, scratching and chewing.

Cerebrocortical control is used for voluntary, complex and learned movements such as hunting or the pet offering its paw to be shaken. Primates and humans have a much greater dependence on cortical motor centres of the forebrain for all movement including gait. In comparison, the spinal reflexes in domestic mammals, are the basic functional unit that underpins all posture and locomotion on which is superimposed, supraspinal input originating largely in the brainstem. As such, forebrain lesions can result in hemiparesis/plegia in humans, but do not compromise significantly locomotion in domestic mammals.

Spinal reflexes

Key points

■ Reflexes are hard-wired into the nervous system and most are polysynaptic.
■ Reflexes can be ipsilateral, contralateral, intrasegmental or intersegmental, somatic or autonomic.
■ Muscle spindles detect stretching of muscle. They provide sensory input to the CNS using 1a afferent fibres and their intrafusal fibres receive motor input from the CNS via γ-efferent fibres. α-LMN innervate the extrafusal muscle fibres.
■ The myotatic ('stretch') reflex has a significant role in maintaining body posture. Gravity causes muscle stretching, stimulating muscle spindles that induce reflex contraction of the muscle.
■ The Golgi tendon organ inverse myotatic reflex protects the skeletal muscle from excessive contraction by causing reflex muscle relaxation.
■ Muscle tone is controlled by activity of α and γ-LMN; these LMNs are stimulated by muscle spindles and specific UMN tracts.

A reflex is defined as a stereotypical response produced by a specific stimulus. The reflex arc involves receptors and nerves of the PNS (sensory and motor) and a region of the CNS in which the sensory input connects to the motor output. This CNS region is in the brain for cranial nerve reflexes and in the spinal cord for limb and body reflexes. Reflexes are 'hard-wired', meaning that the neuronal connections are established during embryonic development and are present at birth. Conversely, neural responses (e.g. the menace response) have to be learned. Their 'wiring' develops postnatally as a consequence of experience. The reflex is the functional unit of the nervous system as compared with the morphological unit that is the neuron.

That the reflex is the most basic functional unit of the nervous system is evidenced by its presence in simple metazoan animals. In vertebrates, incoming sensory input into the dorsal horn can synapse directly with LMNs in the ventral horn of that spinal cord segment and stimulate a motor output. This simplest reflex is called a monosynaptic reflex and is exemplified by the patellar reflex. Most other reflexes involve interneurons interposed between the input and output side. Interneurons permit divergence (see Fig. 4.9) so that the input can be distributed to a wider

population of output neurons. Thus one type of input can stimulate both agonist muscle contraction and antagonist muscle relaxation, e.g. the patellar reflex can stimulate quadriceps muscle contraction and hamstring muscle relaxation (see Fig. 4.4).

There are a number of different types of reflexes including:

(a) Somatic reflexes that permit the animal to respond to the external environment. An example of this is the palpebral reflex, where stimulation around the eyelids causes blinking to protect the eyeball.
(b) Autonomic reflexes that permit the animal to respond to changes in its internal environment. An example of this is the increase in heart rate in response to reduced blood pressure.

Reflex arcs can be ipsilateral, contralateral due to decussation of the fibres, intrasegmental located within one spinal cord segment, or intersegmental involving a number of different spinal cord segments.

Muscle spindles
Muscle spindles are spindle/fusiform-shaped receptors located within striated/skeletal muscles. They are called stretch receptors as they detect stretching of the muscle. Muscle spindles comprise modified muscle cells called intrafusal fibres that have contractile elements at the ends of the spindle and sensory receptors in the middle. The surrounding normal muscle fibres are referred to as extrafusal. Muscle spindles are located in parallel with the extrafusal muscle fibres and, consequently, are stretched when the muscle is stretched. The contractile elements of muscle spindles are innervated by γ-motor neurons that, when stimulated, cause contraction at the ends of the spindle, thus stretching the centre of the spindle. The intrafusal fibres and the γ-motor neuron comprise the fusimotor system. Stretching of the muscle spindle causes firing of the sensory receptors in the spindle and stimulation of the 1a afferent nerve fibres. Sensory impulses travel via the spinal nerve to the spinal cord, or, if arising from head muscles, via cranial nerves to the brainstem. In the CNS the 1a afferent fibre synapses with α-LMNs resulting in stimulation of extrafusal fibres and muscle contraction. The extrafusal fibre plus the α-LMN is the skeletomotor system (Fig. 5.1).

The myotatic reflex
The myotatic ('stretch') reflex arc is a feature of limb and trunk muscles especially. It uses the stimulus of muscle stretching to generate nerve impulses in the 1a afferent fibre. The impulses travel to the spinal cord, synapse (usually via interneurons) onto the α-LMN supplying that same muscle, stimulating nerve impulses in that α-LMN. This causes contraction of the extrafusal fibres surrounding the muscle spindle, thereby shortening the muscle and reducing the stretch of the muscle spindle. Thus, activity in the 1a afferent nerve fibre stimulates agonist muscle contraction. Simultaneously, it also causes reciprocal inhibition; that is, it inhibits contraction in the antagonist muscle. For example, the effect of gravity on the weight-bearing stifle joint is to make it collapse (stifle flexion), thereby stretching the quadriceps muscle and its muscle spindles. Spindle stretching causes reflex contraction of the quadriceps muscle and stifle extension to support

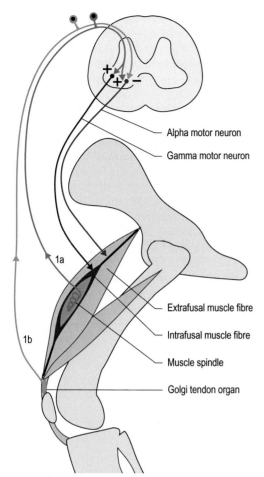

- Alpha motor neuron
- Gamma motor neuron

- Extrafusal muscle fibre
- Intrafusal muscle fibre
- Muscle spindle
- Golgi tendon organ

Fig. 5.1 **Muscle spindles are in parallel with the extrafusal fibres and are stretched when the muscle is stretched. Golgi tendon organs are in series with the extrafusal fibres and are stretched when the muscle shortens due to contraction.**

the animal's weight. Simultaneously, the stifle flexors (hamstring muscles such as the semimembranosus and semitendinosus muscles) will be inhibited. The input from the 1a afferent is also forwarded to the brain to provide proprioceptive information that is essential for planned and coordinated motor function (see Chapter 6).

Different types of 1a fibres are stimulated by static versus dynamic stretching. Stretching of the muscle spindle and stimulation of 1a afferents can be caused by the following.

(a) The effect of gravity causing the joint to flex and passively stretching the extensor muscles. This causes reflex contraction of α-LMN and is used to sustain posture (see 'Posture and the myotatic reflex' in this chapter).

(b) Stretching of tendon and hence the muscle, by tapping of the tendon. For example, the patellar reflex is elicited clinically by tapping the patellar ligament (the continuation of the quadriceps tendon) with a patella hammer, or plexor (see Fig. 4.4 and 13.9).

(c) By activation of γ-LMNs causing intrafusal muscle fibres to contract. This is the mechanism by which many descending UMNs ultimately cause contraction in the muscles – they stimulate the γ-motor neuron, which reflexively causes stimulation of the α-LMNs and amplification of the action.

Within the spinal cord the input from the 1a afferent fibres can link to LMNs in the same spinal cord segment or in different spinal cord segments, ipsi- or contralaterally

(see Fig. 4.8). The propriospinal tract is a white matter tract immediately surrounding the grey matter of the spinal cord, and conveys axons connecting between spinal cord segments. Thus input from one muscle can influence other muscles acting around that joint, or other joints in the same limb, or other limbs. For example, in the withdrawal reflex, noxious stimulation of the foot causes limb flexion. If the animal is standing at the time, then the other limbs will extend to compensate for the loss of weight-bearing in the stimulated limb. The withdrawal reflex uses multiple spinal cord segments to activate both multiple flexor muscles within the stimulated limb, and extensor muscles of the other limbs.

Golgi tendon organs and the inverse myotatic reflex

Golgi tendon organs are located within the tendon; therefore they are in series with the muscle. They are stimulated by the stretching when extrafusal muscle fibres contract, causing muscle shortening and increased tension in the tendon.

Their sensory innervation is type 1b afferent fibre; this has a higher threshold to stimulation than the muscle spindle. Significant stretching of the tendon stimulates nerve impulses in 1b afferent fibre; these are projected into the spinal cord. This input stimulates interneurons that inhibit the α-LMN of that muscle, thereby decreasing muscle contraction and reducing the tension in the tendon (see Fig. 5.1). It may also stimulate α-LMNs of the antagonist muscle.

The activity of the Golgi tendon organs functions to prevent over-contraction of the muscle and muscular avulsion (tearing of the muscle fibres or the tendon) from the bone. It also facilitates switching from extensor to flexor activity.

α-γ co-activation

When the α-LMNs are stimulated, the extrafusal fibres contract, reducing the stretch of the intrafusal fibres; this decreases activation of the Ia afferent fibre. This decreased sensory input to the CNS would result in loss of proprioceptive input (Chapter 6). But if the γ-LMN is activated simultaneously with the α-LMN, then the intrafusal fibres contract, causing comparable shortening of the muscle spindle. Thus the relative stretch of the muscle spindle is maintained and the Ia firing is sustained. Therefore when a muscle is stimulated to contract, both α- and γ-LMNs are simultaneously stimulated and proprioceptive input from the muscle about its length and tension is maintained. This is called α-γ co-activation. Functionally, this acts to maintain appropriate muscle tone, despite changes in muscle length, and to maintain continual proprioceptive input to brain, which is essential for normal posture and movement.

Muscle tone

Muscle tone refers to the muscle's resistance to being stretched. Muscle tone is due to several factors including the tonic γ-loop mechanism. Constant activation of the γ-efferents causes low-level stimulation of the Ia afferents, which causes low-level stimulation of the α-LMN and low-level contraction of the extrafusal fibres. This manifests as muscle tone and resistance of the muscle to being stretched. The inherent elasticity in muscle components also contributes to tone. Tone is further enhanced by the effect of specific UMN tracts, facilitating LMNs (α and γ). Clinically, loss of LMN output to muscle will result in loss of tone. Loss of LMNs occurs with either damage to the cell body in the CNS or the axon in the PNS.

Limb muscle tone can be assessed by laying the animal on its side and gently flexing and extending the limbs. Limb flexion will cause stretching of the extensor muscles and extension will cause stretching of the flexor muscles; both activities induce myotatic reflex-induced contraction in stretched muscles. The reflexively induced contraction will cause resistance to flexion and extension, respectively. Assessment of limb muscle tone is an important component of the neurological examination and can help differentiate UMN from LMN signs, thus aiding lesion localisation.

Posture and the myotatic reflex

The myotatic reflex is reflex activity based on muscle spindle input. It is a major mechanism by which the animal maintains posture and supports itself against gravity.

Gravity acts on the animal to cause flexion/collapse of the limb joints, flexion of the cervical vertebral column due to the weight of the head and extension (lordosis) of the thoracolumbar vertebral column due to the weight of the trunk. Thus gravity causes stretching of the muscle spindles in the extensor muscles of the limbs and neck, and flexor muscles of the thoracolumbar vertebral column. The stretching causes firing of the 1a sensory fibres from the spindles, with input via the spinal nerves to the spinal cord, stimulation of the α-LMNs and extension of the limbs and neck and flexion of the vertebral column. Simultaneously, the antagonistic muscles (limb and neck flexors and vertebral extensors) may be inhibited (Fig. 5.2).

Posture is also supported passively by elastic ligaments. For example, the nuchal ligament extending from the dorsal spinous processes of the cranial thoracic vertebrae to cervical vertebrae is analogous to a gigantic rubber band. It is stretched when the head is lowered (neck flexion) and recoils to help raise the head, acting to decrease the work required by the neck extensor muscles.

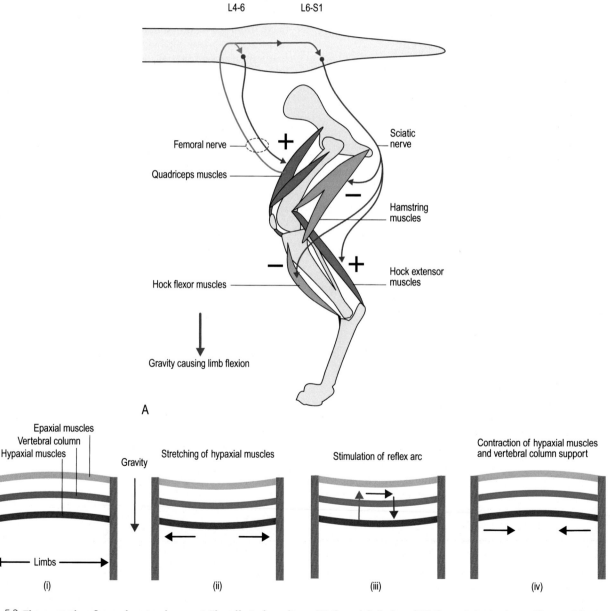

Fig. 5.2 **The myotatic reflex and postural support. The effect of gravity on (A) the pelvic limb and (B) the vertebral column. The quadriceps and hock extensor muscles (A) and hypaxial muscles (B) will be stretched by the effect of gravity, resulting in reflexively stimulated contraction and postural support against the effects of gravity.**

Reflexes in different parts of the body

Clinically, reflexes are tested to evaluate the integrity of the different components of the reflex arc. This includes the sensory input (receptor and spinal or cranial nerve), the CNS region in which input connects to LMN cell body (brain and spinal cord), and the motor output (spinal or cranial nerve, neuromuscular junction and muscle). Disruption of any one of these three components will result in decreased, or loss of, reflex activity. This is most commonly seen with lesions that involve either the region of the CNS in which the LMN cell body is housed, or in the LMN itself. Such a lesion is called a lower motor neuron lesion as it damages the LMN cell body or axon. If the reflex arc is present then the three anatomical components are intact and functioning.

Clinically, observing that a reflex is decreased, can particularly help localise a lesion. The clinician can identify which specific regions of the PNS and the interconnecting CNS have been compromised. For example, loss of the patellar reflex in the dog, means that the femoral nerve (afferent and efferent components of the reflex arc), or spinal cord segments L4–L6 have been compromised. Conversely, an intact reflex arc tells the clinician that the lesion does not involve that area of the CNS or the PNS. This is useful, but does not localise the lesion within the rest of the CNS.

It should be noted that the UMN system has a significant, inhibiting influence on LMNs especially those LMNs supplying extensor (antigravity) muscles. A CNS lesion that is cranial to the area of the CNS involved in the reflex arc may block UMN inhibition of the LMN of the reflex arc. This lesion damages the upper motor neurons, and hence is called an upper motor neuron lesion. Due to loss of the inhibitory influence of the UMN, the reflex may be exaggerated. This exaggerated reflex can indicate the presence of a lesion in the UMN system cranial to the location of the reflex wiring. For example, if there is a lesion in the thoracolumbar spinal cord, then the patellar reflex will be intact and may even be exaggerated.

Clinically, there are a number of reflexes that can be evaluated in the animal. They include limb, trunk and head reflexes and are described in Chapter 13.

Somatic motor systems

General anatomy and function

> ### Key points
>
> - The motor system supports the body against gravity, establishes posture and allows voluntary movement to occur.
> - In general, UMN tracts in the lateral funiculus facilitate flexion, and those in the ventral funiculus facilitate extension. The dorsolateral system of the spinal cord influences skilled and semiskilled movements of the distal limbs and the ventromedial system influences truncal and proximal limb muscles.

The main functions of the somatic motor system are to:

(a) maintain tone to support the body against the effects of gravity;

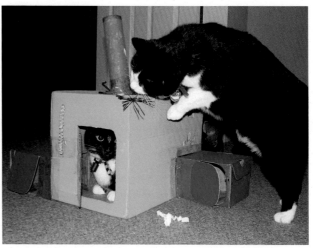

Fig. 5.3 **Hector (inside the box) using somatic motor systems to perform function 'a', especially for the neck muscles, while Harriet is doing all three functions as she explores outside the box.**

(b) provide a stable postural background against which movement can occur;

(c) initiate, modify and terminate voluntary movement (Fig. 5.3).

The UMN system functions to initiate, regulate, modify and terminate the activity of the LMN. In turn, the UMNs are controlled by the executives of the motor system (Chapter 4), which plan and coordinate static and dynamic motor function. The UMNs of primary importance in quadrupeds arise from nuclei in the brainstem and the motor cortex of the forebrain. They influence LMNs supplying striated muscle of the head, body and limbs using cranial and spinal nerves.

The UMNs may stimulate or inhibit the LMNs. The LMNs connect to flexor or extensor muscles. In the spinal cord, UMN tracts are found in the lateral and ventral funiculi. As a general rule, UMN tracts in the lateral funiculus facilitate flexion and those in the ventral funiculus facilitate extension. An alternative nomenclature for spinal cord motor tracts is the dorsolateral and ventromedial systems based on their location in the spinal cord. The dorsolateral system (corticospinal and rubrospinal tracts) influences skilled and semiskilled movements, especially of the distal limb muscles, and these are primarily flexor muscle although the lateral corticospinal tract influences both extensors and flexor muscles of the distal limb. The ventromedial system (vestibulospinal, reticulospinal and tectospinal tracts) influences truncal and proximal limb muscles; these are primarily extensors (see Fig. 4.5).

UMN: Pyramidal and extrapyramidal systems

> ### Key points
>
> - UMN systems of the spinal cord are classified anatomically into the extrapyramidal and pyramidal systems.
> - Extrapyramidal fibres, originating from UMN nuclei located throughout the brain, do not pass through the pyramids of the medulla oblongata. They influence LMNs of cranial and spinal nerves and function primarily to regulate posture and rhythmical,

semi-automatic motor movements. The extrapyramidal system is the dominant system in domestic animals.
- Pyramidal fibres, originating in the motor cortex of the cerebrum, pass through the pyramids into the spinal cord forming the corticospinal tract. Corticonuclear fibres arise in the motor cortex and synapse on cranial nerve nuclei in the brainstem. These tracts are responsible for complex, learned, voluntary movements. These pathways are more important in primates and humans than quadrupeds.
- With the exception of the vestibulospinal tract, both systems decussate and principally innervate γ-LMN.

Functionally and anatomically, UMN systems are divided based on their origin, into those systems originating from the motor cortex and those originating from other UMN centres throughout the brain. Fibres originating from the motor cortex and synapsing on LMN (corticonuclear and corticospinal tracts) are used for learned, skilled movement, whereas the other UMN systems are more important in posture, locomotion and semi-automatic movements such as breathing. Both systems influence cranial nerve nuclei of the brainstem and travel caudally into the spinal cord. The continuation of the corticospinal tract in the medulla oblongata is through the pyramids; the tracts originating from other brain areas do not pass through the pyramids. This has given rise to classifying the two systems into pyramidal and extrapyramidal, however, most corticonuclear fibres do not pass through the pyramids, thus the nomenclature is not precise.

The output from the motor cortex travels via the corona radiata, internal capsule and crus cerebri to the brainstem (see Figs. 1.13, A3, A15-18). There the corticonuclear fibres synapse on cranial nerve nuclei (CN III–VII, IX–XII) in the midbrain, pons and medulla oblongata. The remaining fibres form the corticospinal tract and continue caudally as two longitudinal bands of axons on the ventral surface of the medulla oblongata. In cross-section, these bilateral bands are somewhat triangular in shape, especially in humans, and are known as the pyramids, hence 'pyramidal system' (see Figs. A3, A21-25). The corticospinal/corticonuclear system functions in skilled, voluntary movement and hence dexterity in a species is related to its degree of pyramidal development. Corticospinal fibres account for 20–30% of the total spinal cord white in primates but only about 10% in carnivores. The corticospinal tract is also well developed in raccoons, an animal noted for its dexterity, and the horse has a well-developed corticonuclear system synapsing in the facial nucleus, for lip movement.

The extrapyramidal system comprises diverse tracts originating from UMN nuclei located throughout the brain. The extrapyramidal system functions to stimulate postural muscles for tonic support against the effects of gravity (aiding stretch reflexes), to generate a stable postural platform against which other movement can occur, and recruit spinal reflex circuitry for voluntary movement. It can also initiate, modulate and terminate voluntary movement (e.g. locomotion) and controls muscular activity associated with visceral activities such as cardiac and respiratory function and urination. In animals of traditional veterinary interest, the extrapyramidal system is far more important for motor function than is the pyramidal system (Fig. 5.4).

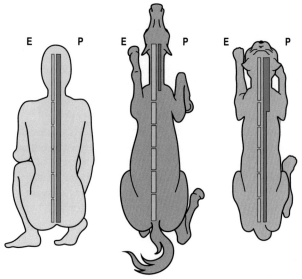

Fig. 5.4 **The degree of development of the extrapyramidal and pyramidal tracts varies markedly in the human, horse and cat. The dashed line represents the extrapyramidal tract (E) on the left in each figure, while the solid line represents the pyramidal tract (P) on the right in each figure (redrawn with permission from Figure 8.50, Dyce, Sack and Wensing, *Textbook of Veterinary Anatomy*, Fourth Edition, Saunders).**

Note that the red nucleus of the midbrain receives direct input from the ipsilateral motor cortex and projects the length of the spinal cord as the rubrospinal tract in the lateral funiculus, adjacent to the corticospinal tract. It is of major importance in domestic species. In dogs, it is considered to be the main tract controlling voluntary movement and acts as an indirect corticospinal tract.

In summary, the extrapyramidal system is responsible for maintaining and changing posture, rhythmical activities such as locomotion and chewing, and semi-automatic activities such as feeding. The rubrospinal tract also appears to have a role in semi-skilled movements of the distal limb. The pyramidal system is responsible for complex, learned, voluntary movements, such as the kitten playing with the Christmas tree ornament or feather (see Fig. 9.2). These voluntary movements are superimposed on an appropriate postural platform that is coordinated by the cerebellum and enacted by the extrapyramidal system.

Termination of UMN tracts on LMN: Descending UMN tracts usually synapse on interneurons, most of which then connect to γ-LMNs. The vestibulospinal tract also connects to α-LMN. Stimulation of the γ-LMNs increases the stretch of the muscle spindle causing firing of the 1a afferents; this stimulates the α-LMNs causing the muscle to contract. Significant amplification of the descending UMN input occurs via γ-1a-α circuit activation. It has been suggested that in dogs only 10–20% of descending UMN pathways need to be intact after a severe spinal cord lesion for locomotion to occur. Thus, animals with chronic, severe spinal cord compression, as in Fig. 5.5 may still be able to ambulate.

Tract decussation
Many motor tracts (e.g. corticospinal, rubrospinal, tectospinal) decussate as they travel between the origin and termination, thereby influencing the contralateral side of the body. The vestibulospinal tract is largely ipsilateral in that it stimulates the ipsilateral α-LMNs supplying extensor

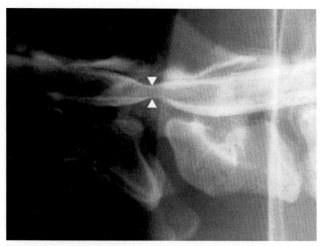

Fig. 5.5 **Dog, cervical spinal cord. Myelogram in which the spinal cord is outlined by radio-opaque contrast agent; there is marked compression of the C6–C7 spinal cord. This dog was still walking quite well despite the lesion; it did, however have moderate proprioceptive deficits.**

muscles, but it also inhibits contralateral extensor tone. The reticulospinal tracts are considered to influence both sides by some authors, or be mainly ipsilateral.

Inhibition versus excitation

The inhibitory pathways tend to dominate the excitatory/facilitatory pathways. This is necessary to decrease the effect of extensor (antigravity) muscle dominance over the flexor muscles, especially in the limbs. The main inhibitory pathway is the medullary reticulospinal tract. This tract exerts a massive inhibitory influence on γ-LMNs and hence indirectly on α-LMNs. The vestibulospinal, tectospinal, pontine reticulospinal and rubrospinal tracts are facilitatory to LMNs (see Table. 4.3). Severe spinal cord lesions can block the influence of descending inhibition, thus the animal may exhibit some spasticity/increased extensor muscle tone and exaggerated spinal reflexes (see Fig. 4.2).

UMN tracts

Table 5.1 lists the tracts of the non-cortical (extrapyramidal) and cortical (pyramidal) systems, their pathways and their functions.

Both the extrapyramidal and pyramidal spinal pathways usually have three neurons. Neuron one is the motor command centre (motor cortex or motor nuclei of the brainstem); neuron two is a short interneuron in the grey matter; neuron three is a ventral horn neuron, which are mostly γ-LMN, but some tracts (e.g. vestibulospinal) may stimulate α-LMN.

Additional comments on certain motor tracts are listed below.

1. Lateral vestibulospinal tract: This is a phylogenetically ancient tract, and facilitates extensor (antigravity) muscle activation. Such activation had to occur as soon as animals became subject to prominent forces of gravity, i.e. land-dwellers. The lateral vestibular nucleus receives input from sacculus and utriculus of the inner ear, which sense static head position. As vestibular input from the sacculus and utriculus is constant, so is the outflow via this tract. Thus the vestibulospinal tract plays a significant role in maintenance of posture against the effects of gravity and activation of extensor

muscles to cope with changes in posture. It is usually strongly inhibited by the cerebellum and the cerebrum. Unsuppressed function of the lateral vestibulospinal tract is partly responsible for the limb and spinal extension observed in decerebrate rigidity.

2. Rubrospinal tract: Phylogenetically, this is the youngest of the extrapyramidal tracts, but older than the corticospinal tract. It is somatopically organised within the cord with the pelvic limbs being lateral to the thoracic limbs. In dogs, it is the most important pathway for the execution of voluntary movement. In the decerebrate animal, if the red nucleus is preserved, then sitting, crouching, walking, climbing and the righting reflex can still occur. In humans, the rubrospinal tract is responsible for infants crawling and adults swinging their arms while walking; irregular arm swing is a prominent symptom in humans with dysfunction of the extrapyramidal system (Parkinson's disease).

3. The corticonuclear/corticospinal systems: The pyramidal system is only present in mammals; it is not found in birds, reptiles, amphibians or fish. Within mammals there is a great deal of variation in its development and location. In cats the tract extends the length of the cord, but in ungulates it ends in the cervical region. Its greater development in humans and primates reflects the fact that, phylogenetically, it is the youngest tract. Like the motor cortex, it is somatopically organised.

This is a three-neuron system in animals. The first neuron is in the motor cortex, which is located just rostral to the cruciate sulcus. In humans two additional motor areas are also present. The supplementary and second motor areas are located on the medial surface of the cerebral hemisphere adjacent to the primary motor area. The cat also has a supplementary motor area. The primary motor areas are somatopically arranged, giving rise to the homunculus in humans and felunculus in cats (see Fig. 4.14). The second neuron is an interneuron usually located in the base of the dorsal horn in the spinal cord, or within the motor nucleus of brainstem cranial nerve nuclei. The third neuron is located within the cranial nerve motor nucleus or the ventral horn of the spinal cord. This neuron is usually a γ-LMN but may occasionally be an α-LMN. The interneuron may be missing in the primate corticospinal tract controlling hand and foot movement, resulting in a two-neuron system with shorter conduction times. This suggests a trend to greater specialisation and is reflected clinically. Damage to the corticospinal system will have more profound effects on animals that have well-developed, two-neuron systems, such as humans and primates (see Fig. 4.9).

The corticonuclear tract projects to midbrain, pontine and medullary nuclei associated with cranial nerve motor function. Decussation occurs just before the fibres reach the motor nucleus. It influences all cranial nerve nuclei innervating striated muscle, controlling voluntary movement of the eyes, face, tongue, jaws, pharynx and larynx.

The corticospinal tract functions in voluntary movement of the limbs, trunk and tail. The tract is facilitatory to both flexors and extensors and used for fine distal control of the digits.

Lateral corticospinal tract: In the dog, 75% of fibres cross in the pyramidal decussation at the medulla/spinal

Table 5.1 **Motor tracts of the pyramidal and extrapyramidal systems**

Tract	Function
Extrapyramidal tracts	These tracts form the bulk of the caudally directed fibres in domestic animals
1. Rubrospinal tract (LF) Originates in the red nucleus (midbrain), axons decussate immediately and pass through the brain stem, synapsing on cranial nerve nuclei (V, VII and nucleus ambiguus). The tracts continue into the lateral funiculus extending the length of the spinal cord	Facilitatory to flexor muscles. It functions in semi-skilled movements in cats (less so in dogs) and humans, and in postural control (e.g. squatting/sitting) and locomotion (limb protraction) in other domestic animals
2. Medullary reticulospinal tract (LF) Originates from the medial medullary reticular formation. The fibres mostly decussate within the reticular formation and descend in the lateral funiculus to terminate on interneurons along the length of the spinal cord	Strongly inhibitory to γ-LMNs of extensor muscles (ipsilateral and contralateral). This tract functions to suppress standing and other antigravity activities
3. Pontine reticulospinal tract (VF) Originates in the pontine reticular formation, with ipsilateral projection throughout the ventral funiculus of the spinal cord terminating on interneurons	Facilitatory to ipsilateral γ-LMNs of anti-gravity/extensor muscles to maintain standing posture
4. Lateral vestibulospinal tract (VF) Originates primarily from the lateral vestibular nucleus, descends ipsilaterally in the ventral funiculus to all levels of the spinal cord terminating on interneurons especially at the intumescences. Some fibres decussate to inhibit contralateral LMNs	Facilitatory to ipsilateral extensors (α- and γ-LMNs), inhibitory to ipsilateral flexors and contralateral extensors It is always active as there constant input to the vestibular nuclei about static head position from the sacculus and utriculus (see Chapter 8)
5. Medial vestibulospinal tract (VF) Originates primarily from the other three vestibular nuclei (medial, rostral and caudal), the tract descends in the medial aspect of ventral funiculus and the medial longitudinal fasciculus of the VF, primarily to cervical and cranial thoracic segments	The neurons of this tract are activated by angular acceleration of the head, which is detected in the ampullae of the semi-circular ducts. Stimulation reinforces activity in the cervical and thoracic limb muscles helping to maintain posture despite changing positions of head
6. Medial longitudinal fasciculus (VF) Originates from all four vestibular nuclei (and other nuclei including CNN nuclei). It descends in the ventral funiculus terminating on interneurons at different cord levels. For example, in the cervical and cranial thoracic cord (cat) or extends the length of the cord (dog)	Functions in conjunction with the medial vestibulospinal tract to co-ordinate trunk and limb movement with head and eye movement
7. Lateral tectotegmentospinal tract (LF) Originates from the rostral colliculus of the midbrain tectum, travels ventrally into the tegmentum through brainstem into lateral funiculus of the spinal cord, terminating in the intermediate horn of C8-L4 segments	Functions as UMN to sympathetic innervation supplying smooth muscle of the head, and the eye for pupillary dilation
8. Medial tectospinal tract (VF) Originates from the rostral and caudal colliculi of the midbrain, decussates and travels in the ventral funiculus to terminate in the cervical segments	Function: the tectal neurons receive input from visual and auditory pathways and their output is involved in reflex postural movements of head and neck in response to auditory and visual stimuli
Pyramidal tracts	These tracts comprise only a small proportion of motor tracts in non-primates
1. Corticonuclear tract Originates in the motor cortex of the cerebrum, travels via the internal capsule, crus cerebri, longitudinal fibres of the pons, without synapsing to terminate on brain stem motor nuclei (III, IV, V, VI, VII, and nucleus ambiguus (IX, X, XI) and XII, usually bilaterally	Function: primarily involved in discrete/skilled voluntary movement affecting the head, limbs, neck and trunk The corticonuclear tract is related to discrete movements of the facial muscles. It is well developed in animals such as horses in which it aids skilled lip movement
2. Corticospinal tract (LF, VF, DF) Originates as above and descends without synapsing via the medullary pyramids into the spinal cord, travelling via the named funiculus, to terminate on spinal cord grey matter. May synapse directly onto α-LMNs. (a) lateral corticospinal tract (70–90% of pyramidal fibres) (b) ventral corticospinal tracts (of much less importance and species variable) (c) a small dorsal corticospinal tract is found in some types of animals (e.g. rodents) extending as far caudally as C5	Lateral CST: Fibres facilitating skilled, discrete movement of the extremities are located in the lateral aspect of the lateral CST. These may act in conjunction with the rubrospinal tract. In primates/humans this system is responsible for fine digital movement. The lateral CST is not well developed in most quadrupeds except for highly dexterous animals like raccoons Ventral CST: Fibres mediating neck and trunk movements (including urinary bladder function) are usually located in the ventral CST. In the absence of a ventral CST, they are located in the medial aspect of the lateral CST

LF = lateral funiculus; VF = ventral funiculus.
See also Fig. 4.5 for tract location in the spinal cord and Table 4.3.

cord junction to form the lateral corticospinal tract in the lateral funiculus (see Figs. A24-25). This tract has overlapping distribution with rubrospinal tract. The lateral corticospinal tract projects throughout the spinal cord, but is concentrated in the cranial region.

Ventral corticospinal tract: The remaining 25% of fibres from the medullary pyramids travel ipsilaterally in the ventral funiculus as far as the mid-thoracic region and decussate just before terminating.

A dorsal corticospinal tract is found in some ungulates and rodents.

Clinical signs of disease in the pyramidal system. In humans, damage to the pyramidal system is much more significant than in domestic mammals. We are prone to ischaemic lesions affecting the motor cortex or internal capsule (e.g. cerebrovascular accident or 'stroke'), which can result in contralateral paresis/paralysis. In domestic mammals, ischaemic lesions are much less common and

pyramidal function is less important. Experimentally, destruction of the motor cortex in animals results in signs that are relatively mild, but may include stumbling, dysmetria and altered tone on the contralateral side. Dogs had no deficit in the gait after experimental removal of the motor area, but did have deficits in contralateral postural reactions. Experimental sectioning of crus cerebri or pyramids in dogs had no effect on gait.

4. Other caudally directed tracts in the spinal cord
   (a) Fibres from the locus ceruleus in the pons travel caudally in the lateral funiculus synapsing in both the dorsal and ventral horns. The fibres release norepinephrine at the termination, which inhibits neuronal function, especially that created by noxious stimuli.
   (b) Fibres from the raphe magnus nucleus in the rostral medulla oblongata travel caudally in the lateral

funiculus to synapse in the dorsal horn. They release serotonin which increases the threshold of response to noxious stimuli.

Dysfunction of UMNs and LMNs

> ## Key points
>
> - UMNs are the managers and may be considered as 'central motor neurons' due to their location. LMNs are the workers and may be considered as 'peripheral motor neurons'.
> - Clinically, the loss of LMNs may be prognostically worse than loss of UMNs.
> - The different clinical signs resulting from UMN and LMN dysfunction can be remembered by the mnemonic the 'Neuro **RAT**': **R**eflexes, **A**trophy and **T**one.

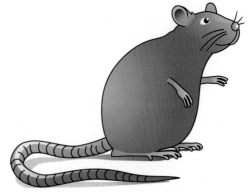

Fig. 5.6 **The 'Neuro RAT' is a useful mnemonic for remembering the differences between upper and lower motor neuron signs: Reflexes, Atrophy, Tone.**

The LMN is regarded as the final common pathway. Upper motor neurons of many tracts may influence a LMN, but the final manifestation of their activity is mediated through that LMN. The LMN can be either inhibited or stimulated, causing the decreased or increased muscle contraction, respectively. The concept of the LMN being the final common pathway is clinically relevant. A lesion that is cranial to the location of the LMN damages UMN tracts affecting that LMN. Even if many of the UMN tracts are lost, the LMN and neuromuscular junction is still intact, therefore the muscle can be stimulated to contract. The number of interneuronal connections to that LMN is vast, thus UMNs can influence it by diverse routes (see Fig. 4.9). However, if the LMN is lost, then the NMJ will degenerate and the muscle will not contract, even if the UMN circuitry is intact. Thus LMN disease usually has a worse prognosis than UMN disease.

UMN versus LMN signs

When a nerve is badly damaged, then distal to the site of the lesion, the axon and its synaptic connections will degenerate. A lesion in the thoracolumbar spinal cord can cause neurological signs in the pelvic limbs by damaging cranially directed sensory tracts and caudally directed UMN tracts. The animal will show proprioceptive deficits, somatic sensory deficits and paresis or paralysis, depending on the lesion severity. A lesion in the lumbosacral spinal cord will also cause sensory and motor deficits in the pelvic limbs, but certain motor signs will be different to those arising from thoracolumbar lesions. The thoracolumbar lesion will damage UMN tracts causing UMN signs to the pelvic limbs while the lumbosacral lesion will damage LMNs causing LMN signs to the pelvic limbs. The distinction between UMN and LMN signs is critical for localising a spinal cord lesion (Fig. 5.6 and Table 5.2).

Affected limbs in animals with neurological disease may be described as having upper motor neuron signs or lower motor neuron signs. This classification means that there is damage to either the UMNs or the LMNs, respectively.

Upper motor neuron signs

The UMN tracts are excitatory or inhibitory to LMNs, and LMNs innervate either extensor (antigravity) or flexor muscles. In animals extensor (anti-gravity) muscles are

Table 5.2 **Clinical signs due to UMN versus LMN lesions – remember the 'Neuro RAT'. Note: thinking of UMNs as central motor neurons and LMNs as peripheral motor neurons may facilitate understanding where a lesion is sited and how that lesion may cause dysfunction**

Sign	UMN disease (damage to the UMNs)	LMN disease (damage to the LMNs)
Reflexes	Normal to increased	Decreased to absent
Atrophy	Disuse: Mild, generalised	Neurogenic: severe, specific muscles
Tone	Normal to increased	Decreased to absent

stronger than flexor muscles, therefore loss of UMN inhibition after a lesion can result in increased tone and reflex activity in the limbs caudal to the lesion (see Fig. 4.2). Characteristically, UMN lesions may cause exaggerated stifle extension in the patellar reflex, especially with chronic lesions. Loss of other UMN tracts that facilitate LMNs and recruit spinal reflex circuitry for locomotion results in reduced or complete loss of movement (paresis or paralysis). In animals, such as horses, in which it is difficult to assess the patellar reflex, UMN paresis is assessed by testing the ability of the horse to resist pulling on the tail. Horses with acute UMN lesions are commonly profoundly paretic, far more so than an ambulant horse with a LMN lesion; if a horse had such profound LMN paresis, it would be recumbent (Fig. 5.7). Increased muscle tone and reflex activity are two cardinal signs of UMN dysfunction. The third sign used to differentiate UMN and LMN lesions is the type of muscle atrophy in the affected limbs. The atrophy in UMN disease is due to disuse. Thus it is generalised caudal to the lesion and is usually mild. Note that lameness in horses and loss of correct weight-bearing may also result in marked disuse atrophy; this atrophy needs to be distinguished from atrophy due to UMN lesions.

Lower motor neuron signs

Dysfunction of LMNs can occur either due to damage to the neuronal cell body in the CNS, or due to damage to the axon in the periphery. Distal to the lesion, both the axon and the neural termination at the neuromuscular junction will degenerate. The efferent portion of any reflex arcs involving these muscles is lost, resulting in decreased or absent reflexes. Due to degeneration of the neuromuscular junction, acetylcholine will not be released from the nerve terminal, and the muscle fibres will not be stimulated to contract. Muscle tone will be reduced or

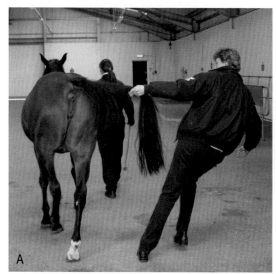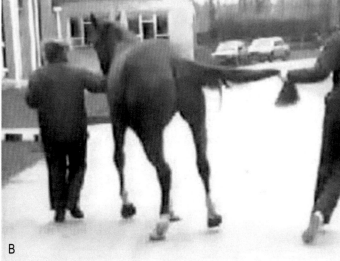

Fig. 5.7 **(A) Normal horse, (B) horse with UMN paresis. Pulling the tail while the horse is moving should result in ipsilateral pelvic limb extension, as is demonstrated by the horse in (A). Horses with UMN dysfunction (B) are unable to achieve this and can easily be pulled to the side. Horses with LMN paresis that are still strong enough to ambulate are able to resist this tail pull better than horses with UMN dysfunction.**

absent (depending on how many axons are lost) due to loss of γ-LMN activation. Denervation of muscles usually results in rapid, severe muscle atrophy. Atrophy may cause as much as 50% of muscle bulk being lost within 2–4 weeks of injury. This is called LMN or neurogenic atrophy and will affect only those muscles that have lost their LMN input. Identifying the specific muscles that are atrophied can be used to identify precisely the involved nerves and/or spinal cord segments. For example, damage to LMN in the suprascapular nerve, supplying the supraspinatus muscle can occur with lesions affecting the caudal cervical spinal cord segments or the cranial brachial plexus (see Figs 5.8, 4.7A and 13.4).

Executive motor function

The neural circuitry involved in planning motor activity is located in the forebrain. This executive manager of the motor system draws on a variety of sensory inputs (from association areas) as well as the limbic system and cerebellum that deal with behaviour and movement coordination (Chapter 7 and 11). It also draws on memory centres of the limbic system and parietal lobe. The motor planning centres also have a database in the basal nuclei which are thought to store fragments of complex, ritual-like motor programmes. Thus the motor planning centres have a number of neural loops that connect to different areas of the brain. It uses the loops to access information from those diverse regions and bring that information back to the executive management for use in planning motor activity.

The cerebral cortex has two main feedback loops to the cerebellum that ultimately influence UMN function. The first loop involves the corticopontocerebellar pathway and is used specifically for motor function that will be expressed via the corticonuclear/corticospinal tracts. Consequently, the development of this system is much greater in humans and primates than in domestic mammals. Output from the cerebral cortex, travelling through the internal capsule and crus cerebri, synapses in nuclei of the pons. The second neurons in this corticopontocerebellar pathway decussate and ascend via the middle cerebellar peduncle into the cerebellum. The return pathway from the cerebellar cortex synapses in the cerebellar nuclei (e.g. lateral nucleus).

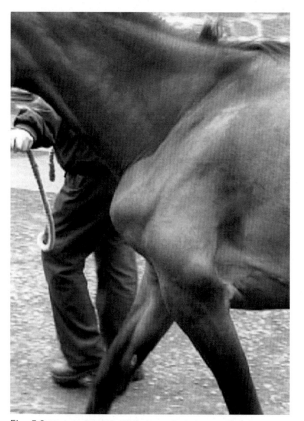

Fig. 5.8 **Horse with brachial plexus lesion secondary to trauma resulting in LMN signs and neurogenic atrophy of the musculature of the proximal thoracic limb and shoulder. The limb was abnormally abducted and had severe, specific muscle atrophy.**

Post-synaptic fibres decussate and exit the cerebellum via the rostral cerebellar peduncle, travel rostrally to the synapse in the thalamus and then to the cerebral cortex.

The second loop from the motor planning centres to the cerebellum ultimately influences extrapyramidal function. It travels to the olivary nucleus in the medulla oblongata, via the caudal cerebellar peduncle to the cerebellum and back via the thalamus to the cerebral cortex or basal nuclei. Again, these pathways decussate twice. The functions of these feedback loops are covered in Chapter 7 on the cerebellum.

Basal nuclei and corpus striatum

> ### Key point
>
> ■ Basal nuclei comprise grey matter deep in the forebrain and midbrain. They function in feedback circuits with the cerebrum to modify cortex output.

Most of the grey matter of the cerebrum is superficially located in the cerebral cortex; the basal nuclei form some of the deeply located, telencephalic grey matter. The basal nuclei comprise structures located in the forebrain and midbrain, but the main components are the caudate and lentiform nuclei (globus pallidus and putamen) in the cerebrum. The caudate nuclei are prominent and bulge into the ventrolateral aspect of the lateral ventricles (Fig. 5.9).

The basal nuclei and intervening white matter are arranged from medial to lateral, as the caudate nucleus, the internal capsule (white matter tracts comprising both afferent and efferent fibres connecting between the cerebral cortex and the brainstem), the lentiform nuclei, the external capsule and the claustrum. This alternating arrangement of grey and white matter is called the corpus striatum (L = striated body).

Inputs to the basal nuclei originate mainly in the cerebrum, the thalamus and the midbrain and most are delivered to the caudate nucleus. The globus pallidus is the only basal nuclear component from which efferent fibres leave to connect with other areas of the brain.

Despite their size and prominence, the functions of the basal nuclei are not clearly defined in animals. They seem to function in feedback circuits with the cerebrum (via the thalamus) ultimately modifying motor cortex output. They may also be involved in arranging complex movements that

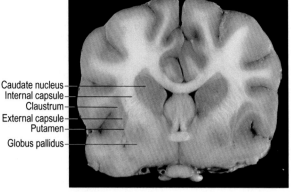

Fig. 5.9 **Transverse section of the canine brain at the level of the rostral commissure (see Figs. A14-16).**

are in frequent use (e.g. feeding or territorial behaviour) and may be considered to store fragments of programmes used for running motor functions that have a specified sequence (ritual) of movements. Unlike the situation in humans and primates, the subcortical centres in domesticated animals can function to a greater extent without cortical input, thus the functional impact of even large motor cortex lesions may be negligible in those species. Additionally, primary lesions in the basal nuclei causing clinical dysfunction are not commonly recognised in animals compared with humans (e.g. Parkinson's disease). However, dysfunction of connections between the basal nuclei and cerebrum may cause circling and propulsive activity in animals with forebrain lesions (see Fig. 4.10). In horses, ingestion of plants of the Centaurea family causes severe necrosis of the basal nuclei; this results in devastating rigidity of muscles associated with eating and swallowing.

Chapter 6
Ascending somatic sensory tracts and conscious sensory systems

Key points

- Sensory information is received from exteroceptors, interoceptors and proprioceptors and is projected to specific regions of the forebrain for conscious perception. Proprioceptive input is also projected to the cerebellum for subconscious processing. Most sensory inputs are also projected to the brainstem ascending reticular activating system for arousal (see Chapter 11).
- Projection to the cerebral cortex utilises a three-neuron pathway between the peripheral receptor and the somatosensory cortex.
- General proprioception is the sense of the relative positions of body parts.
- Conscious proprioception projects to the contralateral cerebral cortex; subconscious proprioception projects to the ipsilateral cerebellum.
- A deficit in general proprioception results in ataxia due to loss of spatial awareness of the body, limbs and/or head. It may also cause a change in the rate, range and force of movement.

A wide variety of sensory modalities are projected to the cerebral cortex (Table 6.1). The stimuli are collected by a plethora of sensory receptors that are classified as exteroceptors, interoceptors and proprioceptors.

Receptors

Animals have a variety of receptor types that detect different stimuli (thermal, mechanical, chemical and photo stimuli); receptors detect changes in both the animal's external and internal environments.

Receptors may be encapsulated in connective tissue or non-encapsulated and have bare dendrites. They are designed to respond preferentially to a certain type of stimulus, but will usually respond to several different forms of energy. Regardless of stimulus type, it is transduced as an electrical impulse.

Exteroceptors are activated by stimuli in the immediate external environment such as temperature and touch. They include both encapsulated (Pacinian corpuscles and Ruffini endings) and free nerve endings that respond to pressure, vibration and distortion of the tissue. They may adapt to a constant stimulus either rapidly or slowly. Exteroceptors also include those receptors concerned with special sensations, such as audition, vision and gustation (taste) (see Chapter 10).

Interoceptors detect the internal, visceral environment of the body. Conscious perception of the viscera is mainly via nociceptors, which are stimulated by distension of visceral walls or ischaemia.

Proprioceptors include receptors such as the muscle spindle fibres and Golgi tendon organs located in muscles, tendons or joints and also tactile/pressure receptors. They detect muscle stretch, tension, position and movement of joints.

Nociceptors respond to many types of stimuli but have a high threshold; that is the stimulus must be of sufficient intensity to cause tissue damage.

Pathway: Most conscious sensory systems share a common format that comprises a three-stage system:

1. A receptor and an axon with a cell body in the ganglion in the PNS;
2. A relay section in the CNS comprising a central pathway that has one, or more, synapses in specific nuclei. It eventually joins, or runs adjacent to, a pathway called the medial lemniscus through the brainstem to the thalamus;
3. Thalamocortical projection to the somatosensory cortex of the cerebrum.

Sensory modalities that do not fit this three-stage structure include olfaction, vision and some nociceptive pathways.

General proprioception

Proprioception (*proprius* – L = one's own, *capere* – L = to receive) is the sense of the relative position of parts of the body. Proprioception indicates whether and how joints, muscles and tendons are moving based on input from

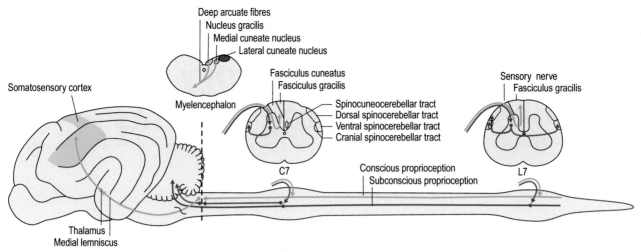

Fig. 6.1 **Proprioceptive tracts to the brain from the body. C7 = 7ᵗʰ cervical spinal cord segment, L7 = 7ᵗʰ lumbar spinal cord segment.**

Modality	Tract	Location
Nociception	Fasciculus gracilis and fasciculus cuneatus (skin)	DF
	Spinocervicothalamic tract (skin)	LF
	Spinothalamic tract (skin, viscera and body)	LF
	Spinoreticular tract (viscera and body)	VF
	Spinomesencephalic tract	VF
Temperature	Spinothalamic tract (viscera and body)	LF
Discriminative touch, pressure and conscious proprioception	Fasciculus cuneatus and spinocuneocerebellar tract (kinaesthesia) from the body cranial to T8 (from the body cranial to T8)	DF
	Fasciculus gracilis and dorsal spinocerebellar tract (kinaesthesia) from the body caudal to T8	DF and LF, respectively
Arousal and behaviour	Spinothalamic tract	LF
	Spinoreticular tract	VF
	Spinomesencephalic tract	VF
Subconscious proprioception and cerebellar input	Dorsal and ventral spinocerebellar tract (from the caudal half of body)	LF
	Spinocuneocerebellar and cranial spinocerebellar tracts (from the cranial half of body)	DF and LF, respectively
	Spinoreticular tract	VF
	Spinopontine tract	VF
	Spinovestibular (from the neck)	VF
	Spino-olivary tract	VF

Table 6.1 **Ascending tracts, their functions and locations in the spinal cord**

DF = dorsal funiculus, LF = lateral funiculus, VF = ventral funiculus.
See also Fig. 2.5.

muscle spindles, Golgi tendon organs and joint receptors. It also indicates where various parts of the body are located in relation to each other. Tactile and mechanoreceptors, especially on the feet, contribute to proprioception, especially conscious proprioception, while hair cells in the vestibular apparatus of the inner ear supply information about head position and movement.

Proprioceptive information from peripheral receptors travels via spinal nerves, the dorsal roots and spinal cord (dorsal and lateral funiculi) to the brain (Fig. 6.1). Proprioception of the head, its muscles and joints, uses mainly cranial nerves VIII and V to reach the appropriate brainstem nuclei. The information that terminates in the somatosensory cortex of contralateral cerebrum is

used in conscious proprioception while that terminating in the ipsilateral cerebellum is used in subconscious proprioception. Conscious proprioception is the conscious awareness of body position and movement of body parts. It enables the cerebral cortex to plan and refine voluntary, learned movements. Subconscious proprioception is based around stretch and tension of muscles, tendons and ligaments, at rest and during movement, and spatial orientation of the body. The cerebellum needs this information to coordinate posture and locomotion. The vestibular system provides proprioceptive information (conscious and subconscious) about head position and movement. This input is fundamental for setting the balance and posture of the whole animal.

Subconscious proprioception from the head (vestibular input), neck, trunk and limbs (spinal input) is essential for normal posture and gait. Subconscious proprioceptive deficits result in the clinical sign of ataxia. Ataxia can be defined functionally as incoordinated movement. It presents as changes in the rate, range and force of movement. Ataxia does not mean that the animal is paretic (weak), however, cases of spinal cord disease usually present with both ataxia and UMN paresis due to compression of the adjacent general proprioceptive and UMN tracts.

Both conscious and subconscious proprioceptive systems are essential for normal posture and gait and it can be difficult to rigorously separate conscious from subconscious proprioceptive deficits when presented with an ataxic patient. However in dogs and cats, subconscious proprioceptive deficits usually perturb posture and gait more than conscious proprioceptive deficits. This is evidenced by observing the effect of lesions located at the termination of subconscious versus conscious proprioceptive pathways. For example, ataxia is more pronounced with lesions in the cerebellum than lesions affecting the somatosensory cortex in the forebrain. Subconscious proprioceptive deficits due to cerebellar lesions may present with truncal sway, base wide or narrow posture and limb movement, and delays in initiating or terminating movement. In dogs and cats with lesions affecting the somatosensory cortex where conscious proprioceptive pathways terminate, only mild stumbling, or a tendency to stand on the dorsum of the paw, may be observed. Gait and posture may otherwise be reasonably normal.

Conscious proprioception

> ### Key points
>
> ■ Conscious proprioception is the information about the position of the head, body and limbs that is received in the contralateral somatosensory cortex of the cerebrum and is used particularly for executing voluntary, skilled movement.
> ■ Information from the neck, trunk and limbs is transmitted via the spinal nerves and spinal cord.
> ■ Information from the head is transmitted via CN V (somatic sensation and muscle proprioception) and CN VIII (head position and movement).
> ■ Conscious proprioception utilises sensory inputs from touch, pressure, muscle and joint receptors. Hair cells of the vestibular apparatus transmit information about head position and movement.

Non-painful, conscious sensations can broadly be divided into two categories that share functional and anatomical features. One group comprises touch and pressure, and the other is composed of joint and muscle/tendon proprioception. Both are principally transmitted to the cerebral cortex via the dorsal column–medial lemniscal system involving primarily the dorsal funiculus of the spinal cord with some transmission in the lateral funiculus (see Fig. 4.5). The dorsal funiculus is also known as the dorsal column and it continues as the medial lemniscus in the brainstem.

Axons conveying this information enter the dorsal funiculus and join the fasciculus cuneatus (from the body cranial to T8) or fasciculus gracilis (caudal to T8). Fibres in the fasciculus cuneatus convey proprioceptive and discriminative touch. They synapse in the medial cuneate nucleus located in the caudal medulla oblongata (see Figs. 6.1, A24–28). Only about one-quarter of the fasciculus gracilis fibres synapse in the nucleus gracilis in the medulla oblongata. Thus the dorsal funiculus is relatively unimportant in transmitting proprioception from the pelvic limbs in quadrupeds; it is important in humans. The majority of fibres entering the fasciculus gracilis leave it in the cranial lumbar region to synapse in the grey matter on interneurons, or relay neurons of other pathways, or even LMNs. Fibres arising from synapses at the base of the dorsal horn (e.g. the nucleus thoracicus (see Table 4.2) may continue cranially in the dorsal spinocerebellar tract (with collateral fibres travelling in the adjacent spinomedullary tract) to synapse near the nucleus gracilis (in nucleus Z) (Figs. A24, A27, A28). Post-synaptic fibres from these proprioceptive relay nuclei (gracile, medial cuneate and Z) decussate in the deep arcuate fibres of the medulla oblongata and continue rostrally in the medial lemniscus to the thalamus where they synapse. They are projected to the contralateral somatosensory cortex of the cerebrum via the internal capsule.

The role of the lateral funiculus in conveying pelvic limb proprioception to the cerebrum may be one explanation why cervical spinal cord compression can produce particularly marked pelvic limb ataxia. This is illustrated in Fig. 6.3 on 'Wobbler' horses and dogs (see accompanying text).

The dorsal column–medial lemniscal system is highly organised topographically and is quite specific with respect to the transmission of sensory and discriminatory information. In other words, there is little convergence (input) of other pathways onto the relay nuclei; this enables the animal to localise precisely a stimulus from the skin, e.g. the horse biting at a fly on its body. Similarly, the somatosensory cortex is somatopically arranged and the size of each area reflects the density of innervation (see Fig. 4.14).

The dorsal funiculus comprises a greater percentage of white matter in carnivores and primates than in other animals; this reflects higher sensory discrimination from the digits, especially compared with ungulates.

There are two kinds of proprioceptive input from the head – that associated with head position and movement (see Chapter 8) and proprioception due to receptors associated with muscles of mastication, facial expression and eye movement. Muscle proprioception is also conveyed by a three-neuron system via all three branches of CN V (trigeminal nerve). The trigeminal ganglion at the base of the neurocranium is the equivalent of a spinal ganglion, containing somatosensory neuronal cell bodies. However, uniquely, the cell bodies of the primary afferent neurons concerned with muscle proprioception are found in the CNS, in the mesencephalic nucleus of V. The axons of the second neurons decussate, travel rostrally in the contralateral trigeminal lemniscus to the thalamus and on to the somatosensory cortex. The proprioceptive fibres in the mesencephalic nucleus of CN V also connect to other cranial nerve motor nuclei for reflex function. Sensory fibres from tongue musculature (intrinsic and extrinsic) have their cell bodies located in the trigeminal, C1 and distal vagal ganglia.

Subconscious proprioception

> ### Key points
>
> ■ Subconscious proprioception is information about the position of the head, neck, trunk and limbs that is received in the cerebellum and is used for coordinating posture, locomotion and semi-automatic movement.
> ■ It is transmitted from receptors such as muscle spindles and Golgi tendon organs of the body musculature, or the vestibular apparatus of the head, to the ipsilateral cerebellum.

Subconscious proprioceptive information is received by the ipsilateral cerebellum and is used for coordinating posture and movement. Receptors involved in subconscious proprioception are primarily muscle spindles and Golgi tendon organs, and the vestibular system of the head. Conscious awareness of this type of proprioceptive information is not required for normal function. However, collateral axons also project to the cerebrum contributing to conscious proprioception and awareness of movement (kinaesthesia).

Subconscious proprioceptive pathways inform the cerebellum about location, status (tension and length) and movement of the skeletal musculature throughout the body (i.e. head, neck, limbs and trunk). The cerebellum also receives copies of planned motor activity from the motor cortex and UMN centres. Thus it compares incoming proprioceptive sensory information with the motor plans and generates an output back to motor centres to adjust and perfect the muscular activity (see Chapter 7).

Spinocerebellar pathways comprise two neurons, compared with the three-neuron pathway involved in conscious proprioception. The first neuron originates at the peripheral receptor and has its cell body in the spinal ganglia. It synapses in the base of the dorsal horn and post-synaptic fibres project via the lateral funiculus to the cerebellum. The exception to this is the spinocuneocerebellar tract, fibres of which pass through the dorsal horn into the fasciculus cuneatus and synapse in the lateral cuneate nucleus of the medulla oblongata and post-synaptic neurons project to the cerebellum. Note that the lateral cuneate nucleus and superficial arcuate fibres are associated with subconscious proprioception, while the medial cuneate nucleus and deep arcuate fibres function in conscious proprioception.

Information from the caudal half of the body travels cranially in the dorsal and ventral spinocerebellar tracts. The dorsal spinocerebellar tract (DSCT) arises from the nucleus thoracicus at the base of the dorsal horn (see Fig. 4.5 and Table. 4.2) located from C8–L4. Fibres enter the lateral funiculus, and travel cranially to the medulla oblongata, into the caudal cerebellar peduncle and terminate in the ipsilateral vermis and paravermis (see Chapter 7). Therefore the DSCT serves both to project to the cerebellum as well as to the sensory area of the cerebral (see the previous page and next column).

The ventral spinocerebellar tract (VSCT) also arises from the nucleus thoracicus, but the fibres decussate to contralateral lateral funiculus and course cranially to the rostral cerebellar peduncle. Here fibres decussate again to end up in the cerebellum ipsilateral to the side of the stimulus.

Information from the neck, forelimbs and cranial half of the trunk (T8–C1) is conveyed cranially by three routes. The spinocuneocerebellar tract travels cranially in the fasciculus cuneatus to synapse in the medulla oblongata (lateral cuneate nucleus), then via the caudal cerebellar peduncle to the ipsilateral cerebellum. The cranial spinocerebellar tract (CSCT) arises from neurons at the base of the dorsal horn, and travels in the ipsilateral lateral funiculus entering the cerebellum via both the rostral and caudal cerebellar peduncles. The cervicospinocerebellar tract relays information concerned with proprioception of the neck which is essential for whole body postural control (see Chapter 8).

There is variation in these tracts between the species, reflecting the species' specific movement capabilities. The dorsal and ventral spinocerebellar tracts are well developed in ungulates. Cats also have the cranial spinocerebellar tracts and spinocuneocerebellar tracts, which enables them to have highly coordinated function of the thoracic limb and forepaw.

Subconscious proprioception from the body is represented ipsilaterally in the cerebellum. Tracts that decussate en route to the cerebellum, like the ventral spinocerebellar tract, decussate again once inside the cerebellum. Fibres involved in vestibular–cerebellar connections always remain ipsilateral. Conversely, input to the cerebellum from the motor planning and UMN centres is represented contralaterally, but cerebellar output to these centres also decussates, thus influencing the original side.

In humans, kinaesthesia is the conscious awareness of body position and movement. We can assume it occurs in animals, such that an animal is aware of its body position and movement, but not of the specific action of each muscle. Proprioceptive information used in kinaesthesia arises from collaterals of subconscious proprioceptive pathways. Collateral information from the caudal half of the body travelling in the dorsal spinocerebellar tract, synapses in the medulla oblongata (nucleus Z). Similarly, collateral information from the cranial half of the body travelling in the spinocuneocerebellar pathway, synapses in the medulla oblongata near the lateral cuneate nucleus (nucleus X). From nucleus Z and nucleus X, fibres join the medial lemniscus for projection to the contralateral thalamus and then to the cerebral cortex.

Conscious and subconscious proprioception in posture and gait

Key points

- Conscious proprioceptive deficits are typified by the animal bearing weight on an abnormal part of the foot – e.g. on the dorsum of the paw.
- Subconscious proprioceptive deficits are typified by an abnormal position of the limbs (props) with respect to the centre of gravity, at rest and during locomotion.

A key concept in clinical neurology is that similar neurological deficits will be produced regardless of where a lesion is located along a neural pathway – origin, midway or the termination. Applying this concept can help illustrate the role of conscious versus subconscious proprioception in dogs and cats, by considering what proprioceptive deficits may be present in an animal with a lesion affecting the termination of the conscious versus subconscious proprioceptive pathway. What happens when proprioceptive information is not received at the somatosensory cortex or at the cerebellum? With somatosensory cortex lesions, the gait is often quite coordinated with minimal ataxia. The limbs are placed in a weight-bearing position under the body at rest and during movement. However the animal may stumble and come to rest standing on the dorsum of the paw ('knuckling') (Fig. 6.2); these signs will be contralateral to the side of the lesion due to decussation of the sensory pathway in the medulla oblongata (see Fig. 4.10). Deficits reflect loss of input especially from tactile and joint angle receptors. Conversely, the animal with cerebellar lesions may show pronounced subconscious proprioceptive deficits in which the limbs will not be placed in a good weight-bearing position under the centre of gravity. At rest the animal may have a base wide or narrow stance, and during locomotion, the limbs may be abducted, adducted or cross over. These signs reflect failure to receive and process input, especially from muscle spindles of the proximal limb, and in particular, from the extrinsic limb muscles (those that attach the limb to the trunk). Extrinsic muscles provide information about the angle the limb makes with the body. Conversely, a spinal cord lesion may compromise both conscious and subconscious proprioceptive pathways: thus the animal is ataxic and has deficits in the paw position response and may stand knuckled.

Clinically, tests that specifically assess conscious proprioception (along with motor function) stimulate the

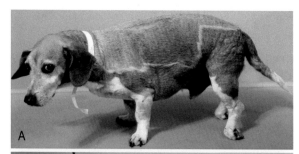

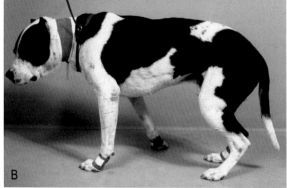

Fig. 6.2 **(A) Dog with a lumbar spinal cord lesion resulting in abnormal paw position sense and 'knuckling'; this sign is characteristic of involvement of the conscious proprioceptive pathways. (B) The limbs are not under the centre of gravity in this dog; this sign is characteristic of dysfunction of the subconscious proprioceptive pathways.**

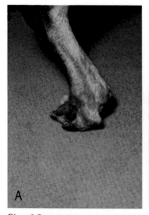

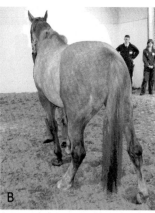

Fig. 6.3 **Wobbler animals with proprioceptive deficits: (A) dog with delayed paw position response and in (B) the horse that would stand base wide for prolonged periods.**

tactile receptors in the foot. Thus the paw position response ('knuckling') and hopping are useful tests. Hopping also stimulates muscle spindle receptors throughout the limb, while the paw position response test stimulates those in distal extensor/flexor muscles in the foot. For subconscious proprioceptive testing, tests that change muscle and tendon inputs by altering the relative position of the limbs under the centre of gravity are useful and include hopping, and reflex stepping (see Chapter 13).

Note: to clinically make an absolute distinction between the two types of proprioception may not be possible and, for spinal cases, is not necessary. Also note that an animal must have a functioning motor system to demonstrate normal proprioception. For example, it must be able to move its foot after the paw is turned over, or lift the limb and place it in a new weight-bearing position during the hopping test. If the animal has significant motor dysfunction (UMN or LMN) it may not be able to perform the test even if the proprioceptive tracts are intact. Thus lesions that disrupt motor systems may lead to apparent proprioceptive dysfunction. Differentiating between proprioceptive versus motor dysfunction is discussed in Chapter 13.

Spinal lesions can compromise the proprioceptive input from the limbs and also from the trunk and neck. The cerebellum needs proprioceptive input from the axial muscles to coordinate contraction of spinal agonists and antagonists. Loss of subconscious proprioceptive input from the trunk explains the difference in the clinical signs observed in a cranial thoracic versus mid-lumbar lesion. In both cases, the animal will have deficits in pelvic limb function. However, with the cranial thoracic cord lesions there may also be truncal ataxia, and the body may list to the side. Such lesions may also affect motor systems resulting in paresis of the trunk muscles.

The effect of spinal cord lesions on general proprioception is illustrated in horses and dogs with 'wobbler syndrome' caused by compressive lesions in the cervical spinal cord. Characteristically, gait deficits and ataxia are more marked in the pelvic limbs, compared with the thoracic limbs. In part this is because the dorsal spinocerebellar tracts from the pelvic limbs are usually more severely compressed than those tracts in the dorsal funiculus conveying proprioception from the thoracic limbs. Loss of general proprioceptive input results in the typical, wobbly gait. With loss of conscious proprioception, the dog may stand on the dorsum of the paw (Fig. 6.3A) or the horse, when turned in a tight circle, may spin on the hoof rather than stepping around in a circle. Wobbler animals also exhibit ataxia, failing to keep the limbs in a good weight-bearing position under the centre of gravity either at rest or during locomotion (Fig. 6.3B). This sign is typical of subconscious proprioceptive deficits. These cervical lesions often affect UMN tracts also, resulting in paresis. Caudal cervical lesions can compromise LMN innervation to the shoulder muscles, resulting in a shortened stride in the thoracic limbs due to reduced shoulder extension. It may also cause prominent, specific atrophy of the affected muscles; this is called neurogenic atrophy as it arises due to loss of peripheral motor neuron (LMN) innervation (Chapter 5).

Nociception

Key points

- A noxious stimulus may be sensed by specific nociceptors, or non-specifically by other receptor types.
- A noxious stimulus may stimulate reflex activity, or it may be transmitted to the brain by pathways in all funiculi and on both sides of the cord.
- Pain is the conscious perception of a noxious stimulus; it is accompanied by an unpleasant emotional response.
- Loss of conscious perception of noxious stimuli in the body caudal to a spinal cord lesion implies severe damage to the spinal cord.

- Noxious stimuli in the head are conveyed by CN V to the pontine nucleus of CN V for reflex function. Fibres also decussate and travel rostrally to the contralateral somatosensory cortex for conscious perception.
- Noxious stimuli from the viscera are transmitted to the CNS primarily via visceral afferent axons traveling within sympathetic and parasympathetic fibres. They may induce local reflex activity, autonomically mediated changes and conscious perception.

Nociception (*nocere* – L = to injure), is defined as the sensory modality that is preferentially triggered by a noxious stimulus that has the potential to damage tissue. The stimulus can be chemical, thermal or mechanical. It may trigger a variety of somatic or autonomic responses and reflexes, and may also result in what humans interpret as pain.

Pain is defined by the International Association for the Study of Pain (http://www.iasp-pain.org) as 'An unpleasant sensory and emotional experience associated with actual or potential tissue damage…'.

Noxious stimuli generate action potentials in a variety of sensory pathways, but only when those stimuli are received and integrated in the cerebrum, and associated with an unpleasant emotional status, may they be considered to be causing pain. Thus nociception has both a sensory and emotional component.

'The inability to communicate verbally does not negate the possibility that an individual is experiencing pain' (http://www.iasp-pain.org). The non-verbal animal's way of conveying pain is through pain-related behaviour such as avoiding the noxious stimulus, depression/withdrawal or self-selection of analgesic therapies as observed in laboratory animals.

Noxious stimuli may stimulate a variety of receptors, some of which respond specifically to noxious (tissue-damaging) stimuli. Other receptors, such as tactile mechanoreceptors, primarily respond to mechanical distortion by non-noxious stimuli, but will also respond to the higher-intensity, noxious stimuli.

Nociceptive input from neck, trunk, limbs and tail
Approximately 50% of afferent axons in cutaneous nerves are associated with nociception. Noxious stimuli are transmitted via two types of fibres in the PNS. Aδ-fibres transmit pinprick fine nociceptive stimuli. They are myelinated, rapidly conducting and transmit 'fast pain'. Transmitted stimuli are localisable to a body area, warn the brain of the potential for tissue damage and cause rapid responses by the brain, for example, promoting activities that remove the body from the noxious stimulus. C-fibres also transmit noxious stimuli, but much more slowly as they are non-myelinated. In humans, C-fibre stimulation causes the aversive aspects of pain described as dull, aching, throbbing, burning, depression or nausea. Such nociception causes the individual to withdraw and rest aiming to promote healing. Clinical examples of Aδ-fibre transmitted stimuli are pin prick or light squeezing of the skin using haemostats whereas C-fibres are stimulated by the crushing pain that can be produced by squeezing the digits with a strong pair of haemostats. Aδ-fibre stimuli are readily localised, whereas C-fibre stimuli may be poorly localised by the brain.

Both fibre types enter via the dorsal root and synapse in the dorsal horn. From there, connections are made within or between segments, for reflex activity such as the withdrawal reflex, in which the animal withdraws the limb from the noxious stimulus. Simultaneously, in the standing animal, the contralateral limb will be stimulated reflexively to extend, but in the normal, recumbent animal, the crossed extension reflex is suppressed (see Fig. 13.10).

The noxious stimulus will also be transmitted cranially in a variety of pathways found in all funiculi. For conscious perception, the tracts ultimately project via the thalamus to the somatosensory cortex. Localisation of pinprick stimuli to the body surface may involve the post-synaptic tract in the dorsal funiculus. This tract conveys both noxious and non-noxious stimuli from the skin and arises from incoming sensory nerves that have synapsed in the dorsal horn. Fibres run cranially mingled with those conveying discriminative touch in the fasciculus gracilis and fasciculus cuneatus. Other types of noxious stimuli causing stimulation of Aδ- or C-fibres may use tracts in the lateral or ventral funiculi such as the spinothalamic tract, spinocervicothalamic, spinoreticular or spinomesencephalic tracts (see Fig. 4.5 and Table 4.3). Some of the tracts are bilateral, some are primarily contralateral. Some synapse in the grey matter several times en route. The key point is that there are multiple, bilaterally represented pathways for conveying noxious stimuli to the brain; this is clinically significant. For a spinal cord lesion to cause loss of nociception caudal to the lesion, there must be extensive destruction across the width of the cord to disrupt all the tracts. Therefore, clinically, loss of nociception is a poor prognostic sign in animals with severe spinal cord lesions (Fig. 6.4).

In the normal animal, a noxious stimulus should cause a conscious response such that the animal whines, or looks at the site of the stimulus, as well as pulling the foot away reflexively (see Fig. 13.10). The withdrawal reflex will occur as long as the reflex wiring comprising the peripheral input, central spinal connections and the LMN to the flexor muscles is intact. Thus an animal with a complete spinal cord transection at the thoracolumbar junction (cranial to the lumbar intumescence) should have an intact flexor withdrawal reflex in the pelvic limbs, but will not demonstrate signs of pain (i.e. conscious perception).

The mechanisms of acupuncture
A-δ fibre input into the dorsal horn activates an enkephalinergic interneuron that inhibits C-fibre input into the same dorsal horn. Thus by stimulating the fast pain fibres, C-fibre input can be diminished. This is called the segmental effect as it acts within the stimulated spinal cord segment. Additionally, stimulation of ascending tracts triggers the release of a variety of neurotransmitters including β-endorphin, noradrenaline and serotonin from the brainstem, and oxytocin and adrenocorticotrophic hormone from the pituitary gland. Neurotransmitters can either act humerally or activate a descending analgesic system in the brain stem that decreases ascending pain signals. For example, nociceptive activation of the spinomesencephalic tract, may stimulate the periaqueductal grey matter of the midbrain, which then activates a descending inhibitory (analgesic) neural system.

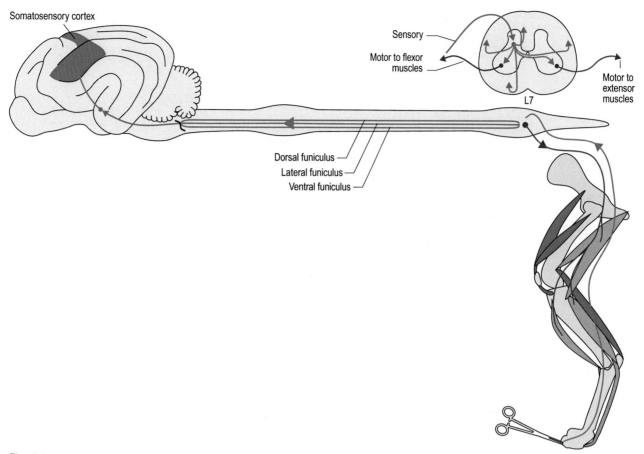

Fig. 6.4 **Nociceptive input from the limbs and body induces local reflex functions and travels cranially in a number of different tracts, in the dorsal, lateral and ventral funiculi. Extensor muscles are red and flexor muscles are orange.**

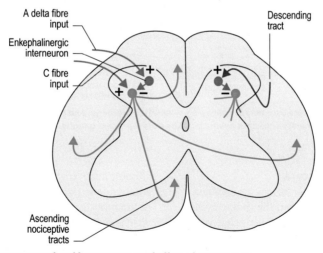

Fig. 6.5 **Mechanisms underlying the segmental and heterosegmental effect of acupuncture.**

These are the heterosegmental effects as they are more generalised. Both the segmental and heterosegmental effects are most potent in the dorsal horn that is being stimulated (Fig. 6.5). Therefore pain relief is best achieved by needling as close as possible to the source of pain.

Nociceptive input from head

All three branches of the trigeminal nerve convey nociceptive information into the brainstem where they synapse in the spinal nucleus of CN V in the medulla oblongata (see Chapter 10). Cranial nerves VII, IX and X, from the ear and oral cavity, also project to this nucleus (Fig. 6.6). Incoming

fibres can then activate other brainstem nuclei for reflex function. In the palpebral reflex, for example, a noxious stimulus travels via CN V to the spinal nucleus of V; interneurons project to CN VII facial nucleus stimulating eyelid closure. For conscious perception afferent axons from the nucleus of V, decussate and travel rostrally with medial lemniscus as the trigeminal lemniscus. They synapse in thalamus and are distributed to the somatosensory cortex. Thus the projection of nociception from the head is primarily contralateral, therefore unilateral lesions of forebrain will cause mainly contralateral hypalgesia of the face.

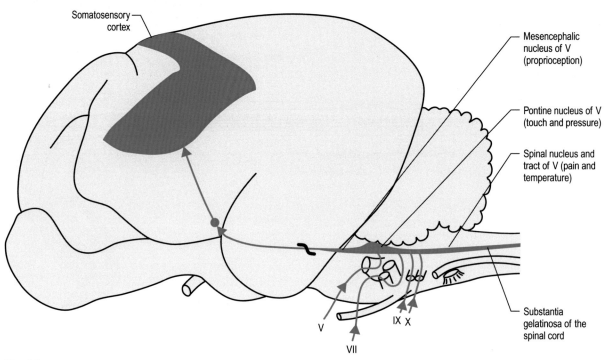

Fig. 6.6 **Nociceptive input from the head. The thick black wavy line represents decussation of the tract.**

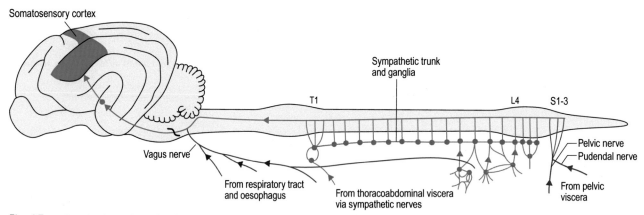

Fig. 6.7 **Nociceptive input from the viscera uses nerves conveying sympathetic (orange) and parasympathetic (purple) fibres. Such input may induce autonomic reflex activity or stimulate conscious awareness. The dots represent ganglia.**

Nociceptive input from the viscera

Noxious visceral stimuli (see Chapter 12) are transmitted to the CNS via sympathetic nerves from the thoracic and abdominal viscera, and pelvic nerves from the pelvic viscera. Input from the respiratory tract and oesophagus is via the vagus nerve. Inputs via the sympathetic fibres will stimulate visceral reflexes such as accelerated heart rate and respiration (sympathetic response). Conversely, afferent fibres travelling in parasympathetic nerves may stimulate the parasympathetic system responses resulting in bradycardia and hypotension. Other inputs, for example distension of the gut wall, may stimulate reflex changes in gut activity, locally using the local autonomic plexi in the gut wall. Noxious stimuli from the viscera are also conveyed to the forebrain for conscious perception, but are often poorly localised (Fig. 6.7).

Chapter 7
The cerebellum

Key points

- The cerebellum receives subconscious proproprioceptive input from Golgi tendon organs and muscle spindles and the hair cells of the vestibular apparatus.
- It coordinates tone and movement of the body (head, neck, trunk and limbs) by modulating activity of UMNs affecting agonist and antagonist muscles.
- It feeds back proprioceptive information to motor planning centres of the forebrain and is involved in setting the postural platform.
- The grey matter consists of a three-layered cortex (granule cells, Purkinje cells and molecular layer) and three pairs of cerebellar nuclei.
- The branching white matter forms the arbor vitae and is connected to the brainstem by three pairs of cerebellar peduncles.
- The neonatal animal's ability to move in a coordinated manner correlates with the amount of cerebellar development at birth.
- The cerebellar nuclei facilitate somatic UMNs and are inhibited by the only efferents from the cerebellar cortex, the gabaminergic Purkinje cells.
- Spinocerebellar pathways, conveying subconscious proprioception, comprise two neurons, compared with the three-neuron pathway involved in conscious proprioception.
- Clinical signs of cerebellar dysfunction may include ataxia, hypermetria, spasticity and tremor, but not paresis.

'The cerebellum is the head ganglion of the proprioceptive system.'
(Charles Sherrington, 1947)

The cerebellum, derived from the Latin meaning 'little brain', comprises just 10% of the brain's volume but contains at least 50% of its neurons. Although it develops as a dorsal outgrowth from the metencephalon, it is not part of the brainstem. The cerebellum receives subconscious proprioceptive information from the body, limbs and head. That sensory input is used to modify and coordinate muscle action for posture and movement.

General anatomy

The cerebellum is sited in the caudal cranial fossa of the neurocranium, and is separated from the cerebral hemispheres by the osseous tentorium and the tentorium cerebelli (see Fig. 3.11).

The cerebellum has a large body that is separated from the small ventral flocculonodular lobe by the uvulonodular fissure. The body of the cerebellum is divided into rostral and caudal lobes by the dorsally located, primary fissure. The flocculonodular lobe comprises a midline nodulus, on either side of which are small, paired lobules called flocculi. The flocculonodular lobe is also known as the vestibulocerebellum as it processes proprioceptive input from the vestibular system (Chapter 8). Dorsal to the flocculus on each side is the paraflocculus. The cerebellum is divided longitudinally into the midline vermis, with its nine lobules and the paired cerebellar hemispheres (Figs. 7.1, A8, A20–A24).

The surface of the cerebellum is corrugated by long, thin folds called folia. Folia comprise superficial cortex (grey matter) and central laminae (white matter); they are separated from each other by sulci. The laminae connect to a deeper mass of white matter called the cerebellar medulla. The branching appearance of the white matter on median section gave rise to the name, 'arbor vitae' (Latin = tree of life) (Fig. 7.1).

The grey matter forms the three layered superficial cerebellar cortex and the three pairs of cerebellar nuclei located deep in the cerebellar medulla. From lateral to medial these are the lateral ('dentate' nucleus in humans), interpositial and fastigial nuclei. Each nucleus receives input from the overlying cerebellar cortex as well as collateral branches of cerebellar afferent fibres. Hence the cortex of the hemisphere, the paravermis and vermis supply the lateral, interpositial and fastigial nuclei, respectively (Figs. 7.2, A21, A22).

Cerebellar peduncles
Three pairs of cerebellar peduncles attach the cerebellum to the brainstem; these are the rostral, middle and caudal cerebellar peduncles. They are named for their site of attachment to the brainstem.

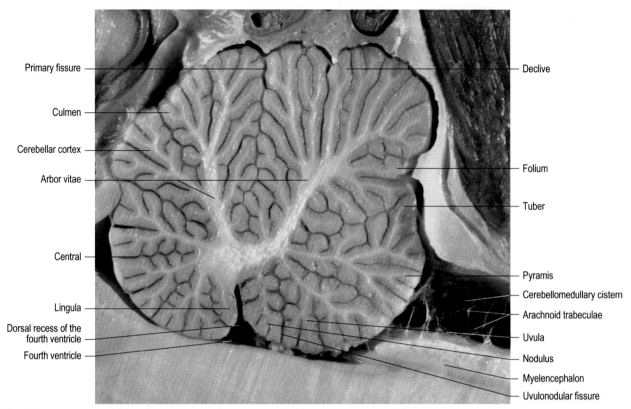

Fig. 7.1 **Lobules of the cerebellum, dog brain, median section. (Specimen courtesy of Mr. Allan Nutman, IVABS, Massey University.)**

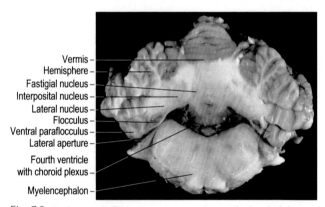

Fig. 7.2 **Canine cerebellum, transverse section at the level of the lateral apertures. (See also A22).**

The rostral cerebellar peduncle contains mainly cerebellar efferents connecting the cerebellum with the midbrain, but also has one afferent tract, the ventral spinocerebellar tract.

The middle cerebellar peduncle has afferent fibres only. These arise from the pons and are part of the corticopontocerebellar pathway (see 'Cerebellar connections' this chapter).

The caudal cerebellar peduncle has both afferent and efferent fibres. The afferent input includes the dorsal spinocerebellar, reticulocerebellar, olivocerebellar, cuneocerebellar and vestibulocerebellar tracts. Efferent fibres are located on the medial aspect of the peduncle and include cerebellovestibular and cerebelloreticular tracts, which connect to the medulla oblongata (Figs. 7.3A, B, A5, A20-23, A29, A30).

Evolutionary and functional anatomy

Phylogenetically, the cerebellum is divided into three longitudinal zones. Functionally, these zones coordinate muscles in different body regions (Fig. 7.4A).

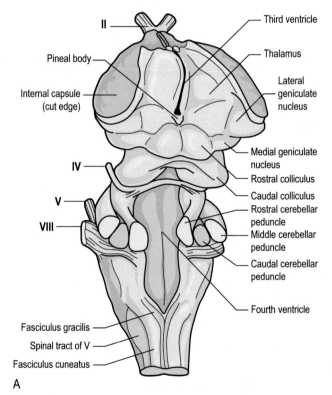

A

Fig. 7.3A **Dorsal aspect of the canine brainstem depicting the cerebellar peduncles. (Figure redrawn with permission from Miller's Anatomy of the Dog, Evans HE, 3rd Edition, Saunders, 1993)**

1. Archicerebellum/vestibulocerebellum: The ventromedial zone consists of the flocculonodular lobe. It receives input from, and functions in conjunction with, the vestibular system to regulate equilibrium/balance and posture. This zone appeared first in fish.
2. Paleocerebellum/spinocerebellum: This zone comprises most of the vermis and the paraflocculus. It is where

the major spinocerebellar afferent tracts terminate and coordinates truncal and limb movements. This zone appeared first in amphibians.

3. Neocerebellum/pontocerebellum: This more lateral zone comprises the lateral hemispheres and caudodorsal vermis of the caudal lobe. It receives cerebral input via the pontine nuclei and regulates skilled movement.

Species differences

The size and shape of the cerebellum correlates with the type of movement and posture of the animal. Those animals with mainly trunk musculature and symmetrical limb movement (e.g. reptiles, fish and flightless birds) have a well-developed medial portion and small lateral hemispheres (Fig. 7.4B). Animals with well-developed limbs and independent limb movement have better developed lateral hemispheres, e.g. mammals and flying birds. Primates and humans, which have upright posture and complex, skilled limb movements, have highly developed lateral hemispheres and corticopontocerebellar systems. (The corticopontocerebellar system influences pyramidal tract function (Chapter 5), which is also highly developed in these species.) Additionally, the lingula, the lobule of the vermis located just rostral to the nodulus, is well developed in animals with large tails (e.g. the rat compared with the pig) and the paraflocculus is bigger in animals with well-synchronised movements of the axial and appendicular musculature.

Cerebellar development in the neonatal animal

The ability of a neonatal animal to move in a coordinated manner correlates with the amount of cerebellar development at birth (Fig. 7.5). In precocious movers, such as herbivores that can ambulate within hours of being born, then cerebellar development is almost complete at birth. It is essential that such animals can get up and run with the herd, thus they must be able to coordinate activity of muscles used for posture and locomotion. In altricial animals, such as humans, many predators, or burrow-born prey species (e.g. rabbits and rodents) cell division and migration are still occurring for several weeks after birth, and the cerebellum will not be fully functional for some time. This is reflected in their limited ability to move in a coordinated fashion in those first few weeks. Such animals are usually born into a protected environment such as a den or burrow.

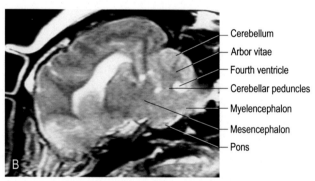

Cerebellum
Arbor vitae
Fourth ventricle
Cerebellar peduncles
Myelencephalon
Mesencephalon
Pons

Fig. 7.3B **Sagittal, T2-weighted, MRI scan dog brain, illustrating the cerebellar peduncles.**

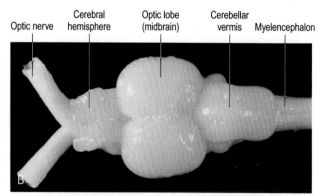

Optic nerve | Cerebral hemisphere | Optic lobe (midbrain) | Cerebellar vermis | Myelencephalon

Fig. 7.4B **Trout brain, dorsal aspect. Note the well-developed cerebellar vermis but no hemispheres. Cerebellar length = 6 mm.**

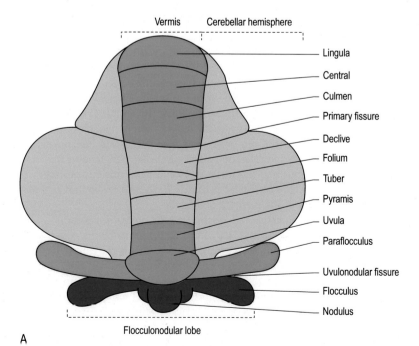

Vermis   Cerebellar hemisphere

Lingula
Central
Culmen
Primary fissure
Declive
Folium
Tuber
Pyramis
Uvula
Paraflocculus
Uvulonodular fissure
Flocculus
Nodulus

Flocculonodular lobe

A

Fig. 7.4A **The cerebellum as if it has been rolled out flat and viewed from the dorsal aspect. The different phyologenetic areas of the cerebellum are depicted: spinocerebellum = midgreen, vestibulocerebellum = dark green, pontocerebellum = light green.**

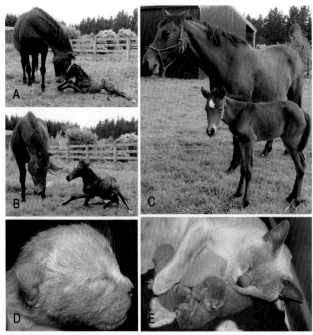

Fig. 7.5 **The cat is an altricial animal, while the horse is precocial. The difference in mobility is largely related to the degree of cerebellar development at birth. Both the kittens and foal are less than 24 hours old. (Cat photos courtesy of Ms. Genevieve Rogerson, Cahill Veterinary Clinic, Palmerston North. Horse photos courtesy of Dr. Debbie Prattley, IVABS, Massey University.)**

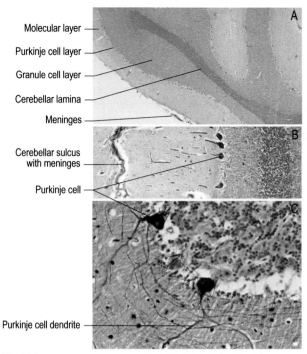

Fig. 7.6 **Histological sections of the cerebellum at different magnifications. (A, B) haemotoxylin and eosin stain, (C) Bielschowsky silver stain (from the Mervyn Birtle histology collection, IVABS, Massey University).**

Histology of the cerebellum

The cerebellum comprises distinct histological layers. Grey matter is found both superficially forming the cerebellar cortex, and in the three pairs of the cerebellar nuclei located just dorsal to the fourth ventricle.

In the folia, the molecular layer is the most superficial. It is relatively acellular, being mainly cell processes, such as axons and terminations of afferent cells (e.g. granule cells, climbing fibres) and the dendrites of the efferent, Purkinje cells.

The Purkinje cells (also known as cerebellar piriform or pyramidal neurons) form the next layer. These cells have a large, pear-shaped cell body with a single axon projecting into the granule cell layer and multiple dendrites in the molecular layer. The cell bodies form a distinct line at the border between the molecular and granule cell layers. The cell density is higher at the tip of the folium than at the base of the folium. Purkinje cells are nestled in a layer of specialised astrocytes called Bergmann glia.

The third layer is the granule cell layer which is composed of numerous, small-bodied neurons. It is a dense cell layer comprising 3–7 million granule cells/mm^3. The thickness varies, being 5–6 cell layers at the bottom of the folium and 15–20 at the top of the folium.

Deep to the granule cell layer is white matter forming the lamina of the folium. It connects to the deeper white matter mass of the cerebellar medulla, in which are sited the cerebellar nuclei, dorsal to the roof of the fourth ventricle. (Fig. 7.6 and 7.2, A21, A22).

The functional histology of the cerebellum is complex, but in essence it comprises a system that receives afferent input from proprioceptors throughout the body (head, neck, trunk and limbs), and also from the motor planning centres of the forebrain.

Afferent fibres to the cerebellum send collateral branches to synapse on, and excite, the cerebellar nuclei; afferent

input also travels to the cerebellar cortex, where they stimulate the Purkinje cells or, they stimulate interneurons that inhibit Purkinje cells. Incoming fibres are descriptively named for their morphology and form mossy fibres (majority of fibres) or climbing fibres. Both mossy fibres and climbing fibres send collateral axons to the cerebellar nuclei as they ascend through the cerebellum to reach the cerebellar cortex. Mossy fibres are named for their mossy-like spreading appearance. They originate in brainstem nuclei and the spinal cord and ultimately synapse in the granule cell layer. The climbing fibres originate in the olivary nucleus of the medulla oblongata. They decussate and climb all the way to the cerebellar cortex (molecular layer) before synapsing.

The output from the cerebellum is to motor planning centres in the forebrain, or to UMN centres of the motor cortex, or the UMN nuclei located throughout the brain. The output is largely from the cerebellar nuclei, which are facilitatory to the motor systems. However, Purkinje cells may inhibit the cerebellar nuclei, thereby blocking their facilitation of motor systems. The lateral and interposital nuclei project via the rostral cerebellar peduncle to the thalamus and red nucleus. The fastigial nucleus projects via the caudal cerebellar peduncle to the vestibular and reticular nuclei of the medulla oblongata.

The Purkinje cells form the only output from the cerebellar cortex. This output is primarily to the cerebellar nuclei. The exception to this is the output from the vestibulocerebellum (flocculonodular lobe) that projects directly to the vestibular nuclei of the brainstem, inhibiting their function. This arrangement is relevant to the pathogenesis of paradoxical vestibular disease (see Chapter 8). All Purkinje cells are inhibitory at their synaptic termination, mediated by the neurotransmitter GABA.

The functional histology of the cerebellum is summarised in Table 7.1 and Fig. 7.7. Overall, the cerebellum can function

Table 7.1 **The functional histology of the cerebellum**

Afferent fibre and general origin	Specific origin	Excitation at termination	Cerebellar function
Mossy fibres Brainstem and spinal cord Associated with proprioception and input from cerebral motor executive centres	Sensory Vestibular nuclei Spinocerebellar tracts Tectum (auditory and visual systems for head posture) Motor executive Pontine nucleus from forebrain motor executive centres	Cerebellar nuclei Granule cells which project to the molecular layer and excite Purkinje cells Stellate cells which inhibit Purkinje cells, which reduces inhibition of Cerebellar nuclei	1 Cerebellar nuclei are active causing facilitation of UMN centres 2 PC are active causing inhibition of cerebellar nuclei 1 Cerebellar nuclei are active causing facilitation of UMN centres
Climbing fibres Associated with motor executive centres of the forebrain and brainstem	Primarily the olivary nucleus of medulla oblongata	Cerebellar nuclei Purkinje cells	1 Cerebellar nuclei are active causing facilitation of UMN centres 2 PC are active causing inhibition of cerebellar nuclei

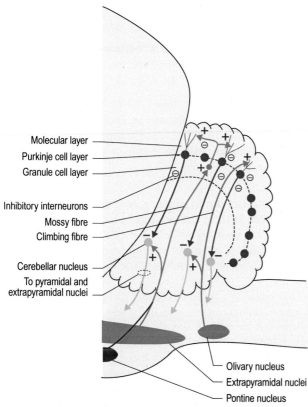

Fig. 7.7 **Functional connections in the cerebellum. The red circles in the molecular and granule cell layers represent inhibitory interneurons that can inhibit Purkinje or granule cells. Note: for simplicity, only some connections with the brainstem are depicted.**

Labels: Molecular layer; Purkinje cell layer; Granule cell layer; Inhibitory interneurons; Mossy fibre; Climbing fibre; Cerebellar nucleus; To pyramidal and extrapyramidal nuclei; Olivary nucleus; Extrapyramidal nuclei; Pontine nucleus

Proprioceptive inputs to the cerebellum are primarily from somatic muscle spindles and Golgi tendon organs, and the vestibular apparatus. These inputs inform cerebellum about the position, status/tension and activity of the skeletal musculature, and the position and movement of the head. The cerebellum also receives copies of planned motor activity from the motor centres. With input about body and head position, and information about planned motor activity, the cerebellum can compare motor intention with action. It modulates motor output to achieve desired postures, and coordinated movement, involving a plethora of agonist and antagonist muscles. Ongoing proprioceptive feedback from the muscles and from the vestibular apparatus, permit constant comparison of the intended and achieved motor function. In mammals there are essentially no direct connections from the cerebellum onto LMN, thus the cerebellum cannot initiate movement. Consequently, in mammals of veterinary interest, cerebellar dysfunction does not cause paresis. However, birds have a prominent cerebellospinal tract and avian spinal cord LMNs depend more on cerebellar than cortical control. While cerebellar dysfunction does not cause paresis in domestic mammals, it does disrupt posture (static and dynamic), and the spatial accuracy and temporal coordination of movement.

Cerebellar connections

Cerebellar afferents convey proprioceptive information, or information relevant to the planning and execution of motor activity (Figs. 7.7, 7.8).

1. Proprioceptive input from limbs, trunk, neck and head is represented ipsilaterally and informs the cerebellum about the distribution/location of body parts and status of muscles and joints. Afferent fibres are projected via the spinocerebellar and vestibulocerebellar tracts.
2. Input about planned motor activity. The cerebellum needs this to establish the appropriate postural platform before the activity is initiated and, then, to regulate and coordinate muscle activity throughout that motor action.
   (a) Input relevant to the coordination of functions originating from the motor cortex (learned, complex voluntary movement) is via the corticopontocerebellar pathway to the contralateral cerebellar hemispheres. There is a direct correlation between the extent of development of this system and the level of development of a species' motor skills. Thus, it is far better developed in primates and human, which have highly developed control of digits, facial muscles (facial expression), tongue and laryngeal

in two ways via the cerebellar nuclei. The nuclei may be stimulated by afferent cerebellar fibres or inhibited by the Purkinje cells. This results in the cerebellar nuclei being either facilitatory to motor systems or having no effect on them; they cannot inhibit them.

Cerebellar function

The function of the cerebellum is to smooth and coordinate motor function for posture and movement. It does this by using subconscious proprioceptive information (see Chapter 6) to modulate motor activity of UMN nuclei and the motor cortex; these then influence LMN activity. The cerebellum compares body position with desired motor output at the initiation, during, and at the termination of movement.

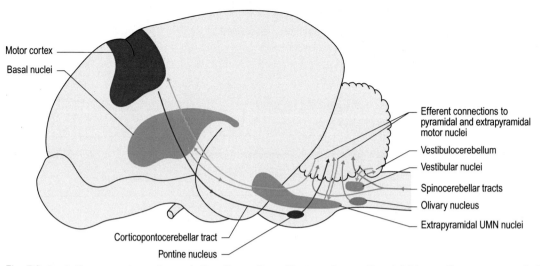

Motor cortex
Basal nuclei
Efferent connections to pyramidal and extrapyramidal motor nuclei
Vestibulocerebellum
Vestibular nuclei
Spinocerebellar tracts
Olivary nucleus
Extrapyramidal UMN nuclei
Corticopontocerebellar tract
Pontine nucleus

Fig. 7.8 **Cerebellar connections. The cerebellar efferent fibres (blue) may have a direct inhibitory effect (e.g. on vestibular nuclei), or have a facilitatory effect on UMN centres; but this latter effect is inhibited by Purkinje cells of the cerebellar cortex.**

musculature for speech. The corticopontocerebellar pathway from the cerebral cortex travels through the internal capsule and the crus cerebri to synapse in nuclei in the pons. Post-synaptic fibres decussate and ascend via the middle cerebellar peduncle into the cerebellum. The return pathway is from the cerebellar cortex to the cerebellar nuclei (e.g. lateral nucleus). Post-synaptic fibres decussate and exit the cerebellum via the rostral cerebellar peduncle, travel rostrally to the synapse in the thalamus and then to the cerebral cortex.

(b) Input relevant to coordination of the extrapyramidal function (semiautomatic movement, posture and locomotion) originates from the cerebrum, thalamus and midbrain, and projects to the olivary nuclei in the medulla oblongata. These nuclei project to the contralateral cerebellum. The cerebellum makes return connections via the cerebellar nuclei to the contralateral extrapyramidal nuclei of the forebrain (cortex and basal nuclei) and brainstem.

Efferent fibres from the cerebellar cortex are from the Purkinje cells. They are inhibitory and the majority synapse on the cerebellar nuclei, inhibiting them. The output from the cerebellar nuclei forms the majority of efferent fibres from the cerebellum; it is facilitatory to motor systems, thus loss of cerebellar cortical output usually results in excess UMN activity and spasticity. Note: output from the vestibulocerebellum (flocculonodular lobe) bypasses the cerebellar nuclei and synapses directly onto the vestibular nuclei.

Summary of cerebellar connections
- All afferent fibres to the cerebellar cortex are excitatory.
- All efferent fibres from the cerebellar cortex (Purkinje cells) are inhibitory.
- Purkinje cells are directly excited by cortical afferents but are also inhibited by interneurons. The output of Purkinje cells depends upon the balance between excitation and inhibition.
- Cerebellar nuclei neurons are all excitatory to nuclei of pyramidal and extrapyramidal systems.
- Cerebellar nuclei are inhibited by Purkinje cells and excited by afferent collaterals of afferent fibres.
- Cerebellar nuclei can be excitatory or silent to motor nuclei, but never inhibitory.

Role of cerebellum in posture, locomotion and movement: Setting the postural platform
Posture is the position of the body or body parts. It results from coordinated activity of extensor and flexor muscles acting around numerous joints of the limbs and vertebral column.

The cerebellum is the centre that coordinates activity in agonist/antagonist muscles acting around the joints throughout the body. But it also has a critical role in establishing the postural platform on which movement is superimposed. For example, a cat cannot catch an object with one paw without first redistributing its weight over the other three legs. Setting the body up to support the movement is called setting the postural platform.

To set the appropriate tone in the postural muscles, the cerebellum must be informed about what movements are being planned by the executive and senior management motor systems. It must also know exactly where the body parts are at that moment and what they are doing with respect to supporting posture. Thus it compares input from the motor planning centres with subconscious proprioceptive input.

The cerebellum then influences output of the UMN to the LMNs controlling postural muscles, to set the postural platform – this may involve redistribution of the weight. Having coordinated that postural adjustment, the cerebellum receives the new proprioceptive input from the activated postural muscles. In turn, the cerebellum feeds back to the motor management systems informing them that the postural platform has been set and the motor activity can go ahead (Fig. 7.9).

If the postural platform is not established, then the movement cannot occur. This is called postural paralysis.

Cerebellar dysfunction
In summary, three different syndromes may occur with lesions in different parts of the cerebellum (Fig. 7.4A). If the

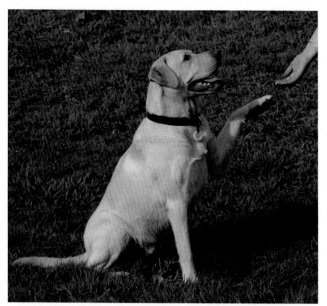

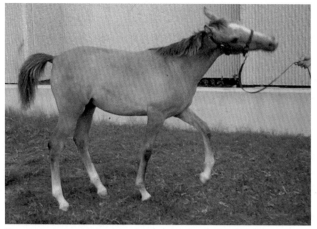

Fig. 7.10 **Hypermetric thoracic limb gait in a young Arabian horse with cerebellar degeneration (courtesy of Prof. Joe Mayhew, IVABS, Massey University).**

Fig. 7.9 **Setting the postural platform. Barney has flexed his left thoracic limb. Before he could do that, he had set the postural platform to permit the movement. He had to unload his body weight from the left thoracic limb and redistribute the weight onto the right thoracic limb, which is in obvious extension. Barney has also shifted his weight caudally onto his seated hindquarters. Additionally, visual input has resulted in a change in the head position, tilting it upwards. This will stimulate the vestibular system (see Chapter 8) and the neck proprioceptors; vestibular stimulation will further facilitate the extension of the thoracic limb. Thus, an apparently simple movement (flexing one limb) actually requires coordination of most of the muscles in the trunk, limbs and neck.**

cerebellum is diffusely affected, then a combination of signs may occur.

1. Vestibulocerebellar signs. The animal has a disturbance of equilibrium with swaying posture, wide-based stance and falling to the side when moving around. It may also have nystagmus and strabismus, but spasticity and tremor are not apparent.
2. Spinocerebellar signs. Hypermetria and hypertonus (spasticity) result in exaggeration of spinal reflexes, gait and postural responses such as hopping, wheelbarrowing, hemiwalking, etc.
3. Pontocerebellar signs. These affect feedback pathways between the cerebellum and the forebrain and can result in asynergia in which there is loss of harmony and synchrony in movements. Signs include dysmetria and overshooting of body parts, such as the head and limbs, and tremor that is exacerbated as the animal attempts to make a voluntary movement; this is known as an 'intention tremor'.

Cerebellar lesions can result in either or both of the following:

- Inadequate processing of incoming proprioceptive information resulting in subconscious proprioceptive deficits
- Inadequate output for modulating motor activity, thus motor activity is usually excessive.

Consequently, the following signs may be seen.
Ataxia is the uncoordinated or inconsistent movement of the trunk, limbs and neck. This is caused by reduced/no processing of proprioceptive input to the cerebellum. Thus the cerebellum does not know the position and status of body parts and cannot coordinate postural and locomotory muscles.

Dysmetria is abnormal rate, range or force of movement. Failure to receive incoming subconscious proprioceptive information results in incorrect postural adjustment and there will be delays in the initiation and termination of movements. Similarly, if the cerebellum cannot continually monitor subconscious proprioceptive input during movement, there will be failure to regulate the rate, range and force of movement. In the case of cerebellar lesions this often results in hypermetria with increased rate, range and force of movement. Hypermetria is characterised by overshooting of body parts during movement, and exaggerated stepping action (goose-stepping) during locomotion in animals. As the diseased cerebellum cannot receive subconscious proprioceptive feedback informing it that adequate movement has occurred, it fails to facilitate termination of movement (Fig. 7.10).

Spasticity occurs because of inadequate inhibition of UMNs. This leads to excessive muscle tone (extensor dominance) and also contributes to hypermetria. Note that paresis is NOT a feature of cerebellar disease. The rostral lobe of cerebellum particularly, exerts an inhibitory effect on antigravity muscles. Thus lesions of the rostral lobe can result in marked extensor activity including opisthotonus and thoracic limb extension.

Tremor arises due to failure to coordinate activity of the contracting agonist and relaxing antagonist muscles acting around a joint. Thus the muscle groups fight each other causing the joint to oscillate between flexion and extension. The classic presentation is known as an 'intention tremor' in which a tremor occurs associated with goal-directed movements such as an animal reaching forward with its head.

Vestibular signs occur due to involvement of the vestibulocerebellar connections or the vestibulocerebellum. The vestibulocerebellum receives proprioceptive input about head proprioception from the vestibular system. Inadequate vestibulocerebellar function results in reduced output from the cortex of the vestibulocerebellum. As this output is from inhibitory Purkinje cells to the vestibular nuclei, there is usually excessive activity of the vestibular nuclei in the brainstem. This occurs with lesions in the flocculonodular lobe or in the caudal cerebellar peduncles that convey connections between the vestibular nuclei and cerebellum. Therefore on the side with the lesion, there will be increased activity in the vestibular nuclei, resulting in increased ipsilateral extensor (anti-gravity) muscle tone and a head tilt to the side opposite to the lesion. This results in the paradoxical vestibular syndrome, which is explained more fully in Chapter 8.

Menace response deficits can occur in cerebellar disease in which, despite normal vision, the animal fails to blink in response to a threatening stimulus. The pathway by which this occurs is unclear but may be due to the visual pathway connecting to CN VII nuclei for blinking, via the cerebellum (corticopontocerebellar tract) or it could be due to failure of cerebellar facilitation to forebrain motor cortex.

Mostly signs of cerebellar dysfunction are ipsilateral, except in paradoxical vestibular syndrome in which the signs suggest a contralateral lesion.

Chapter 8
Vestibular system

Key Points

- Vestibular input helps maintain positions of the eyes, neck, trunk and limbs that are appropriate for the head position.
- The receptors of the vestibular system consist of three semicircular ducts detecting angular accelerations, and the utriculus and sacculus detecting static head position and linear accelerations.
- The vestibular ganglion is located in the petrosal part of the temporal bone. CN VIII enters the cranial cavity through the internal acoustic meatus and vestibular fibres synapse with four pairs of vestibular nuclei located in the rostral medulla oblongata.
- Vestibular nuclei receive additional proprioceptive input from proprioceptors in neck muscles.
- The vestibular system provides the cerebellum with subconscious proprioceptive information and the forebrain with information for conscious awareness about head and neck position.
- The output from the vestibular nuclei is modified by efferent fibres from the cerebellum.
- Lesions in the vestibular system can cause strabismus, pathological nystagmus and loss of extensor muscle tone (usually ipsilateral).

General concepts

The vestibular system (*vestibulum* – L = entrance) is the neural system that sets body equilibrium or balance. Equilibrium is defined as the condition in which all influences acting on a structure are cancelled out by others, resulting in a stable, balanced system. For example, if the head moves to the left, there has to be increased extensor muscle activity on the left side of the body to accommodate the shift in weight. Head movement can be primary (animal turning to look at something) or

secondary due to movement of the body. The latter can be generated by the animal (e.g. sitting, locomotion) or by external forces, such as being pushed by another animal. Head movement is detected by the vestibular system, the input from which results in modification of somatic muscle activity to accommodate the new set of forces acting on the body.

Cephalisation is the concentration of the exteroceptors and neural processing centres at the leading end of the animal. Use of exteroceptors such as vision, audition, olfaction and gustation, as well as tactile receptors, (e.g. whiskers) necessitates precise control of head position and movement. Controlling head position and movement requires detailed proprioceptive input that modifies motor activity in the neck muscles. Changes in head and neck position require postural changes in axial and appendicular muscle activity to provide the correct postural support. This is reflected in increased extensor muscle activity on the side to which the head is turned. Therefore head position dictates tone in muscles through the neck, trunk and limbs. To maintain appropriate visual input requires that the position and movement of the eyes be linked to head position and movement.

The vestibular apparatus, located in the inner ear, houses the receptor organs for detecting head position and movement. Stimulation of the vestibular apparatus provides the major input to the vestibular nuclei in the brainstem. However, the vestibular nuclei also integrate input from the gravity and movement sensors in the inner ear with proprioceptive information from muscles and joints.

The vestibular apparatus on each side consists of five distinct organs. There are receptors in three semicircular ducts, which are sensitive to angular acceleration/head rotation, and in two otolith organs (utriclus and sacculus), which are sensitive to linear accelerations and the influence of gravity in static head positions. The receptors are housed in the inner ear, in a series of membrane-lined, fluid-filled ducts and spaces located in the bony vestibule of the petrous temporal bone.

The receptors that detect head position and movement are hair cells. These are specialised epithelial cells with fine, hair-like processes on top of them. The base of the hair cell synapses with sensory nerves that convey action potentials via the vestibular portion of cranial nerve VIII (vestibulocochlear nerve) to the vestibular nuclei. The cell bodies of these bipolar sensory neurons form the diffuse vestibular ganglion in the petrosal portion of the temporal bone. There are four pairs of vestibular nuclei, located in the brainstem, just ventral to the cerebellum. The vestibular nuclei have five main efferent connections. They give rise to UMN spinal cord tracts that reflexively stimulate ipsilateral extensor muscle activity in the limbs, trunk and neck, inhibit antagonist muscles and contralateral extensor muscles. Rostrally directed output from the vestibular nuclei affects function of the cranial nerve nuclei, III, IV, VI, causing extraocular muscle contraction for eyeball position and movement. The vestibular nuclei send information to the cerebellum and cerebrum about head proprioception for subconscious modulation of postural muscle activity, and for conscious awareness, respectively. The vestibular nuclei also connect to the vomiting centre of the brainstem reticular formation; this is the basis of motion sickness.

The basic mechanism that stimulates the hair cells is similar for the detection of either static, or changing, head position. On each hair cell are 40–80 stereocilia (long microvilli) and a single kinocilium. These processes project into an overlying gelatinous layer, which, when it moves, causes deviation of the cellular processes. This deviation induces changes in membrane potential of the hair cell and may trigger an action potential in the sensory nerve fibre that synapses with the base of the hair cell. Gravity constantly stimulates hair cells that detect static head position. However, hair cells that detect head movement will only do so during acceleration or deceleration of the head, not when the head has reached constant velocity.

Structural and functional anatomy

The vestibular system is divided into peripheral and central components; this segregation has clinical implications. The peripheral vestibular system consists of the vestibular components of the inner ear (receptors and axons of CN VIII), while the central vestibular system comprises the vestibular nuclei and their output.

The inner ear is housed in the petrous temporal bone bilaterally. It contains a number of canals and cavities forming the bony labyrinth. On each side there are three semicircular canals, the bases of which connect to the bony vestibule. Ventral to the vestibule is the sculpted spiral canal that houses the cochlear with its auditory receptors (see Chapter 10). The semicircular canals arise from the vestibule, curve around and connect back to the vestibule. At one end of those connections the canal is dilated to form the ampulla. The bony canals and cavities are lined with membranes forming the membranous labyrinth (e.g. semicircular ducts). Perilymph is the fluid located between the membrane and the bone while endolymph fills the membranous (Fig. 8.1).

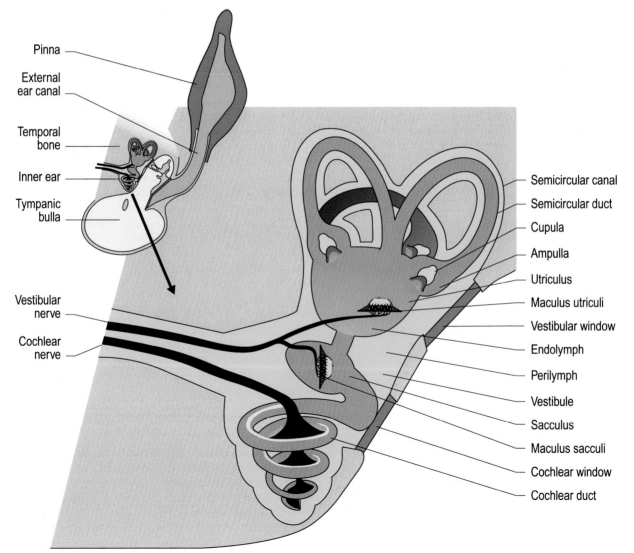

Fig. 8.1 **The vestibular system of the inner ear.**

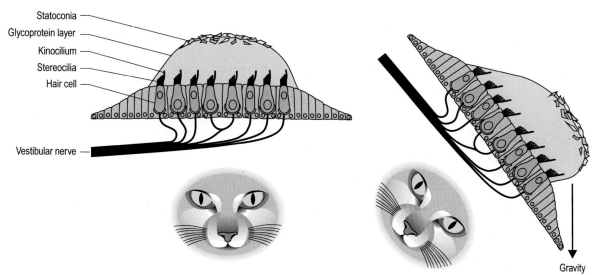

Fig. 8.2 **Macula of either the utriculus or sacculus. Regardless of head position gravity will be acting on the mass of the statoconia (otoliths) in one or both maculae. This force pulls on the glycoprotein gel and deflects the stereocilia towards, or away from, the kinocilium stimulating or inhibiting, respectively, nerve cells at the base of the hair cells.**

Static position, linear acceleration and deceleration of the head

Located within the vestibule are expanded portions of the membranous labyrinth, called the utriculus and the sacculus (Fig. 8.1). These membrane-bound portions of the vestibular system each have a region called a macula; this is where the hair cells are located. The stereocilia and kinocilium of each cell project into an overlying gelatinous matrix called the otolithic membrane. Embedded in the membrane are calcareous crystals called otoliths that, having sufficient mass, move under the effect of gravity, pulling on the otolithic membrane and causing deflection of the stereocilia and kinocilium. The macula in the utriculus is oriented in the horizontal plane, whereas in the sacculus it is oriented vertically. Thus no matter what position the head is in, gravity will be acting on one or both sets of otoliths causing deflection of the cell processes on the hair cells and stimulating the sensory nerves at their base. The stimulation is constant due to the ongoing effect of gravity on the mass of the otoliths (Fig. 8.2). Linear acceleration or deceleration will also affect otolith position.

Angular acceleration and deceleration of the head

The three semicircular canals and their membranous ducts are located at right angles to each other (in the x, y and z directions) with the anterior and posterior canals being vertically oriented and the horizontal canal being laterally oriented. The semicircular ducts on each side of the head function as synergic pairs. Turning the head in one direction will cause endolymph to flow towards the ampulla on that side, but away from the ampulla in the paired duct on the opposite side. This causes stimulation of hair cells on the first side, but inhibition on the opposite side. Thus the input received by the vestibular nuclei of the brainstem is unequal. Unequal input from paired semicircular ducts is interpreted as head movement. Note that if there is disease in the vestibular system on one side, then even at rest the brain will receive uneven input and thus, it is perceived that the animal's head is moving. The uneven input from the two sides will be interpreted as head movement inducing the reflex changes in posture and eyeball position/movement (see Clinical dysfunction) that result in clinical signs of vestibular disease.

Like the semicircular canal, the semicircular duct is dilated at one end forming the ampulla. The hair cells that perceive head movement are located on a ridge of tissue (crista ampullaris) in the ampulla of the semicircular ducts. Numerous stereocilia and a single kinocilium project from the surface of the hair cells into a gelatinous matrix called the cupula; this projects into the endolymph.

As the head moves, so will the petrosal part of the temporal bone, and the associated semicircular ducts and hair cells (Fig. 8.3 and 8.4). However, due to inertia, movement of the endolymph inside the ducts lags behind. The endolymph presses on the cupula, which deflects the stereocilia towards or away from the kinocilium, resulting in stimulation or inhibition of the vestibular neurons, respectively.

If the head continues to rotate in the same direction at the same speed, endolymph movement will catch up with the movement of the ducts and hair cells. As it no longer exerts pressure on the cupula, the stereocilia will not be deflected and the vestibular neurons will not be stimulated or inhibited. Thus there is minimal detection of head movement, via the semicircular ducts, when the head is moving at constant velocity.

When the animal stops rotating, the duct and hair cells cease moving, but again, due to inertia, the endolymph continues to move, but in the opposite direction relative to the membranous labyrinth. The cupulas in the synergic ducts are deflected in the opposite direction. Again there is uneven input to the vestibular nuclei and this is interpreted as head rotation but in the opposite direction. This causes the sensation of dizziness that humans perceive.

Effect of stimulating the vestibular nuclei

The cell bodies of the bipolar, vestibular neurons are located in the vestibular ganglion in the petrosal part of the temporal bone. The efferent axons from these neurons join with those from the cochlear portion to form the vestibulocochlear nerve (CN VIII). CN VIII enters the cranial cavity through the internal acoustic meatus. It attaches to the lateral aspect of the medulla oblongata just caudal to the caudal cerebellar peduncle (See Figs. A21, A22, A29).

There are four vestibular nuclei (rostral, medial, lateral and caudal) located near the caudal cerebellar peduncle on

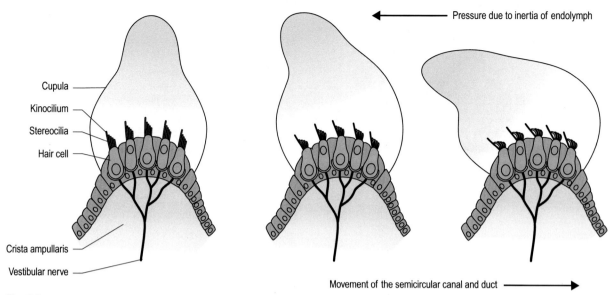

Fig. 8.3 **Deflection of processes on hair cells in the ampulla of the semicircular duct, by endolymph pushing on the cupula during head movement.**

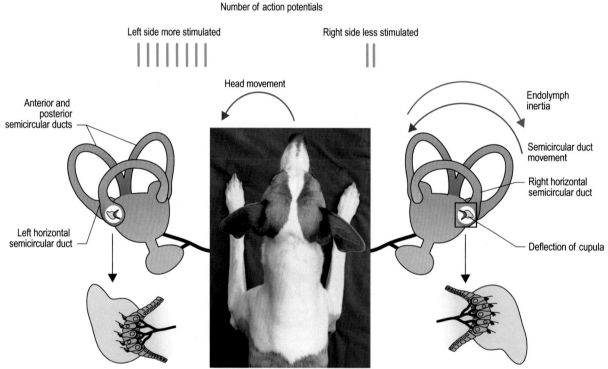

Fig. 8.4 **As Timmy turns his head to the left, endolymph in the paired horizontal canals flows in opposite directions, causing stimulation in the left canal and inhibition in the right canal. The brain receives uneven input from the two canals and this is interpreted as angular movement of head to the left.**

each side of the brainstem (see Figs. A21-23, A29). Outputs from the vestibular nuclei project to the spinal cord, cerebellum, brainstem and forebrain (Fig. 8.5).

An animal turning its head to the left illustrates the effects of these outputs.

1. Posture. Vestibular nuclear projections to the spinal cord are via the vestibulospinal tracts and medial longitudinal fasciculus in the ventral funiculus. The fibres terminate directly, or indirectly, on LMNs that facilitate ipsilateral extensor muscles and inhibit ipsilateral flexors (See Figs. 4.5, A30 and Table 5.1). Fibres also decussate to inhibit contralateral extensor muscle activity. Vestibulospinal tracts facilitate spinal reflexes, especially those involved in maintaining the posture (antigravity/extensor

muscles). Turning the head to the left causes a shift in the distribution of body mass to the left; this shift in mass is supported by increased extension on the left side. The extension is reflexively induced involving both the myotatic (see Chapter 5) and vestibular reflexes. Extension on the right side is reduced, thereby minimising the animal's weight transfer to the left (Fig. 8.6). The vestibulospinal (and reticulospinal) tracts are powerful facilitators of the antigravity/extensor muscles. This influence is demonstrated by the rigidity observed in decerebrate animals in which there is loss of inhibition of the vestibular (and reticular) nuclei.

2. Subconscious proprioception. Vestibulocerebellar tracts project to the cerebellum and convey information about head position and movement. The portion of the

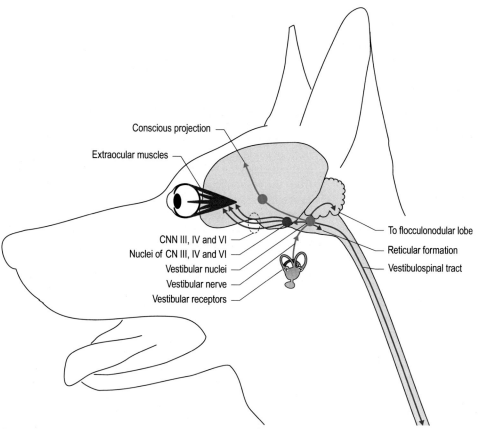

Fig. 8.5 **Neural connections arising from the vestibular nuclei of the brainstem.**

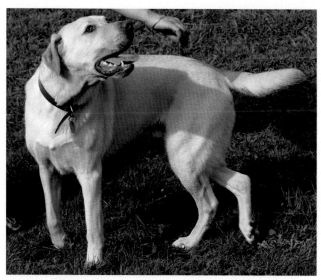

Fig. 8.6 **As Barney turns to the left, uneven stimulation of the vestibular nuclei results in ipsilateral extension, inhibition of ipsilateral flexion and contralateral extension. Thus a change in posture supports the shift in the centre of gravity.**

cerebellum that receives vestibular input is called the vestibulocerebellum and is sited caudoventrally in the flocculonodular lobe (see Chapter 7). The cerebellum uses this information about head proprioception (both static and dynamic), in conjunction with proprioceptive input from the neck, trunk and limbs, to modify and coordinate motor output from UMN centres of the brainstem and forebrain, to maintain static and dynamic posture of the whole body.

3. Eyeball position and movement. Fibres from the vestibular nuclei project rostrally (in the medial longitudinal fasciculus/vestibulomesencephalic tract (see Figs. A17-19, A30) to synapse on cranial nerve nuclei III, IV and VI that supply LMN to the extraocular muscles (Chapter 10). This wiring is the basis of the vestibulo-ocular reflex in which head movement cause reflex changes in eyeball position, and sets the position of the globes in the bony orbits at the end of head movement. During head movement the eyeballs move reflexively in a jerky fashion, called physiological nystagmus. The jerky movement is due to fixation of the gaze on a spot for a moment before flicking rapidly to a new position. Physiological nystagmus enables the animal to maintain a useful visual input during head movement. If the eyeballs remained centred in the orbit during movement, then the visual field would become blurred. For example, an animal is gazing at a spot in front of it, but then begins to move its head to the left. Its gaze remains fixated on that first spot, thus both eyes deviate to the right as the head moves to the left. The left lateral rectus muscle and right medial rectus muscle of the eyes are increasingly stretched until suddenly, and reflexively, they are stimulated to contract; this moves the eyes abruptly to the left. The gaze is fixated on a new position, the head continues to turn, muscles are stretched and rapid eyeball movement to the left occurs again, etc. Thus the animal's eyes deviate slowly in the opposite direction to which the head is turning and then make a rapid, active movement in the direction that the head is turning (see Fig. 13.7). This rhythmical, reflexive eyeball movement is called physiological nystagmus. Similarly, if the animal moves its head up or down, vertical nystagmus is induced with the fast phase of eyeball movement in the direction that the head is moving. The input from the vestibular system

and output to CNN nuclei III, IV and VI also set the position of the eyes at the end of head movement. The position of the eyes will be centred in the orbit after horizontal movement, but after vertical movement the default position will depend on whether it is a predator or prey species. In carnivores, the eyes will be centred in the orbit, thus if the head is tilted upwards, the eyes will also be looking upwards. In herbivores, with an elevated head position, the eyes will be directed downwards as the default normal position. Professor R. Le Couteur, UC Davis, teaches a useful way of remembering this. As the big cat is chasing the herbivore in the wild and is going to leap for the throat, the cat has its head tilted upwards and is looking forward (eyeballs centred in orbit) at that luscious target of the throat. The herbivore has its head tilted up as far out of reach as possible, but is looking down at the slavering jaws of the predator snapping below it.

4. Conscious awareness. Other rostrally directed fibres travel bilaterally, synapsing in the medial geniculate nucleus of the diencephalon, and then via the internal capsule to the temporal lobe for conscious awareness of head position.

5. Motion sickness. Local projections from the vestibular nuclei into the brainstem connect to the vomiting centre of the reticular formation. This is the pathway by which head movement may trigger motion sickness, which occurs when visual and vestibular inputs do not correlate with each other.

Note that there is also input to the vestibular nuclei from the first three cervical segments of the spinal cord utilising the spinovestibular tract in the ventral funiculus. The input conveys proprioceptive information about head position from muscles at the head–neck junction to the caudal vestibular nucleus. Thus, damage to the first three cervical vertebral spinal cord segments, or their dorsal roots, can also result in dramatic vestibular signs.

Also note that in the cat and other types of mammal, up to 20% of fibres in the vestibular nerve have been described

as efferent, originating from a variety of regions in the medulla oblongata, including the reticular formation and the vestibular nuclei. Their role may include facilitation, or inhibition, of vestibular receptors in the membranous labyrinth.

Relationship between the vestibular apparatus and neck reflexes

There is an intimate relationship between head position, neck position and limb position. If head position alters, without changing the head–neck angle, the primary input is from the vestibular apparatus, which induces reflex activity in the limbs and trunk; these are called vestibular reflexes. Changes in head–neck junction angles are detected by proprioceptors in the neck muscles. The resulting reflex changes in the limbs are induced by neck reflexes.

Neck muscles at the head–neck junction, such as the rectus and obliquus capitus muscles, are rich in muscle spindles with five times the number of muscle spindles per gram compared with a large, postural muscle like the gluteals. Input from these and other neck muscles, travel cranially in the spinal cord via the spinovestibular tract to the caudal vestibular nuclei. Spinovestibular fibres are intermingled with the lateral vestibulospinal tract fibres in the ventral funiculus. The overall effect of vestibular and neck reflexes on limb flexion and extension is summarised in Fig. 8.7.

Clinical dysfunction

Disturbance of the vestibular system produces a series of characteristic signs that reflect derangement of the functions described in the preceding section. Lesions may be located in the inner ear (semicircular ducts, utriculus or sacculus) the vestibular portion of CN VIII, the vestibular nuclei, the caudal cerebellar peduncle, the vestibulocerebellum or, potentially, the cranial cervical spinal cord. The key point to understanding vestibular dysfunction is to recall that during normal function, the

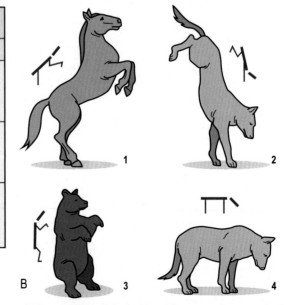

Neck	Labyrinth		
	Head up	**Head normal**	**Head down**
Extended	A	B	C
Normal	D	E	F
Flexed	G	H	I

A

B

Fig. 8.7 **Limb position is reflexively induced by sensory input from both the vestibular apparatus (labyrinth) and from proprioceptors in the muscles at the head neck junction. Hence an animal's limb posture will be dependent on whether the head is tilted or neutral, and whether there is flexion or extension at the head-neck junction. (Figure redrawn with permission from Roberts TDM, *Understanding Balance, The Mechanics of Posture and Locomotion.* Chapman & Hall, London, 1995).**

brain interprets unmatched input from the vestibular apparatus as indicating head movement. This unbalanced input will then induce changes in postural muscle tone, eyeball position and movement. If the normal animal moves its head to the left as in Fig. 8.4, there will be increased input from the left horizontal canal and decreased input from the right horizontal canal. This causes increased extension in the limb, trunk and neck muscles on the animal's left side and decreased extension on the right side. The animal's eyes will jerk in a rapid fashion to the left. The adjustments of limb position and head position will be coordinated by the cerebellum.

If the animal had a lesion in the right side of the vestibular system then the vestibular nuclei would have decreased input from the right but sustained input from the left, that is, unbalanced input with left side input being greater than the right. In this diseased animal, the unbalanced input occurs when the animal is at rest, not moving as described in the preceding paragraph for the normal animal. The brain would interpret the unbalanced input as indicating that the head is turning to the left. At rest, the animal would have increased anti-gravity extensor tone on the left, and decreased muscle tone on the right side. Thus the animal with a right-sided vestibular lesion would have decreased tone in the right-sided postural muscles compared with the left. This would present as decreased neck muscle tone on the right resulting in a head tilt to the right. There would be excess extensor tone on the left side of the body and decreased extensor tone on the right, thereby pushing the animal to the right. Thus the animal would tilt, stagger, drift, circle or, in severe cases, roll to the right (Figs. 8.8 and 8.9).

The animal tries to compensate for the altered posture but due to abnormal output from the vestibular nuclei to the cerebellum (subconscious proprioception of the head),

coordination of limb position and stepping movements would be perturbed. Thus the animal would be ataxic with wide- or narrow-based postures and uncoordinated movement.

The brain perceives the animal to be turning to the left due to the unbalanced input, thus at rest, the eyes make rapid jerky movements to the left, before drifting back across the orbit again. This abnormal movement of the eyeballs is called pathological nystagmus and may occur in the horizontal, vertical or rotatory direction, depending on which semicircular duct inputs (x, y or z direction) have been disturbed by the lesion. Acutely affected dogs may appear nauseous or vomit (motion sickness) due to unbalanced input to the reticular formation.

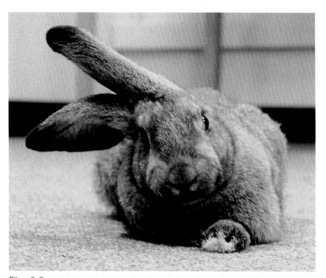

Fig. 8.8 **Rabbit with right-sided peripheral vestibular disease resulting in ipsilateral head tilt and loss of extensor muscle tone in the neck and trunk and limbs. See also Fig. 1.14.**

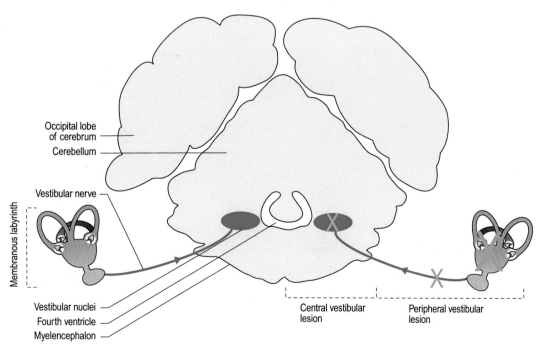

Fig. 8.9 **The caudal brainstem in transverse section, showing the sites of peripheral and central vestibular system lesions (green crosses) and their effect on vestibular stimulation when the head is in a resting, neutral position (see Figs. A21-23).**

Location of lesion and clinical signs

Classical vestibular signs include head tilt, staggering and ataxia, circling and pathological nystagmus. They may arise from lesions in the periphery in the inner ear or the vestibular portion of the vestibulocochlear nerve (CN VIII). Or they may arise centrally in the brainstem, the vestibular portions of the cerebellum or the cranial spinal cord (Fig. 8.9). Thus vestibular disease is called peripheral or central, respectively.

Differentiating the location of the lesion is important for diagnosis and prognosis. Lesion localisation follows the golden rule of identifying which other neural functions are compromised and which neural functions are normal (see Fig. 13.1).

Any lesion in the nervous system, peripheral or central, may also compromise nearby structures. A disease causing peripheral vestibular lesions in the inner ear may also affect the facial nerve running beside the middle ear. In small animals, but not in large animals, the sympathetic supply to the head passes adjacent to the middle ear and can also be compromised. Respectively, this collateral damage can cause ipsilateral facial paresis and Horners syndrome (miosis, ptosis, enophthalmos and protrusion of the third eyelid (see Fig. 12.6) or changes in ipsilateral sweating. Lesions affecting the site of attachment of CN V, VII and VIII to the pons and rostral medulla oblongata can result in signs of masticatory muscle atrophy as well as facial hypalgesia and paresis, and vestibular signs.

Lesions affecting the vestibular nuclei (central disease) are highly likely to also affect nearby brainstem tracts and structures. These include adjacent proprioceptive pathways, UMN nuclei, sensory input from the head (CN V), facial nucleus (CN VII) and the ascending reticular activating system (ARAS) (Chapter 11). Thus central vestibular lesions may also cause ataxia, due to general and vestibular proprioceptive deficits, UMN paresis, facial hypalgesia and paresis, and decreased awareness, but not Horner

syndrome. The second dog in Fig. 10.12 (B and C) presented initially with CN V signs and subsequently developed facial paresis (CN VII), head tilt and pathological nystagmus (CN VIII). The presence of these clinical signs indicates that the lesion is likely to be where CNV, VII and VIII attach to the brainstem.

Vestibular signs can also occur with lesions affecting the vestibulocerebellum. If the lesion in the cerebellum is quite extensive it may be accompanied by other signs of cerebellar disease (tremor, spasticity, dysmetria, see Chapter 7) but the animal will not be paretic (as the UMN nuclei are not involved). It will be bright, alert and responsive (no involvement of the ARAS) and will not have other CNN deficits (CN V and VII) or Horners syndrome.

Rarely, lesions in C1–3 spinal cord segments may affect the proprioceptive input from the muscles such as the obliquus and rectus capitis, and result in vestibular-like signs. Pathological nystagmus may be observed with such lesions.

Paradoxical vestibular disease

Lesions may also occur in the area of the caudal cerebellar peduncle, which conveys the afferent subconscious proprioceptive fibres going to the cerebellum tracts and the efferent fibres from the vestibulocerebellum (flocculonodular lobe) to the brainstem. Lesions affecting the caudal cerebellar peduncle produce paradoxical vestibular signs. The signs are paradoxical because they seem to indicate that the lesion is on the contralateral side of the CNS. Note: paradoxical vestibular disease is far less common than other forms of vestibular disease.

In typical vestibular disease (peripheral or central) the head tilt and circling will be towards the side of the lesion, while the fast phase of pathological nystagmus will be away from the side of the lesion (e.g. right-sided lesion, will result in a head tilt to the right and the fast phase of nystagmus to the left). In paradoxical vestibular disease, the

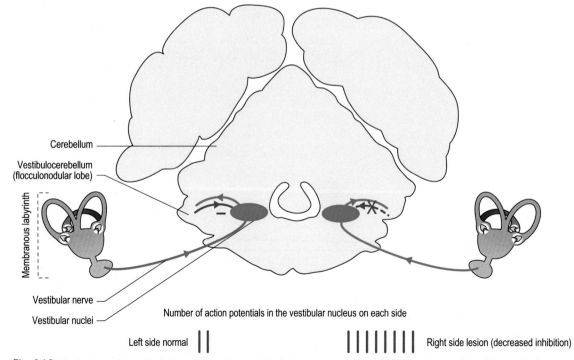

Fig. 8.10 **Mechanism of paradoxical vestibular disease. The lesion causes reduced inhibition by the right-side vestibulocerebellum on the ipsilateral vestibular nuclei.**

head tilt and circling is to the opposite side of the lesion and the fast phase of the nystagmus is towards the side of the lesion.

The explanation for this rests in the primary concept that the output from the vestibulocerebellum is direct (not via the deep cerebellar nuclei) and hence, is inhibitory to the vestibular nuclei. Thus on the side with the lesion, there will be decreased inhibition to the vestibular nuclei. These nuclei will have more activity than the vestibular nuclei on the normal side. The brain perceives from this unbalanced input that the animal must be turning to the side of the lesion (Fig. 8.10).

For example, if the right-side caudal cerebellar peduncle is damaged, as by a tumour or inflammatory mass, there will be decreased cerebellar cortical inhibition of the ipsilateral vestibular nuclei. Therefore, there will be increased activity of the vestibular nuclei on the right side. The uneven activity in the left- and right-side nuclei will be interpreted as the animal turning to the right. There will be increased reflex output down the right-side vestibulospinal tract, thus the right side extends while left-sided extension is inhibited. The animal tilts, staggers and drifts to the left (contralateral to the side of the lesion). At the same time, the apparent perception of turning to the right means that the eyeballs flick rapidly to the right as they would if the animal was truly turning to the right.

Identifying that the lesion is causing paradoxical signs involves identifying what other neural functions are compromised. Many proprioceptive fibres from the limbs and body (spinocerebellar tracts) travel via the caudal cerebellar peduncle into the cerebellum, thus such lesions can also compromise ipsilateral proprioception. In the example above the animal would have right-sided proprioceptive deficits. Due to the proximity of brainstem UMN nuclei, such lesions may also cause ipsilateral paresis.

Differentiating central versus peripheral vestibular disease

Identifying whether the lesion is located in the central vestibular apparatus (brainstem) or in the peripheral apparatus (inner ear or vestibular portion of CN VIII) is important for aetiological, treatment and prognostic reasons. The prognosis is usually less favourable with a central lesion due both to the difficulty of treating the lesion effectively, and the involvement of other neural structures in the brainstem.

Lesion localisation follows the same principles as outlined at the end of chapter 1 and Figures 1.14 and 13.1. That is, the clinician needs to identify those neural structures

that are dysfunctional **and** those that are still functioning normally. The brainstem is associated with many neural functions all crowded closely together, thus a small lesion can cause a variety of neural signs (see also chapter 13 and figure 13.14). Conversely, there are only a few other neural structures that are associated with the inner ear and may become collaterally damaged by an inner ear lesion. Such structures include the facial nerve, CN VII and the sympathetic supply to the face. Table 8.1 summarises the signs that may be seen with lesions in different portions of the vestibular system.

Sign	Central vestibular disease	Peripheral vestibular disease
Head tilt	Yes	Yes
Nystagmus	Yes	Yes
Circling	Yes	Yes
Strabismus	Yes	Yes
Perturbed vestibulo-ocular reflex	Yes	Yes
Long tract signs ■ proprioceptive deficits ■ motor deficits (paresis)	Yes	No
Decreased mentation/arousal	Yes	No
Other cranial nerve deficits ■ CN V ■ CN VII ■ CN IX–XII	 ■ Yes ■ Yes ■ Potentially yes	 ■ No ■ Yes ■ No
Horner's syndrome (see chapter 12)	No	Yes

Notes:

1) Circling is usually towards the side of the lesion except in paradoxical vestibular disease. Circles are usually small in diameter in vestibular disease, while in forebrain disease, they are often larger and do not have a head tilt (see Chapter 9).

2) Pathological nystagmus is usually seen with both central and peripheral vestibular disease. It may be horizontal, vertical or rotatory. Vertical nystagmus may indicate central disease, but is not pathognomonic.

3) If the lesion is located in the vestibulocerebellum, and involves other portions of the cerebellum, other signs of cerebellar disease may also be apparent, for example, tremor, spasticity and hypermetria (see chapter 7).

4) As noted previously in this chapter, damage to the cranial cervical cord can perturb proprioceptive input about head position and result in vestibular signs.

It is also worth noting, that with either cause, blindfolding may exacerbate subtle signs due to loss of visual input compensating for loss of head proprioception.

Chapter 9
Posture and movement in quadrupeds

Key points

- In veterinary species, the extrapyramidal motor system is most important for gait and movement. Output from the motor cortex, through the pyramidal system, influences voluntary, skilled movement but has minimal influence on gait.
- Alternation between extension and flexion for locomotion is largely generated by spinal cord reflexes; such patterns are triggered and sustained by central pattern generators.
- UMN tracts primarily responsible for the support phase are the vestibulospinal and pontine reticulospinal tracts facilitating extensor muscles. The flexor phase is controlled by the medullary reticulospinal and the rubrospinal tracts.
- Some UMN nuclei in the brainstem work as locomotive trigger centres and initiate or terminate ambulation.
- Forebrain lesions in non-primates can cause postural reaction deficits and mild motor signs.
- Brainstem lesions can cause opisthotonus due to loss of cerebral inhibition of the UMN nuclei that facilitate extensor muscle activity. Or lesions may cause paresis due to loss of UMNs facilitating locomotory activity.
- Cerebellar lesions can cause ataxia without paresis.
- UMN and LMN lesions result in disparate types of paresis distinguishable by the Neuro 'RAT' – (reflexes, atrophy and tone). The signs are also determined by lesion location and severity, and the number of tracts that have been compromised.

Motor function in quadrupeds compared to primates

In quadrupedal animals of veterinary interest, the main UMN tracts that influence locomotion originate in the brainstem, whereas the motor cortex/corticospinal system has minimal influence on gait; this is different to primates and humans. After experimental removal of the motor cortex of quadrupeds, gait is relatively normal. In contrast to this, damage to the motor cortex in humans can result in marked hemiparesis; this is exemplified by cerebrovascular accidents, or 'strokes'.

Integration of neural functions for locomotion and movement
Basic stepping movements and control systems
Stepping, and the oscillation between extension and flexion of limbs, trunk and neck, weight bearing and non-weight bearing, is based primarily on reflex circuitry within the spinal cord; it also involves central pattern generators. The flexion of one limb can induce reflex extension in the other limbs, both of the same limb girdle and the other limb girdle (see Fig. 9.1); this utilises the crossed extension reflex. Note that in the normal animal, when recumbent, the crossed extensor reflex is inhibited. In recumbent animals with UMN lesions, active flexion of one limb (e.g. withdrawal reflex) can result in the contralateral limb extending. This is abnormal and indicates loss of caudally directed UMN pathways that inhibit crossed extension reflexes.

The extensor postural thrust reflex is utilised when the foot makes contact with the ground, and the limb joints begin to flex under the effect of gravity. This activates the muscle spindles in extensor muscles, inducing reflex extension and thrust is generated against the ground, resulting in support for the body. This reflex utilises the same circuitry as the mytotatic reflex.

Input, integration and output of the reflexes: Sensory input for the reflexes comes from muscle spindles, Golgi tendon organs, joint and tactile receptors. Integration of that input in the spinal cord causes inhibition or excitation of LMNs, as appropriate, in that same limb, in the opposite limb or the limbs of the other girdle. The activity of the epaxial and hypaxial muscles of the trunk, neck and tail are also interlinked. For example, look at how a cat uses its tail to maintain its balance by offsetting muscle activity in the trunk when it is 'tight-rope walking' along the top of a narrow fence. Integration of neural activity between the muscles of the limbs, trunk, neck and tail is done primarily using spinospinal tracts such as the propriospinal tract. This tract connects between spinal cord segments and is located in all funiculi immediately surrounding the grey matter (see Fig. 4.5). Constant proprioceptive input from muscles of the entire body both activates the reflexes and sends sensory information to the cerebellum for use in coordination of motor activity. Proprioceptive input to the forebrain gives rise to conscious awareness of posture and movement; this is called kinaesthesia (see Chapter 6).

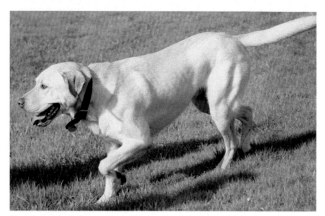

Fig. 9.1 **Extension and flexion of alternate limbs is mediated largely by reflex circuitry within the spinal cord, but supraspinal input is required for locomotion.**

The LMNs are stimulated or inhibited by both reflex connections and the input from the UMN system. The UMN tracts stimulate, or inhibit, muscle activity of the body. In quadrupeds, UMN nuclei of the brain stem are the nuclei primarily responsible for locomotion; there is minimal input from the motor cortex of the cerebrum. Via spinal cord UMN tracts, UMN nuclei recruit spinal reflex circuitry for locomotion. Their input initiates, regulates, modulates, coordinates and terminates activity in the reflex circuits and in specific LMNs. There are specific locomotive trigger centres in the brainstem. When stimulated, ambulation is triggered. When inhibited, ambulation is terminated.

The UMN tracts primarily responsible for the protraction and support phase are the vestibulospinal and pontine reticulospinal tracts facilitating extensor muscles. For the retraction/flexor phase, extensor muscle activity must be inhibited and flexor muscle LMNs must be stimulated utilising the medullary reticulospinal and the rubrospinal tracts (Table 4.3). At the end of retraction, extension and subsequently, the support phase, occurs again.

Coordination of locomotion

The overall function of the cerebellum is to coordinate agonistic/antagonistic muscle activity to permit posture and to create movement that occurs at the correct rate, range and force (see Chapter 7).

1. Posture. The cerebellum has an important role in coordinating overall posture.

   As described previously, increased load on individual muscles stretches muscle spindles causing reflex contraction of postural muscles, mediated through local spinal circuits. But posture involves the contraction–relaxation of many muscles around numerous joints and that requires overall coordination. The cerebellum's role is to coordinate the contraction–relaxation of all muscles in the body used for maintaining posture both at rest and during movement.

   The postural platform. The cerebellum has a critical role in establishing the postural platform (see Chapter 7). Failure to do so prevents normal, coordinated movement from occurring.

2. During movement.

   The cerebellum coordinates the initiation of movement, the actual movement itself and the termination of movement; it cannot initiate movement per se. Throughout movement, proprioceptive input

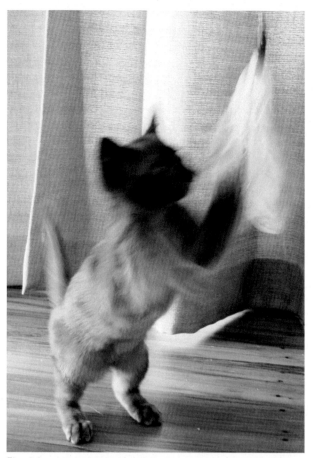

Fig. 9.2 **In this fast-moving kitten, the cerebellum has coordinated complex activity in postural muscles to achieve a postural platform that permits use of both forelimbs for a new type of motor function.**

from the head, neck, trunk, tail and limbs, continually informs the cerebellum how much movement has occurred, how fast it is occurring and how forceful the movement is. The cerebellum compares the achieved movement with the planning information it received about that movement. Based on constant proprioceptive feedback, it determines whether the movement is being performed adequately with the correct rate and force. It determines when the correct range of movement has been achieved, and thus when the action should be terminated. The output from the cerebellar cortex is inhibitory. Thus lesions causing loss of cerebellar output often result in increased rate, range and force of movement. This is called hypermetria.

Complex motor activity

For voluntary, learned movement (e.g. capturing 'prey' as in Fig. 9.2 or pawing, Fig. 9.3) the planning occurs in the executive motor planning areas of the forebrain. The executive centres draw on integration/interpretation areas associated with a variety of sensory receiving areas (e.g. visual cortex and somatosensory cortex), and memory and behaviour centres of the parietal and temporal lobes. A copy of the planned movement is sent to the cerebellum, which then establishes the appropriate postural platforms. The cerebellum feeds back to the motor planning centres informing them that the posture has been established. The executive centres then direct the senior motor system hierarchy (pyramidal and extrapyramidal systems) and movement is initiated. Throughout movement, the cerebellum, using constant proprioceptive input, monitors the rate, range and force of movement and sends modifying

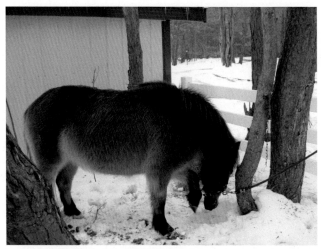

Fig. 9.3 **Pawing is an example of a complex voluntary movement** (courtesy of Dr. Katherine Houpt, Cornell University).

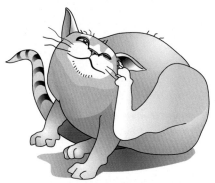

Fig. 9.4 **Rhythmical movements, such as scratching, breathing and locomotion, use spinal cord reflex circuits and are controlled by central pattern generators in the brainstem.**

commands to the UMN centres and constant feedback to the motor planning centres as to how the movement is progressing (see Fig. 7.8).

Repetitive movements and central pattern generators

The CNS contains many neural networks that produce oscillatory outputs used for controlling rhythmical motor activity such as locomotion, scratching, chewing, micturition and breathing. Such neural networks are called central pattern generators (CPGs); they contain excitatory and inhibitory neurons.

The CPGs associated with locomotion and scratching have local neural circuits in the spinal cord intumescences. Located in the brainstem are control centres that, via UMN tracts, initiate and terminate the rhythmical activity. Activation of the brainstem centres is like pushing the start button to run a modular programme of neural activity. Once activated, the local (e.g. spinal cord) circuitry produces contraction/relaxation of multiple flexors and extensors in specified spatiotemporal patterns; this results in repetitive activities like locomotion (Fig. 9.4). Within the spinal cord, the CPG networks are bilaterally symmetrical; there are also interconnections between circuits controlling paired thoracic and pelvic limbs. Spinal cord CPGs can act in isolation from brain and may result in stepping movements; this is called spinal walking and may be seen in animals with chronic spinal cord transection. Spinally generated stepping movements do not produce useful, purposeful locomotion. Input from supraspinal centres in the brain is required for

balance, coordination, initiation, regulation, modulation and termination of locomotion.

The CPGs associated with the rhythmical movements of the thoracic wall and diaphragm for respiration are located in the brainstem with output to local circuits in the cervical and thoracic spinal cord. The CPG for chewing is also located in the brainstem.

The final common pathway

In summary, influencing the output of the LMN, are incoming peripheral sensory fibres, interneurons from many spinal cord segments, UMN, and, indirectly, the cerebellum and executive motor centres of the forebrain. There is a complex system of checks and balances, whereby the senior and executive components of the motor system facilitate or inhibit the LMN activity. These influences act directly on individual groups of LMNs or indirectly by activating reflex circuits.

The following points are given to illustrate some of the complexities that are used to achieve optimal motor function.

Facilitation of LMNs occurs by output from many areas, including limited areas of the cerebral cortex, the globus pallidus of the basal nuclei, the red, pontine reticular and vestibular nuclei. Indirect facilitation also occurs by inhibition of inhibitory pathways. For example, the medial medullary reticular formation gives rise to the medullary reticulospinal tract, which exerts a massive inhibitory effect on LMNs supplying extensor muscles. However, the lateral medullary reticular formation can inhibit it, thereby resulting in indirect facilitation of LMN activity.

The LMNs are directly inhibited by the medullary reticulospinal tract and are also indirectly inhibited by the executive management which can inhibit certain UMN centres of the brainstem. The cerebral cortex also projects to the substantia nigra of the midbrain, which has an inhibitory effect on the basal nuclei, dampening down the stimulatory effect of the globus pallidus on the UMN nuclei of the brainstem.

Ultimately, the activity of motor system hierarchy is expressed as movement through the activation, or inhibition, of α-LMN firing. Again, this often occurs indirectly as a consequence of γ-LMN-1a (see Chapter 5, the myotatic reflex) activity. Thus, the α-LMN is referred to as the final common pathway. Through the α-LMN, a myriad of inputs is finally expressed. The activity of all these inputs is summated and if facilitation exceeds inhibition, the α-LMN is activated and the muscle will contract at a strength that is proportional to the frequency of firing. This is occurring constantly and in hundreds of muscles around the body. Simultaneously, there are changes in the activity of muscles antagonising the contracting muscles. If the antagonist muscle(s) is inhibited, agonist contraction results in joint movement. If the antagonist muscle(s) also contracts, then the joint position is fixed. Isometric contraction of agonists and antagonists and fixing of joint position, is the basis of static posture. The contraction–relaxation of so many muscles is coordinated and regulated by the organising centre, the cerebellum.

Lesion location in the hierarchy and its clinical effect on locomotion

(See Tables 13.4 and 13.5 for all clinical signs associated with lesions in different parts of the nervous system.)

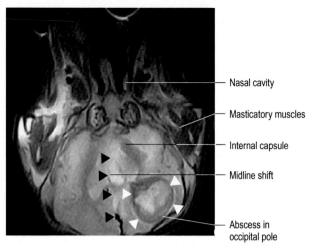

Nasal cavity

Masticatory muscles

Internal capsule

Midline shift

Abscess in occipital pole

Fig. 9.5 **Magnetic resonance image in the dorsal plane of calf brain depicting an abscess in the right forebrain. White arrowheads outline the abscess, and black arrowheads indicate the distortion of the brain, with a shift of the midline towards the left, due to the mass effect of the abscess (courtesy of Dr. Michael Hewetson, University of Finland).**

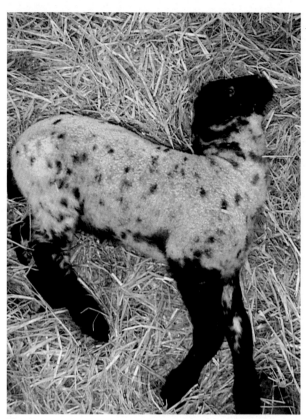

Fig. 9.6 **Lamb with opisthotonus (courtesy of Dr Phil Scott, University of Edinburgh).**

Forebrain lesions in quadrupeds have little effect on basic locomotion as this is primarily directed by senior management in the brainstem. Cortical lesions may result in mild motor signs such as a stumbling gait and contralateral postural reaction deficits ('knuckling') occur if cranially projecting proprioceptive systems are compromised. Walking in wide circles may also be noted due to effects on basal nuclei. Note that circling occurs with forebrain and vestibular disease. With forebrain lesions, circles tend to be large diameter while tighter circles occur with vestibular disease. Additionally, forebrain lesions will not have other signs of vestibular dysfunction, such as head tilt or pathological nystagmus.

For example, a calf was presented walking in large-diameter circles to the right, displaying, left-sided visual deficits and reduced awareness (see Chapter 11). The function of cranial nerves III–XII were normal, and the spinal cord reflexes were intact. These findings indicate that the brainstem and spinal cord were not affected (see Fig. 13.1). The signs of dysfunction point to a lesion in the forebrain, specifically the right cerebral hemisphere, accounting for the reduced awareness, circling, and the left-sided visual deficits (the optic pathways decussate en route to the visual cortex.) An abscess in the right occipital cortex was confirmed on MRI scan (Fig. 9.5).

Lesions involving basal nuclei often have minimal effect on voluntary movement and do not usually lead to adventitious (unexpected) movements such as seen in humans. Occasionally, lesions may cause the animal to have torticollis and be curved to one side or circle to one side, or have bizarre, complex movements with dystonia and chorea (involuntary, jerky, uncoordinated movements). Experimentally, lesions in the caudate nucleus and putamen can result in hyperactivity, whereas lesions in the globus pallidus can cause hypoactivity. For example, bilateral lesions of the putamen may result in obstinate progression with the animal trying to continue to walk even when it has come up against a wall ('head-pressing'). Unilateral lesions can result in hyper activity on one side only, so the animal takes bigger strides on one side and walk in circles. Bilateral lesions of

the globus pallidus can result in the animal remaining in a fixed posture for prolonged periods even if the posture is abnormal.

Lesions in the midbrain can cause decerebrate rigidity by disconnecting the forebrain from the caudal brainstem. The UMN nuclei facilitating extensor activity (e.g. pontine reticular formation and vestibular nuclei) are released from cerebral inhibition, while the UMN nuclei facilitating flexor activity are no longer facilitated by cerebral input. The animal will have opisthotonus with hyperextended limbs, trunk and neck (Fig. 9.6).

Lesions in the cerebellum will affect motor coordination, specifically the rate, range and force of movement. However, executive and senior management of the motor systems are still functioning. The UMN centres can still talk to junior management (spinal interneuronal circuitry) and the workers (LMNs) so movement is strong and purposeful, but it lacks coordination and is ataxic. Failure of coordination of agonist–antagonist muscle function may result in tremor. Spasticity may occur due to loss of the cerebellum's inhibitory influence on UMN nuclei of the brainstem. This results in excessive output from UMN nuclei and extensor dominance. Lesions in the vestibulocerebellum or caudal cerebellar peduncle can result in vestibular signs (see Chapter 8).

Paresis is reduced voluntary movement, whilst paralysis is loss of voluntary movement. Paresis/paralysis occurs due to loss of motor systems associated with initiation and facilitation of movement (UMNs) or due to the loss of LMNs and neuromuscular unit that carries out the movement.

Lesions in the brainstem affecting UMN nuclei will result in paresis in the limbs and trunk and perturbed

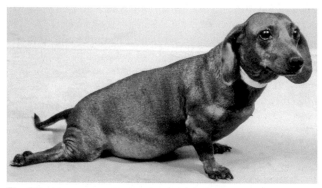

Fig. 9.7 **This paralysed dog had severe spinal cord damage, such that an extensive area of the TL cord had been destroyed by a process called ascending/descending myelomalacia. The destruction of LMNs in the TL region has caused LMN signs to the abdominal wall muscles. This is evidenced by loss of tone in the abdominal wall and the resulting pot belly. The lesion also progressively destroyed the LMN supplying the pelvic limbs.**

locomotion. Bilateral lesions of caudal brain stem can cause tetraparesis/plegia.

Paresis/paralysis due to spinal cord lesions is usually described based on the character of the clinical signs; these signs differentiate into upper or lower motor neuron lesions. Damage to UMNs causes UMN signs, and loss of LMNs causes LMN signs (compare Figs. 9.7 and 4.2). The two types of lesions are differentiated by the Neuro RAT (**R**eflexes, **A**trophy, **T**one) (see Fig. 5.6 and Table 5.2). With UMN lesions (involving 'central motor neurons'), although the myotatic reflex and other limb reflexes will be intact and extensor muscle activity may dominate, this is not sufficient to support the animal, thus the animal will be paretic or recumbent. Input from supraspinal motor systems is required to achieve sufficient and coordinated activity to maintain balance and posture and to initiate and terminate movement. With LMN lesions (affecting 'peripheral motor neurons'), loss of innervation to the muscles results in reduced muscle tone, loss of reflexes and rapid (neurogenic) atrophy. The animal will be obviously weak in the affected areas (Fig. 9.7).

Tetraparesis/plegia can occur with lesions sited anywhere from caudal brainstem to T2, whereas paraparesis/plegia can occur with lesions sited between T2 and the sacral segments. Unilateral lesions of the spinal cord can result in ipsilateral paresis or paralysis (hemiparesis/plegia).

Table 13.5 lists the specific signs for lesions in the different regions of the spinal cord.

The Schiff-Sherrington syndrome may be seen in animals with severe, acute spinal cord lesions in the thoracolumbar spinal cord. This syndrome is characterised by spasticity of the thoracic limbs when recumbent, although these limbs may function normally when the animal is assisted to stand. The extension is due to loss of inhibitory influences from neurons in the cranial lumbar area that inhibit LMNs supplying thoracic limb extensors. Within the first few hours of sustaining the lesion, the animal may also have reduced tone and reflexes in the pelvic limbs, despite the lesion being cranial to the lumbar intumescence. This is a form of spinal shock, which occurs to a much greater extent in primates and humans than in domestic animals. Schiff-Sherrington syndrome indicates severe damage, but not necessarily permanent loss of function of the spinal cord and usually resolves within 1–2 weeks.

Orchestration of posture and movement

The simplest motor task is the contraction of a muscle. The simplest stimulus driving this contraction is stretching of the muscle as detected by muscle spindles. This myotatic reflex is the simplest reflex and involves stimulation and contraction in the same muscle. In the absence of input from the motor system hierarchy, limb extensor muscle activity tends to be dominant.

Increasing complexity of motor function requires integration in the nervous system, using interneurons (junior management) to recruit other LMN. Recruitment will lead to other reflex effects such as (a) relaxation of the muscles acting around the same joint that antagonise the first muscle, (b) stimulation of muscles with similar or complimentary activity to the first muscle in the same limb, (c) reflex muscle contraction or relaxation in the opposite limb and (d) reflex activity in muscles of the limbs in the other girdle (see Fig. 4.8).

Repetitive activities, such as locomotion, scratching or chewing, use central pattern generators to stimulate local reflex circuits for alternating contraction and relaxation of extensor and flexor muscles.

Movement stimulates muscle spindles and changing proprioceptive input from muscles; this input makes an important contribution to locomotion. The proprioceptive input reflexively induces muscle contraction, but is also sent cranially to the brain to inform coordinating, sensory and ultimately motor centres about the position and movement of body parts.

Superimposed on spinospinal circuitry are caudally directed outputs from the brain's UMN centres (senior management). These supraspinal inputs initiate, modify, regulate, coordinate and terminate the activity generated in the spinal cord. Certain UMN tracts facilitate flexor activity, others facilitate extensor activity. The extrapyramidal system is especially important for posture and locomotion, working with intraspinal circuitry and muscle reflexes. The pyramidal system is especially important for voluntary, learned motor activities. The vestibulospinal output is essential for balance. It does this by facilitating extensor muscle activity of the neck, trunk and limbs resulting in support for head position.

The cerebellum acts to keep the animal's centre of gravity located over its supports (limbs) both at rest and during locomotion. The cerebellum coordinates agonist–antagonist muscle function in the limbs, trunk and neck muscle using continuous proprioceptive input from these muscles (subconscious proprioception). With that input it modulates output from the UMN centres for posture, locomotion and voluntary movement. It also receives input from the executive and UMN motor centres about planned motor activity and compares that input with proprioceptive input from the neck, trunk, limbs and head. By comparing planned movement with where the body parts are located and how they are moving, it can modulate the activity of the senior management UMN centres. It exerts both precontrol over movement which is about to occur (e.g. establishing the postural platform) and regulates movements as they occur.

At the top of this hierarchical spectrum are the executive centres, primarily located in the forebrain. Executive motor management plans motor activity ranging from purposeful gait to voluntary learned movements. The executive uses inputs from sensory areas (e.g. touch, kinaesthesia, thermoreception, nociception, vision, audition, olfaction), and motivation, memory and behaviour areas of the forebrain, including the limbic system (Chapter 12). It also relies on information from integration centres of the cerebellum, forebrain (basal nuclei) and reticular formation. The executive motor planning centres then direct UMN centres of the motor cortex and brainstem, which then utilise LMNs to perform consciously directed, voluntary movement.

Thus, while a significant portion of posture and locomotion is based on local spinal reflexes, coordinated, balanced movement, that starts and stops at the right moment and has the correct rate range and force of movement, requires supraspinal inputs.

Chapter 10
Cranial nerves

- Cranial nerves and their CNS components are bilaterally paired.
- Most cranial nerves, excluding the optic and olfactory nerves, have a peripheral portion that is ensheathed/myelinated by Schwann cells.

The vast majority of vertebrates have 12 pairs of cranial nerves (CNN), but there may be more or less in amphibians and fish. Cranial nerves are numbered, using Roman numerals, for their point of attachment to the brain. The first cranial nerve (CN I) attaches to the most rostral aspect of the forebrain at the olfactory bulb, whilst CN XII is attached to the caudal medulla oblongata (Fig. 10.1). The others attach, in sequence, between these two end points.

Named cranial nerve nuclei III–XII are found in the brainstem; they are bilaterally paired (Fig. 10.1). Their location relative to the sulcus limitans determines their function. Sensory cranial nerve nuclei are located dorsal to the sulcus limitans, parasympathetic (autonomic) nuclei are located lateral to it, and somatic motor nuclei are ventral to it (Figs. 1.7, 2.3A) (Note: an exception to this is the location of the vestibular nuclei, which are sited dorsal and lateral to the sulcus limitans, despite having both sensory and motor functions). Remembering this anatomical arrangement is useful, as when the veterinarian is looking at a cross-section of the brainstem (e.g. MR image or tissue section), they can make an educated assumption about function of grey matter based on its dorsoventral position.

Key points

- Twelve pairs of cranial nerves innervate the head and extend into the neck and body cavities.
- Individual nerves have specific sensory and/or motor (somatic and autonomic) functions.
- Knowledge of the location and action of individual cranial nerves is critical for the interpretation of the neurological examination (Tables 10.1, 10.2).
- Cranial nerves are numbered sequentially from rostral to caudal based on the site of their attachment to the brain. CNN I and II attach to the forebrain; CNN III and IV are associated with the midbrain (rostral brainstem); CN V to XII are associated with the mid and caudal brainstem.
- Neurons of CNN III–XII are arranged in nuclei in the brainstem.

Functional classification of cranial nerve nuclei

A nucleus is a collection of neuronal cell bodies, with similar function, that are clustered together and located in the CNS. Cranial nerve nuclei can have two different names depending on whether their function is somatic or autonomic (there are only parasympathetic nuclei in the brain). For example, the oculomotor nucleus of CN III supplies some of the extraocular muscles, while the parasympathetic nucleus of CN III innervates smooth muscle of the eye. Some nuclei contain neurons of multiple cranial nerves yet all those neurons have a similar function. For example, the nucleus ambiguus, comprising neurons associated with CN IX, X and XI, innervates the striated muscle of the larynx and pharynx.

Table 10.1 **Cranial nerves and their function**

Nerve	Function	Brain attachment	Exit from neurocranium (dog as type animal)
I – olfactory nerve	A = olfaction	Forebrain	Cribiform plate
II – optic nerve	A = vision	Forebrain (diencephalon)	Optic foramen
III – oculomotor nerve	E = pupillary light reflex (parasympathetic) E = extraocular muscles – ventral, medial, dorsal rectus; ventral oblique mm.	Brainstem (midbrain)	Orbital fissure
IV – trochlear nerve	E = extraocular muscles – dorsal oblique m.	Brainstem (dorsal midbrain)	Orbital fissure
V – trigeminal nerve	A = facial sensation Ophthalmic branch – cornea and superior (upper) eyelid Maxillary branch – muzzle and inferior (lower) eyelid Mandibular branch – mandibular skin E = masticatory muscle function (mandibular branch), tensor tympani muscle of the middle ear	Brainstem (pons–medulla oblongata junction)	Ophthalmic branch – orbital fissure Maxillary branch – round foramen Mandibular branch – oval foramen
VI – abducent nerve	E = extraocular muscles – lateral rectus and retractor bulbi mm	Brainstem (medulla oblongata)	Orbital fissure
VII – facial nerve	A = taste on rostral 2/3 of tongue, concave surface of the pinna E = muscles of facial expression, stapedius muscle, parasympathetic to palatine and lacrimal glands, mandibular and sublingual salivary glands	Brainstem (pons–medulla oblongata junction)	Internal acoustic meatus and exits the skull via the stylomastoid foramen
VIII – vestibulocochlear nerve	A = hearing and balance	Brainstem (pons–medulla oblongata junction)	Internal acoustic meatus, (remains within temporal bone and does not exit the skull)
IX – glossopharyngeal nerve	A = pharyngeal and middle ear sensation, taste on caudal third of tongue E = pharyngeal and laryngeal muscles; parasympathetic to the zygomatic and parotid salivary glands	Brainstem (medulla oblongata)	Tympano-occipital fissure
X – vagus nerve	A = pharynx, larynx, external ear canal; taste on root of tongue and epiglottis; general sensory from the viscera E = pharyngeal, laryngeal and oesophageal muscles; parasympathetic to viscera	Brainstem (medulla oblongata)	Tympano-occipital fissure
XI – accessory nerve	E = larynx, parts of the trapezius, brachiocephalicus and sternocephalicus muscles	Brainstem (medulla oblongata)	Tympano-occipital fissure
XII – hypoglossal nerve	E = tongue muscles (extrinsic and intrinsic)	Brainstem (medulla oblongata)	Hypoglossal canal

A = afferent, E = efferent.

Table 10.2 **Cranial nerve testing and sign of dysfunction**

Head function	Innervation	Clinical testing	Dysfunction
Olfaction	Ia	Observation, odourant such as food	Dysosmia
Vision	IIa	Maze test, visual tracking Menace response – IIa and VIIe Pupillary light reflex – IIa and IIIe (parasympathetic)	Blindness, mydriasis (although this can be due to CN III dysfunction)
Pupil size	IIa, IIIe Parasympathetic, e Sympathetic, e	Pupillary light reflex Pharmacological testing	Anisocoria, Mydriasis (↓ CN II or parasympathetic innervation) Miosis (↓ sympathetic innervation). (Note cerebellar lesions and primary ophthalmic lesions can also affect pupil size)
Eyeball position	VIIIa IIIe, IVe, VIe	Visual tracking of moving objects Eyeball position in different head positions Vestibulo-ocular reflex VIIIa and IIIe, IVe, VIe	Strabismus – static (LMN), – dynamic (vestibular)
Facial sensation	Va – all three branches	Tactile stimulation Va – different regions of the face – muzzle, inferior eyelid, superior eyelid, mandible Palpebral reflex – Va and VIIe (superior and inferior eyelids) Auriculo-palpebral reflex Va and VIIe (stimulate skin just in front of the external ear canal)	Facial hypalgesia
Mastication	Ve – mandibular	Jaw tone Assess the bulk of the masticatory muscles, e.g. temporalis and masseter muscles	Muscle atrophy Dropped jaw, if bilateral dysfunction
Facial expression and movement	VIIe	Facial symmetry Palpebral reflex Va and VIIe Auriculo-palpebral reflexes Va and VIIe Movement of muzzle, external nares, eyelids, ears Symmetry of position of lip commissures when head is held up vertically	Facial paresis/paralysis
Vestibular function	VIIIa	Head position Eyeball position (also involves III, IV, VI) Vestibulo-ocular reflex (VIIIa and IIIe, IVe, VIe) Gait and movement	Head tilt, circling, rolling Spontaneous nystagmus Strabismus Deranged body posture and ataxia
Pharyngeal function	IX and X, a and e	Gag reflex (IXa, Xa and IXe, Xe) Swallowing	Dysphagia Drooling of saliva (ptyalism)
Laryngeal function	X and XI, a and e	Phonation Respiration	Dysphonia Respiratory stridor – laryngeal obstruction, aspiration
Tongue	XIIe	Observation – LMN signs, usage Withdrawal from tactile stimulus via CN V	Atrophy, paresis/paralysis – unilateral or bilateral Hypalgesia

a = afferent, e = efferent.

Cranial nerves may have one type of function only, or have several functions. It should be noted that even the 'motor only' nerves (e.g. CN III) may contain proprioceptive afferent fibres. Motor fibres of cranial nerves form the lower motor neurons (LMNs) of the head region (Table 10.3). Note that CN VIII has traditionally been described as purely sensory, however efferent fibres have been described in both the vestibular and cochlear portions of CN VIII

(See also Chapter 8: end of section on 'Effect of stimulating the vestibular nuclei' and Chapter 10, olivocochlear reflex.)

Rather than considering the 12 cranial nerves in isolation, it is useful to group them by function.

Olfaction

Key points

- Odoriferous substances stimulate olfactory neurons. Action potentials pass caudally into the cranial cavity, synapsing in the olfactory bulb. Olfactory tract axons project to both sides of the forebrain for olfactory perception, stimulation of behavioural responses and to the brainstem for reflex function.
- Input from the vomeronasal organ is via the olfactory nerve and may stimulate the Flehmen reaction during sexual activity in some species.

The name olfactory 'nerve' is correct as it is derived from the olfactory placode and not CNS tissue (see page 1), however in humans the olfactory bulb is so diminutive as to resemble a nerve. In veterinary species, the olfactory bulb is prominent (Figs. 10.3, A2, A3, A10).

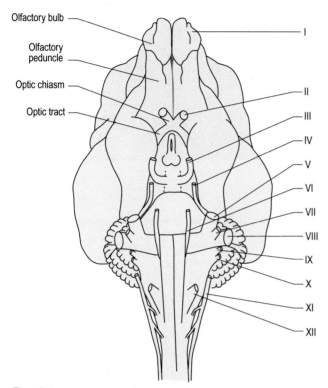

Fig. 10.1 **Ventral aspect of canine brain and cranial cervical spinal cord depicting the attachment of the cranial nerves.**

Table 10.3 **General functions of cranial nerves**	
Sensory only	I, II,
Motor only[†]	III, IV, VI, XI, XII
Mixed sensory and motor	V, VII, VIII*, IX, X,
Autonomic (parasympathetic)	III, VII, IX, X

*efferent components have been described in CN VIII
[†]these nerves may contain proprioceptive sensory fibres

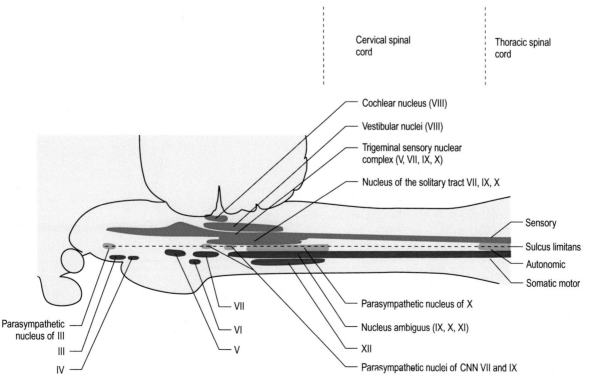

Fig. 10.2 **The functional columns of grey matter in the spinal cord and their fragmentation to form nuclei of the cranial nerves in the brain stem.**

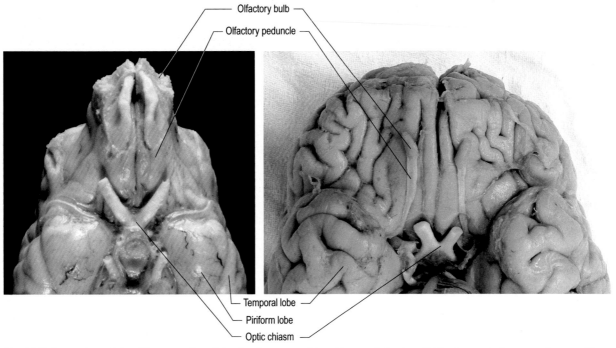

Olfactory bulb
Olfactory peduncle
Temporal lobe
Piriform lobe
Optic chiasm

Fig. 10.3 **Comparison of the olfactory region of the dog (macrosmatic) and human (microsmotic) brains, ventral aspects. (Image of human brain courtesy of Dr. Henry Waldvogel, University of Auckland.)**

The olfactory mucosa is located on the ethmoidal labyrinth and dorsal nasal septum in the dog. Grossly, the olfactory mucosa may be slightly yellowish compared with surrounding mucosa, due to pigment in the sustentacular (supporting) cells. Afferent fibres from the olfactory mucosa and vomeronasal organ contribute to CN I, which is unmyelinated. Olfactory neurons are bipolar cells with 6–8 long cilia that project into the overlying mucus in the caudodorsal part of the nasal cavity. Olfactory receptors are also located in the vomeronasal organ on the rostral floor of the nasal cavity. These receptors may respond to pheromones, which are chemicals that trigger social responses between members of the same species. The vomeronasal organ may mediate the curling of the upper lip, the Flehmen reaction, in males scenting females with respect to mating suitability. Odoriferous substances dissolve in the mucus overlying the olfactory mucosa, or in the vomeronasal organ, stimulating the olfactory neurons. As odoriferous substances can be cytotoxic, olfactory neurons can be renewed from stem cells located at the base of the olfactory mucosa. The potential for harvesting olfactory stem cells and using them as a source of new neurons for a patient is currently an area of active research in neuroscience.

Axons from the olfactory mucosa and the vomeronasal organ pass through the cribiform plate into the cranial cavity and synapse on the olfactory bulb neurons. Post-synaptic axons travel caudally in the olfactory tract of the olfactory peduncle. The tract splits into lateral, intermediate and medial stria (see Fig. A11). The axons of the lateral stria synapse in the olfactory tubercle and pass to the cortex of the piriform lobe for olfactory perception. Fibres also connect to the limbic system (see Chapter 11). More medial fibres pass to the septal nuclei (Fig. A13), which are located between the rostral aspects of the lateral ventricles, and to the hypothalamus and reticular formation of the brainstem. Fibres also decussate via the rostral commissure and pass to the contralateral olfactory bulb.

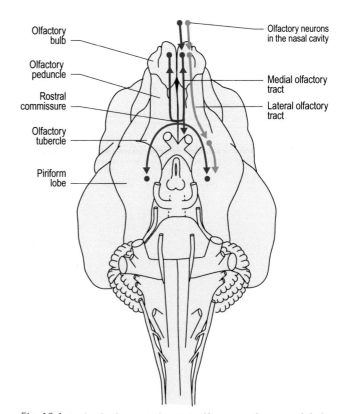

Olfactory bulb
Olfactory peduncle
Rostral commissure
Olfactory tubercle
Piriform lobe
Olfactory neurons in the nasal cavity
Medial olfactory tract
Lateral olfactory tract

Fig. 10.4 **Canine brain, ventral aspect, olfactory pathways and their connections.**

The rostral commissure also interconnects the two piriform lobes (Fig. 10.4). Through the connections to the limbic system, cerebral cortex and hypothalamus, olfaction can be a potent stimulator of behaviour and emotional states. Connections to the brainstem permit olfacto-visceral reflexes such as salivation in response to olfactory stimulation.

Note that olfaction does not pass through the thalamus; this is different to all other afferent information which does pass through the thalamus en route to the cerebral cortex.

Lesions in one olfactory bulb lead to unilateral anosmia; this is hard to detect clinically. Bilateral lesions are required in the olfactory mucosa, or bulbs, peduncles or piriform lobes to cause complete anosmia.

Vision and CN II functions

Key points

- The optic nerve is myelinated by oligodendrocytes. It is the only part of the CNS that can be observed on clinical examination.
- Photoreceptors in the deepest layers of the retina convert light into action potentials. The action potentials are modified by neurons in the more superficial layers of the retina, and exit the retina as axons in the optic nerve.
- The majority of optic nerve axons decussate, but the degree of decussation depends on the type of animal and correlates inversely with the degree of binocular vision.
- Caudal to the optic chiasm the majority of optic nerve axons travel to the lateral geniculate nucleus of the thalamus and then to the visual cortex for visual perception. The remaining axons course to the midbrain for reflex function.

General anatomy

The optic nerve is actually a tract of the CNS as it is myelinated by oligodendroglia, thus the term 'nerve' is a misnomer (p1). It is the only part of the CNS that can be observed on a neurological examination.

Photoreceptors (rods and cones) are the receptors of the visual system and convert light into receptor potentials. Rods are highly sensitive to light, therefore they are used during dim light conditions, while cones are less sensitive to light but respond to specific light frequencies, that is, colours. The presence of 20 times more rods than cones in the canine retina accounts for dogs' good night vision. The vertebrate retina is inverted in the sense that the light-sensing cells sit at the back of the retina, so that light has to pass through layers of neurons before it reaches the photoreceptors. This arrangement ensures that incoming light only stimulates photoreceptors once. If the photoreceptors were at the front of the retina, then some of the incident light would stimulate them, while the remaining light could pass to the back of the retina. There it would be reflected back into the eye at a new angle stimulating different photoreceptors. Thus light from a single visual point would stimulate photoreceptors in different regions (incident versus reflected) causing loss of resolution and visual blurring.

There is a three-stage neuronal system in the retina. The photoreceptors form the deepest layer, the middle layer contains integrating neurons, while the superficial layer contains the multipolar ganglion neurons, the axons of which pass across the retina to collect at the optic disc and form the optic nerve. Thus light passes through the cornea, anterior chamber pupil posterior chamber, ganglion and bipolar layers to reach the photoreceptors. Receptor potentials from the rods and cones undergo

complex processing by integrating neurons of the retina but ultimately result in action potentials in retinal ganglion cells. Several important features of visual perception can be traced to the retinal encoding and processing of light.

In most domestic mammals, axons of retinal neurons are unmyelinated until they coalesce at the optic disc. Thus the opaque nature of myelin does not interrupt the passage of light through the retinal layers to the photoreceptors. However, there are no photoreceptors at the optic disc, resulting in a blind spot in the visual field. Myelination of the optic nerve fibres makes the optic disc appear creamy white on fundic examination. In some species, such as rabbits, there is some myelination of retinal ganglion axons. This may be observed clinically as a white streak extending from the optic disc.

The optic chiasm and decussation

The optic nerve extends caudally from the retina, through the optic canal in the presphenoid bone into the neurocranium. It joins the ventral aspect of the diencephalon at the optic chiasm, just rostral to the hypophysis (pituitary gland). In general, the majority of axons decussate, but the degree of decussation depends on the type of animal. In fishes and birds, all fibres decussate (Fig. 10.10). In mammals, there is partial decussation (ungulates about 80–90%, dogs 75%, cats 65%, primates 50%).

Light also crosses in the lens of the eye, thus axons decussating at the optic chiasm come from the nasal portion of the retina and temporal field of view, while the temporal retinal axons receiving the nasal field of view, remain ipsilateral (see Fig. 10.5).

The visual pathway continues caudal to the optic chiasm as the optic tracts (see Figs. A14, A15). In animals in which there is partial decussation at the optic chiasm, each optic tract contains axons from the contralateral nasal retina and the ipsilateral temporal retina. Thus the optic tract contains axons from retinal areas of the two eyes that are receiving input from the same part of the visual field (Fig. 10.5A).

The placement of the eyes and decussation of the optic chiasm is functionally significant. Animals with laterally placed eyes, e.g. ungulates/prey animals (Fig. 10.5B) have wide fields of view and a high percentage of fibres decussate at the optic chiasm. Thus the majority of visual input is processed in the contralateral visual cortex. A wide field of view permits these animals to see behind them; this is useful to detect danger such as stalking predators. But depth of field/binocular vision requires processing of visual input from both eyes in the same visual cortex, thus prey species have poor binocular vision. Conversely, animals with eyes that face forward, like the cat, have smaller fields of view, but have better binocular vision due to decreased decussation at the optic chiasm. This results in the animal receiving input from each eye on both sides of the brain. For example in Fig. 10.5A, input from the orange diamond located in the left side of the visual field will project to the nasal retina of the left eye and the temporal retina of the right eye. The input from those retinal areas will both end up in the same visual cortex – that is the right side one. Thus the same region of the brain processes two sets of information seen by the separate eyes, about the same object. This dual perspective results in binocular vision which is essential for depth perception. Depth perception is required for accurate judgement of distance and how fast an object is moving, therefore it is essential for predatory

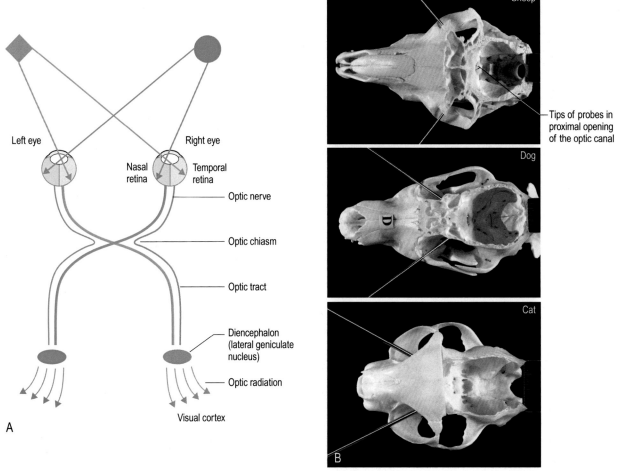

Fig. 10.5 **(A) The optic pathway and transmission of light stimuli to the visual cortex. (B) Examples of optic axes of the sheep, dog and cat, identified using metal probes placed in the optic canals. The angles between the axes for the sheep, dog and cat are 100°, 70° and 58°, respectively; the decreasing angles indicate increasing overlap of the visual fields.**

animals. The ability to perform coordinated, conjugate eye movements, including convergence (focussing both eyes on the same object) is also greater in animals with forward-facing eyes and reduced decussation.

The total field of view combined from both eyes in the horse is approximately 320°. That comprises a field of view for each eye being about 200°s, with about 65° of overlap. The overlapping visual field is especially well developed ventrally for viewing objects on the ground. However, there is not overlap immediately in front of the nose, creating a blind spot. Most dogs have a total visual field of 250°. The degree of binocular overlap is about 75° for long-nosed dogs to 85° for short-nosed breeds. Comparatively, humans have a maximum total horizontal field of view of approximately 180°, 120° of which comprises the binocular field of view, flanked by two uniocular fields of approximately 40°.

Post-chiasmatic visual pathways

From the optic chiasm, axons course caudodorsolaterally in the optic tracts (see Figs. A14, A15). The majority of axons connect to lateral geniculate nucleus (see Fig. A17) of the caudal diencephalon (metathalamus) and then via the optic radiation to the visual cortex for visual perception. Alternatively, axons travel to the midbrain for reflex function (see Visual reflexes, this chapter). Using the cat as an example, approximately 80% of fibres from each eye go to the lateral geniculate nuclei and 20% to the midbrain.

The visual cortex is divided into specific functional regions. In primates, different areas process input

regarding stationary objects, spatial relationships and depth perception, or panoramic vision for movement. The visual cortex also makes connections to adjacent association cortex, motor cortex, midbrain and cerebellum. Connections to the midbrain are essential for normal vision.

Lesions in the visual system rostral to the chiasm (pre-chiasmatic lesions) can result in blindness in one eye, since the optic nerve consists of fibres from only one eye. Post-chiasmatic lesions however, can result in changes in vision from both eyes as the optic tract contains fibres from both eyes.

Eyeball position and movement

Key points

- Seven extraocular muscles control eyeball position and movement; they are specifically innervated by cranial nerves III, IV and VI.
- Head position and movement, sensed by the vestibular apparatus (CN VIII), stimulates cranial nerves III, IV and VI causing reflex positioning of the eyes – the vestibulo-ocular reflex (see Fig. 13.7).

The eyes move in synchrony with each other, but different muscles for each eye are often activated to achieve

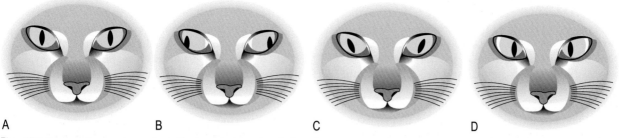

Fig. 10.6 **Extraocular muscles and strabismus. (A) Normal eyeball position, (B) ventrolateral strabismus (CN III dysfunction), (C) extorsional strabismus (CN IV dysfunction), (D) medial strabismus (CN VI dysfunction).**

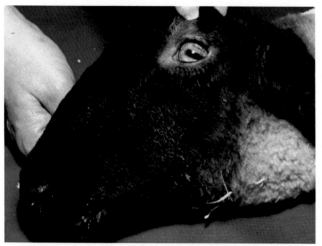

Fig. 10.7 **Polioencephalomalacia showing strabismus secondary to paresis of the trochlear nerves; normally sheep have pupils that are horizontal, lined up with the medial and lateral canthi photo (photo courtesy of Dr Phil Scott, University of Edinburgh).**

conjugal eye movement. For example, moving the eyes to the left requires activation of the left lateral rectus muscle (left CN VI) and the right medial rectus muscle (right CN III). Dysfunction of CNN III, IV and VI results in strabismus (Figs. 10.6, 10.7).

Oculomotor nucleus (CN III)

The location of the oculomotor nucleus is in the ventral aspect of the periaqueductal grey matter in the midbrain. The efferent fibres pass to the ventral surface of the midbrain and form CN III (see Figs. A3, A18, A31). The oculomotor nerve supplies the levator palpabrae superioris muscle for elevation of the upper eyelid and extraocular muscles such as the dorsal, medial and ventral recti, and ventral oblique muscles.

Lesions cause ptosis (drooping of the superior eyelid) and ventrolateral strabismus. The parasympathetic nucleus of CN III and oculomotor nucleus are located adjacent to each other and therefore lesions of that area usually involve both components. Damage to the parasympathetic portion will result in mydriasis and loss of the pupillary light reflex (see Visual reflexes, and Chapter 12).

Trochlear nucleus (CN IV)

The location of the trochlear nucleus is in the midbrain just caudal to the oculomotor nucleus, at the level of the caudal colliculi. The efferent fibres pass lateral and dorsal to the mesencephalic aqueduct to exit on the dorsal aspect of the brain stem. All fibres decussate just ventral to the cerebellum in a thin membrane forming (the rostral

medullary velum) that forms the roof of the fourth ventricle and supply the contralateral dorsal oblique extraocular muscle (see Figs. A5, A7, A19). Lesions cause strabismus with outward rotation of the dorsal aspect of the eye (extorsion).

Abducent nucleus (CN VI)

The location of the abducent nucleus is in the rostral medulla oblongata just dorsal to the trapezoid body. Its efferent fibres supply the lateral rectus and retractor bulbi muscles (see Fig. A3). Therefore lesions cause medial strabismus and failure to retract the globe during eyelid closure as would normally be observed during menace response testing (see Chapter 13).

Visual reflexes

> ### Key points
>
> - Visual reflexes are integrated in the midbrain.
> - The pupillary light reflex is driven by light and results in reflex constriction of the pupils bilaterally. The reflex uses input via CN II (optic) and output via parasympathetic fibres of CN III.
> - The direct (ipsilateral) reflex is stronger than the indirect (contralateral) reflex.
> - Head turning in response to visual stimuli is initiated by the rostral colliculi in the midbrain tectum.

Visual reflexes include head turning in response to visual and auditory stimuli (see Auditory reflexes), and the pupillary light reflex. The stimuli are received and integrated in the midbrain, from which arise connections to other cranial nerve nuclei and the spinal cord.

The pupillary light reflex (PLR)

The majority of afferent fibres travelling in the optic nerves (CN II) decussate at the optic chiasm and most fibres continue to the visual cortex via the lateral geniculate nuclei. A minority of fibres (20% in the cat) peel off the optic tract and synapse in the pretectal nucleus, which is located just rostral to the midbrain tectum between the rostral colliculus and the thalamus. The majority of efferent fibres from the pretectal nucleus decussate again in the caudal commissure, thereby projecting ultimately to the parasympathetic nucleus of III that is ipsilateral to the eye that was stimulated. However, because decussation is incomplete at both the optic chiasm and caudal commissure, a unilateral input will stimulate the parasympathetic nuclei of III bilaterally. Efferent parasympathetic fibres of III travel with the somatic fibres of the oculomotor nerve (CN III) to the orbit. The parasympathetic fibres synapse in the ciliary ganglion just caudal to the eye and postsynaptic fibres innervate the constrictor muscles of the iris. Because of various decussations, light stimuli cause reflex constriction of the ipsilateral pupil (direct reflex) and the contralateral pupil (indirect reflex). Since in domestic mammals the majority of fibres in the pupillary light reflex pathway cross in the optic nerve chiasm and the majority cross back again in the caudal commissure, the direct reflex is stronger than the indirect PLR (Figs. 10.8 and 10.9). In humans 50% of fibres cross each time, so there is no difference in the strength of pupillary constriction between the direct and indirect PLR. Conversely, in animals such as birds, in which there is complete decussation at the optic chiasm, the indirect reflex does not occur.

Note that the pupillary light reflex is a true reflex, not a response. It is incorrect to call it the pupillary light response. By comparison, the menace response is a learned function and it is incorrect to call that the menace reflex.

The midbrain comprises the dorsal tectum associated with primarily sensory function and the cerebral peduncle associated with motor function (see Fig. 1.6B). The paired rostral and caudal colliculi form the tectum (Figs. 10.11, A5, A7, A18-20, A31). The rostral colliculi are associated with visual reflexes; as such they are virtually non-existent in blind species such as the blind mole rat. (For caudal collicular function in auditory reflexes – see next section.) The rostral colliculi also receive input from the visual cortex and are important in vision. Output from the colliculi (tectum) form the tectonuclear tracts that pass into the brainstem providing UMN input to LMNs of CNN nuclei (CNN III, IV, VI). Tectal output also forms the tectospinal tract influencing LMNs supplying the cervical muscles. Thus visual and auditory stimuli can cause reflex turning of the eyes or head, to allow the animal to focus on the stimulus (Fig. 10.9). The tectonuclear tract also connects to CN VII resulting in the protective dazzle reflex, in which bright light shone into the eye causes partial closure of the eyelids.

In higher vertebrates, the colliculi are overshadowed by the occipital lobes, but in some fish, rodents and birds the optic tectum may be more important and is referred to as the optic lobe (Fig. 10.10). In these animals the primary input to the tectum is visual, however, it may also receive auditory, somatosensory and even electroreceptive stimuli. All inputs contribute to spatial mapping of the environment. With increasing development of the cerebral cortex and its connections, the physiological significance of the colliculi decreases.

Each colliculus has many neural links through which visual and auditory functions are integrated. They are connected across the midline by a commissure. The rostral and caudal colliculi are connected rostrally to the lateral and

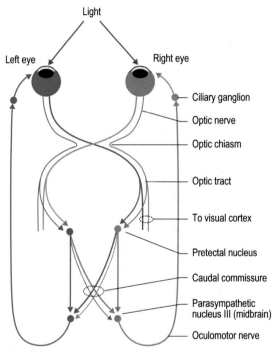

Fig. 10.8 **Pupillary light reflex pathway.**

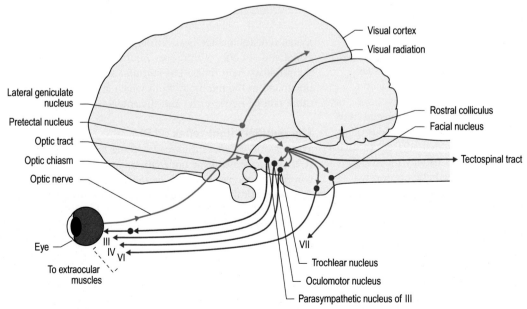

Fig. 10.9 **Pathways involved in visual reflexes. Green = vision and visual processing, violet = interneuronal connections, purple = parasympathetic connections for pupillary light reflex, red = UMN and LMNs for eye, eyelid and head movement.**

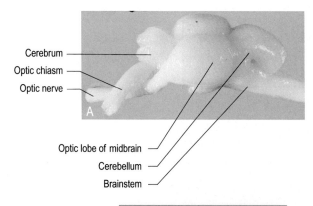

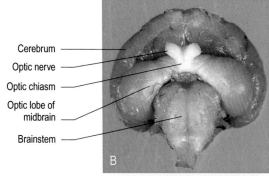

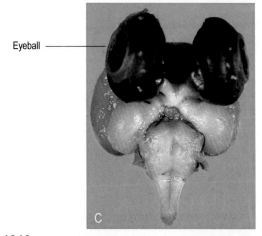

Fig. 10.10 **Comparative brain anatomy. (A) Trout fish brain, dorsolateral aspect and (B, C) zebra finch brain, ventral aspect. Both species have well-developed optic lobes in the midbrain. Note that the optic nerves of the trout brain are completely separate and have 100% cross over at the optic chiasm. (C) The size of the eyes explains the prominent optic nerves and lobe in this species. Note: brains are not to scale with each other.**

medial geniculate nuclei, respectively, and to the pretectum and the thalamus. Caudally, there are bilateral projections via the tectoreticular, tectonuclear and tectospinal tracts.

The rostral colliculi, pretectum and the lateral geniculate nuclei are associated with visual reflexes such as head and eye turning in response to visual stimuli, coordinating eye movements and the pupillary light reflex. The function of the caudal colliculi is covered in the section on auditory reflexes.

Masticatory muscle function

The location of the motor nucleus of CN V is in the mid brainstem at the junction between the pons and

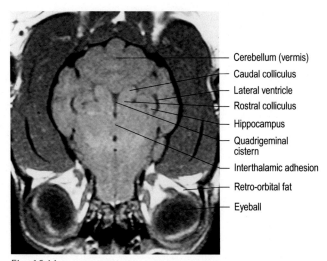

Fig. 10.11 **Dog brain, horizontal plane, T1-weighted magnetic resonance image at the level of the interthalamic adhesion.**

Key point

■ The majority of the masticatory muscles are innervated by the motor nucleus of CN V and the mandibular branch of the trigeminal nerve. The caudal half of the digastricus muscle is innervated by cranial nerve VII.

the medulla oblongata (see Figs. A3, A30). Its efferent fibres travel only in the mandibular branch of the trigeminal nerve CN V and supply the mylohyoideus muscle and the masticatory muscles such as the temporalis, masseter and pterygoid muscles that raise the mandible. It also supplies the tensor tympani muscle, used to protect the ear from loud noise, and the tensor veli palatini muscle which tenses the soft palate. The mandibular branch of CN V supplies the rostral belly of the digastricus muscle which opens the jaws, while the caudal belly is supplied by CN VII. The dual innervation of the digastricus muscle (CNN V and VII) reflects its embryonic origin from the first two pharyngeal arches. The facial nerve (CN VII) also supplies the buccinator muscle of the cheek, which functions to return food from the oral vestibule to the masticatory surface of the teeth.

The most common sign of damage to masticatory muscle innervation is atrophy (Fig. 10.12). This is due to LMN damage, for example, due to a tumour or neuritis. However, primary muscle disease, such as masticatory myositis, can also cause marked muscle atrophy. Lesions of CN V, mandibular branch, need to be bilateral to result in overt loss of jaw muscle tone and a 'dropped jaw'.

Sensory input from the head

Key points

■ All three branches of the trigeminal nerve transmit sensory information from the head to the sensory nucleus of CN V, which extends throughout the brainstem. The trigeminal ganglion is located at the base of the neurocranium.

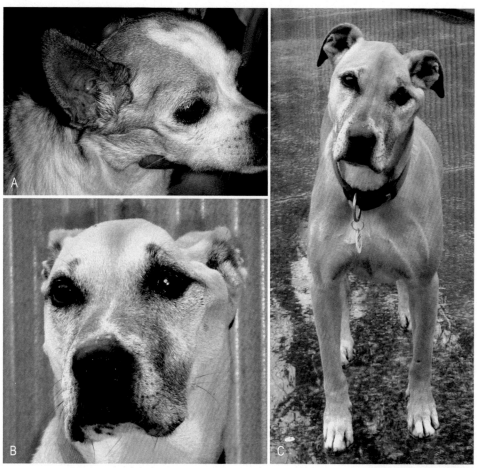

Fig. 10.12 **Loss of LMN (peripheral motor neuron) innervation to the masticatory muscles in these two dogs, resulted in severe atrophy of the temporalis and masseter muscles and prominence of the zygomatic arch. Both dogs had ipsilateral facial hypalgesia. (C) Depicts the same dog as in (B), 2 months later illustrating development of a head tilt. The dog also had pathological nystagmus and ipsilateral facial paresis indicating involvement of CNN VII and CNVIII in the lesion. As CNN V, VII and VIII arise as a cluster from the brainstem (see Figs. 10.1, A.2 and A.3), they can be involved in the same, focal lesion. The dog in (A) had a tumour; the same was presumed for the dog in (B) and (C).**

■ Proprioception, tactile and thermal sensation, and nociception are received by the mesencephalic, pontine and myelencephalic regions of the sensory nucleus of CN V, respectively.
■ Tactile stimulation of the skin of the maxilla, the superior eyelid and the mandible tests the maxillary, ophthalmic and mandibular branches of the trigeminal nerve during the neurological examination.

Tactile, proprioceptive, thermal and nociceptive input from the head is received in the sensory nuclear complex of the trigeminal nerve in the brainstem (Figs. 10.2 and 6.6). All three branches of CN V (mandibular, maxillary and ophthalmic) are associated with sensory input from the face (Fig. 10.13). Sensory input from the external ear is via CNN VII, IX, X and spinal nerves, C1 and C2. Lesions of CN V result in hypoalgesia or anaesthesia of the face. Sensory nerve cell bodies are located in the trigeminal ganglion outside the CNS; this arrangement is similar to sensory input via spinal nerves. Unusually, some somata are also sited in the CNS in the mesencephalic nucleus of V. The trigeminal (Gasserian/semilunar) ganglion is located in the trigeminal canal at the apex of the petrosal part of the temporal bone, inside the neurocranium.

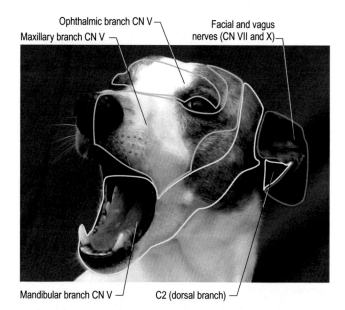

Fig. 10.13 **The autonomous zones of facial sensory innervation. For the branches of the trigeminal nerve (CN V), green outlines the region for the ophthalmic branch, blue for the maxillary branch and yellow for the mandibular branch. The inner and outer aspects of the pinna are innervated by the facial nerve, CN X, and branches of C1 and C2 nerves, respectively.**

Sensory nucleus of CN V

The sensory nucleus of V complex is an elongated grey matter column that extends caudally from the midbrain to the substantia gelatinosa, which caps the dorsal horn of the spinal cord (see Fig. 6.6). The nuclear complex is associated with an adjacent white matter tract forming the spinal tract of V. The complex is divided into mesencephalic, pontine and spinal nuclei and tracts. It receives somatic afferent information (see Figs. A19-31).

Via CN V, the mesencephalic nucleus and tract of V receives proprioceptive input from the muscles of mastication, temporomandibular joint, teeth and, probably, the extraocular, facial and lingual muscles. Efferent axons travel to muscles of mastication and, via the reticular formation, to motor nuclei of the brainstem and cranial spinal cord.

The pontine nucleus and tract of V receives input about touch and pressure (mechanoreception). Collateral axons also project to motor nuclei associated with corneal, palpebral, tongue and salivary reflexes.

The spinal nucleus and tract of V is located, caudal to the attachment of CN V in the medulla oblongata where it is prominent in the dorsolateral area. It receives sensory input related to nociception and temperature from the skin and mucous membranes of the head. The main input comes in via CN V but some input from the ear is delivered via CNN VII, IX and X. The nucleus also contains interneurons connecting the trigeminal nucleus with other nuclei of the brain stem and cervical cord. The spinal nucleus and tract of V continue into the spinal cord as the substantia gelatinosa and dorsolateral fasciculus, which receive input from the rest of the body about noxious and thermal stimuli (see Tables 4.2, 4.3 and Fig. 4.5).

For conscious perception of sensation from the head, axons from the sensory nuclear complex form the trigeminal lemniscus (quintatothalamic tract), decussate, join with the medial lemniscus and travel via the thalamus to the somatosensory cortex (see Fig. 6.1).

Lesions cause hypoalgesia, which is ipsilateral if the lesion is located in the brainstem, but contralateral if the lesion is located in the forebrain (see cases described in Fig. 10.12).

Facial expression

Key points

■ Muscles of facial expression are innervated by the motor nucleus of CN VII sited in the rostral medulla oblongata.
■ The facial nucleus receives inputs for reflex function from other brainstem nuclei, and from the cerebrum for facial expression.

The location of the motor nucleus of CN VII is in the ventrolateral area of the rostral medulla oblongata (see Fig. A29). Afferents to the facial nucleus are used in protective functions involving facial musculature. Examples include, afferents from the spinal nucleus of CN V (trigeminofacial and corneal reflexes – for facial or eyelid movement after a sensory stimulus) and the trapezoid body and cochlear nuclei (acousticofacial reflexes such as closing the eyes

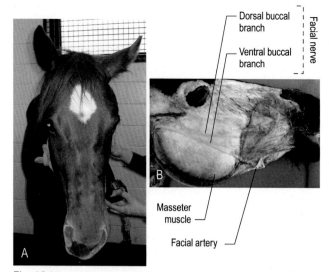

Fig. 10.14 **(A) Left-sided facial paresis secondary to otitis media. (B) Superficial dissection of a horse's face to display the superficial portions of the facial nerve (photo courtesy of Mr. Allan Nutman, Massey University).**

after a loud noise). There is also input from the cerebral cortex (via the corticonuclear tract) for controlling facial expression. From the facial nucleus, the efferent fibres pass dorsorostromedially to loop around the abducent nucleus (CN VI) and then descend to exit the brainstem ventrolaterally. This loop is called the internal genu of the facial nerve. The neurons of the nucleus are topographically arranged so that rostral neurons innervate rostral muscles, caudal neurons supply caudal muscles, but dorsal neurons innervate ventral muscles and vice versa. The facial nerve exits the neurocranium via the internal acoustic meatus and passes through the facial canal in the petrosal portion of the temporal bone. The portion of this canal that lies adjacent to the tympanic cavity of the middle ear lacks a bony wall, and the nerve is separated from the cavity by only a few micrometres of loose connective tissue. Thus lesions in the middle ear may cause dysfunction of CN VII. Once it emerges from the stylomastoid foramen at the base of the external ear canal, it branches and the buccal branches run superficially across the masseter muscle and are often palpable in the intact animal. Its superficial path makes it vulnerable to trauma and pressure such as from harness buckles (see Figs. 10.14 and 13.2). Facial nerve dysfunction results in loss of facial and auricular movement and muscle tone. With unilateral lesions, there is loss of facial symmetry (Fig. 10.14).

Audition

Key points

■ The hearing apparatus consists of the outer, middle and inner ears, the cochlear portion of CN VIII, the auditory pathways in the brainstem and the auditory cortex in the forebrain.
■ Sound waves are converted into mechanical vibrations by the tympanic membrane. In the middle ear, the auditory ossicles transmit and amplify the vibrations.

> The vibrations stimulate pressure waves in the fluid in the inner ear stimulating hair cells in the cochlea. Hair cells transform vibrations into electrical signals that are transmitted by the cochlear nerve to the cochlear nuclei of the brainstem.
> ■ Output from the cochlear nuclei stimulates auditory reflexes and also travels to the forebrain for the conscious perception of sound.

The hearing apparatus consists of the outer, middle and inner ear, the cochlear portion of the vestibulocochlear nerve (CN VIII) and brainstem auditory pathways in the brainstem. These project to the forebrain and terminate in the auditory cortex in the temporal lobe.

The outer ear in domestic mammals is the receiving device for sound. It is mobile, controlled by muscles at the base and can be turned towards the direction of the sound to improve reception. At the base of the external ear canal is the tympanic membrane or eardrum.

The middle ear is the tympanic cavity. It contains the auditory ossicles and is connected to the nasopharynx via the auditory tube (Eustachian tube in humans). This tube permits pressure to be equalised between the enclosed middle ear cavity and nasopharynx, and hence, the external environment. The three auditory ossicles, located in the middle ear, are the smallest bones in the body. From lateral to medial they are the malleus, incus and stapes. They form synovial articulations with each other. The malleus contacts the tympanic membrane. The stapes contacts the vestibular window and thereby interfaces with the fluid-filled inner ear (Fig. 10.15). The stapedius and tensor tympani muscles connect to the stapes and the malleus and function in protective acoustic reflexes (see next section).

The inner ear houses the receptors for hearing in the cochlea, and for balance in the vestibular apparatus (see Chapter 8). The inner ear consists of a series of canals and cavities, forming the bony labyrinth. Membrane-bound ducts line the bony labyrinth forming the membranous labyrinth. Between the bone and membrane is fluid called perilymph, while endolymph fills the membranous labyrinth.

The membranous structures of the inner ear are in communication with the middle ear via membrane-covered vestibular (oval) and cochlear (round) windows.

The cochlea is a hollow, snail-shell-like spiral of bone with a central axis, the modiolus (Fig. 10.16). The cavity of the cochlea spirals around the modiolus and membranes divide it into three longitudinal regions creating the scala vestibuli, the central cochlear duct and scala tympani. Perilymph is found in the scala vestibuli and tympani, and endolymph in the cochlear duct. The latter is separated from the scala vestibuli by the spiral basilar membrane on which hair cells are sited forming the spiral organ. Overlying the hair cells is the tectorial membrane.

The terminals of the cochlear portion of the vestibulocochlear nerve synapse with the hair cells. The microvilli of the hair cells contact the overlying tectorial membrane. Sound arriving at the external ear causes the tympanic membrane to vibrate. This vibration is amplified and carried across the middle ear by the auditory ossicles and results in pressure waves in the fluid of the inner ear. These waves enter the bony cochlea causing vibration of the basilar membrane, which makes the microvilli rub against the tectorial membrane. Deflection of the microvilli on the hair cells results in ion channels opening in the base of the hair cell and depolarisation of the associated nerve endings, generating a nerve impulse.

The composition of the basilar membrane varies along its length, so that specific portions only will vibrate in response to a specific frequency of sound. High-frequency sounds stimulate the basilar membrane at the base of the cochlear, while low-frequency sounds stimulate at the apex. Thus, there is frequency-dependent stimulation of specific fibres within the cochlear nerve and this is translated into pitch perception in the auditory cortex. Different species can

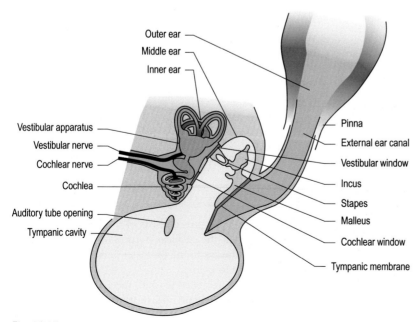

Fig. 10.15 **The canine ear.**

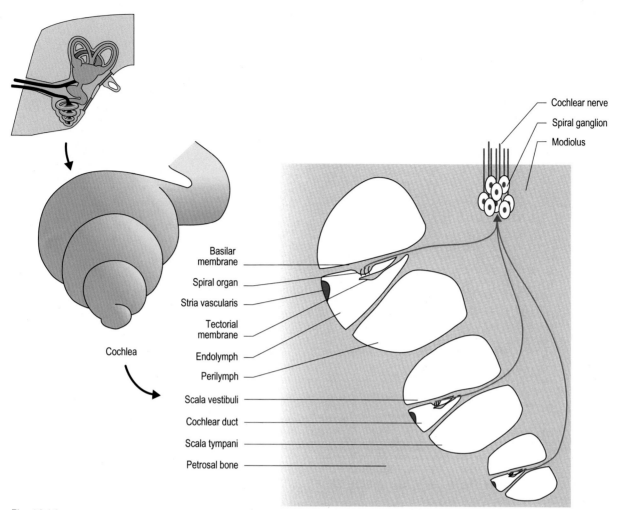

Fig. 10.16 **The cochlea. The top image is stylised to depict the spiral nature of the cochlea while the bottom left image is the shape that would be formed by a cast of the bony labyrinth. The bottom right image is a transverse section through the cochlea.**

perceive different pitches with dogs hearing frequencies in the range of 67–45 000 Hz, while horses can detect 55–33 500 Hz and humans 64–23 000 Hz. The cochlear window acts as a dampener for excess pressure waves within the cochlea dispersing them into the middle ear cavity.

Audition, the conscious perception of sound, shares the same three-stage system that is the template for most sensory systems. The axons of the first neuron in the pathway form the cochlear portion of the vestibulocochlear nerve (CN VIII) and have their nerve cell bodies located in the spiral ganglion inside the cochlea. The cochlear nerve synapses with the neurons in the dorsal and ventral cochlear nuclei located on the dorsolateral aspect of the rostral medulla oblongata (Figs. A21, A22, A29). Efferent axons from the cochlear nuclei travel rostrally, in the lateral lemniscus, to synapse with the third neuron in the medial geniculate nucleus of the diencephalon (metathalamus, see Figs. A30, A20, A19, A17). The output from this nucleus travels, via the internal capsule, to the auditory cortex in the temporal lobe for conscious perception of sound (see Fig. 4.13). The pathway is bilaterally represented.

In addition to this simplified three-neuron pathway many fibres synapse in other nuclei as part of the auditory pathway, or for acoustic reflexes. This includes the nuclei of the trapezoid body (caudal border of the pons), the lateral lemniscus (pons and midbrain) and the caudal colliculus of the midbrain (Figs. 10.17, A3, A7, A19).

Synapses in the caudal colliculus and connections with the tectonuclear/tectospinal pathways, as described for visual reflexes, are used for reflex eye and head movement in response to sound.

Auditory reflexes, and the brainstem auditory evoked response

Acoustic reflexes
Protective acoustic reflex
When loud, potentially damaging noises occur, input from CN VIII reflexively stimulates CNN V and VII that innervate the tensor tympani and stapedius muscles of the middle ear, respectively. The tensor tympani muscle attaches to the malleus while the stapedius muscle attaches to the stapes. Contraction of these muscles reduces movement of the ossicles and so limits transduction of sound to the delicate inner ear. The reflex acts bilaterally even after a unilateral stimulus.

Olivocochlear reflex
Efferent fibres in CN VIII arise from the olivary nucleus of the medulla oblongata and synapse on the hair cells in the cochlear inhibiting their activation. This reflex may be both protective limiting stimulation of hair cells by sound and also aid in hearing by neutralising the background

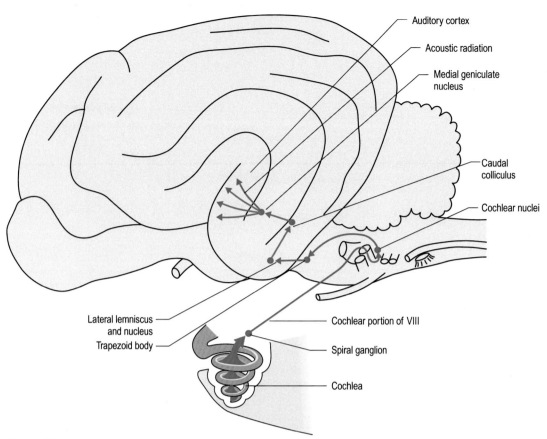

Fig. 10.17 **Neural projections from the spiral ganglion to the auditory cortex.**

noise and enhancing the ability to localise the source of a sound.

Reflex head turning

The caudal colliculi receive input from the rostrally directed auditory pathway. The colliculi function in reflexes such as head turning in response to auditory stimuli.

Brainstem auditory evoked response (BAER)

The BAER is an electrical wave form generated by the transmission of nerve impulses along the auditory pathway. It can be used to evaluate the function of components of the auditory pathway from the cochlea to the auditory cortex. In the normal animal, auditory stimuli applied to the external ear result in sequential electrical events occurring in the cochlea, CN VIII, cochlear nuclei and auditory pathways in the brainstem. These evoked potentials can be recorded using surface electrodes placed over the scalp. However, the potential differences of the electrical activity are small and hard to distinguish from the other electrical activity in the brain. Thus headphones are used to deliver hundreds of auditory stimuli (clicks) and the potentials generated are averaged, thereby eliminating background noise. The resulting wave form has up to seven peaks that are thought to correlate with electrical activity generated in the following structures: I vestibulocochlear nerve, II cochlear nuclei, III nucleus of the trapezoid body, IV lemniscal nuclei, V caudal colliculus, VI medial geniculate nucleus and VII auditory radiations.

Lesions that affect peripheral auditory function or the central pathway passing through the brainstem to the forebrain, will alter the wave form. The test was originally used to assess brainstem function, however this has now advanced imaging techniques are now being used

preferentially. The BAER are robust however, functioning even if there is no electroencephalogram (EEG) activity, for example after a barbiturate overdose, and assessment of BAER activity can be used to determine whether a patient is 'brain dead'. More commonly, it is used to assess whether animals, such as Dalmation puppies, are unilaterally or bilaterally deaf due to developmental sensory neural deafness (Fig. 10.18). The latter is a breed-related disease causing degeneration of the stria vascularis, which supplies blood and endolymph to the cochlea; this ultimately leads to degeneration of the hair cells.

Additionally, hearing may be tested by evaluating otoacoustic emissions. Auditory stimuli produce a hydromechanical energy wave that travels up the cochlear spiral, stimulating hair cells. This energy wave may be partially re-emitted from the cochlea back into middle ear and result in a sound emitting from the external ear canal. Otoacoustic emissions can be spontaneous or evoked; the latter can be used to test function of the hair cells in the cochlea. This testing has been used for some time in human audiology. It can be used in animals and has been successful in documenting hearing dysfunction in dogs.

Balance and the vestibular system

See Chapter 8.

Taste and sensory input from the pharynx and viscera

The solitary tract and its nucleus are located in the pons and the medulla oblongata extending from the level of the facial nucleus to the obex; they are sited (dorso)lateral to

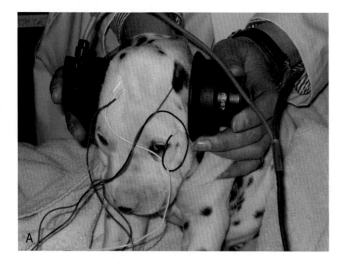

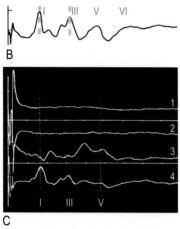

Fig. 10.18 **(A) Dalmatian puppy undergoing BAER testing to determine whether it has sensory neural deafness. (B) BAER from a horse. Roman numerals refer to specific waveform peaks (see text). (C) Traces from a Dalmation dog identified by the BAER as being totally deaf in the left ear (upper two traces). (Courtesy of Professor J. Mayhew, IVABS, Massey Uniersity).**

> ### Key point
>
> - The solitary tract and its nucleus in the caudal brainstem receive visceral inputs from the tongue (taste – CNN VII, IX, X), the carotid sinus (CN IX), thoracic, and abdominal viscera (CN X).

the parasympathetic nucleus of X (see Figs. 4.13, A28, A29). Their appearance is indistinct on gross section. The solitary tract receives visceral afferents from the head to do with taste (via cranial nerves VII, IX, X), blood pressure from the carotid sinus (CN IX), and stretch or chemical changes in the thoracic and abdominal viscera (CN X) and projects them to the medially located, nucleus of the solitary tract. Cranial nerve VII conveys taste from the rostral two-thirds of the tongue, while the glossopharyngeal and vagus nerves convey taste from the caudal third and the base of the epiglottis. The rostral portion of the nucleus, which receives taste sensory input, is also known as the gustatory nucleus.

The nucleus functions as a relay station (interneurons and projection neurons) for sensory input, and is involved in reflexes associated with the auditory tube, pharynx, larynx, oesophagus, trachea, thoracic and abdominal viscera.

Parasympathetic innervation of the eye, head and body cavities

See also Chapter 12.

> ### Key points
>
> - Parasympathetic fibres are found in cranial nerves III, VII, IX and X. They innervate smooth muscle and glands in the head and body.
> - In response to input from the optic nerve, presynaptic axons from the parasympathetic nucleus of III synapse, in the ciliary ganglion, with postsynaptic fibres; these innervate sphincter muscles of the iris.
> - Glands of the head are innervated by parasympathetic fibres in CNN VII and IX.
> - The vagus nerve is the source of parasympathetic motor fibres to the thoracic and abdominal viscera.

Parasympathetic nucleus of the oculomotor nerve

This nucleus is located just medial to the oculomotor nucleus in the ventral midbrain. It forms the efferent portion of the pupillary light reflex (Figs. 10.8 and 10.9).

Parasympathetic nucleus of the facial nerve

This is a small, ill-defined nucleus located within the reticular formation in the ventrolateral area of the rostral medulla oblongata. It receives afferent fibres from the nucleus of the solitary tract and the spinal nucleus of V. Efferent fibres innervate the palatine, lacrimal and nasal glands, the sublingual and mandibular salivary glands and smooth muscle of the nasal and oral cavities resulting, for example, in reflex secretions.

Parasympathetic nucleus of the glossopharyngeal nerve

This nucleus is located at the rostral end of parasympathetic nucleus of X. Its efferent fibres innervate the zygomatic and parotid salivary glands.

Parasympathetic nucleus of the vagus nerve

This long nucleus is located just lateral to the fourth ventricle and the central canal; it extends from just caudal to the trapezoid body to the level of the pyramidal decussation (see Figs. A23, A24, A27, A28). It is the source of autonomic motor fibres that form the vagus nerve and supply the thoracic and abdominal viscera.

Note that the parasympathetic supply to the pelvic viscera arises from the sacral spinal cord (see Chapter 12).

Innervation of the pharynx, larynx and oesophagus

> ### Key points
>
> - Striated muscles of the pharynx, larynx and oesophagus are innervated by fibres from the nucleus ambiguus (CNN IX, X, XI). This nucleus also participates in coughing, swallowing, gagging and vomiting reflexes.

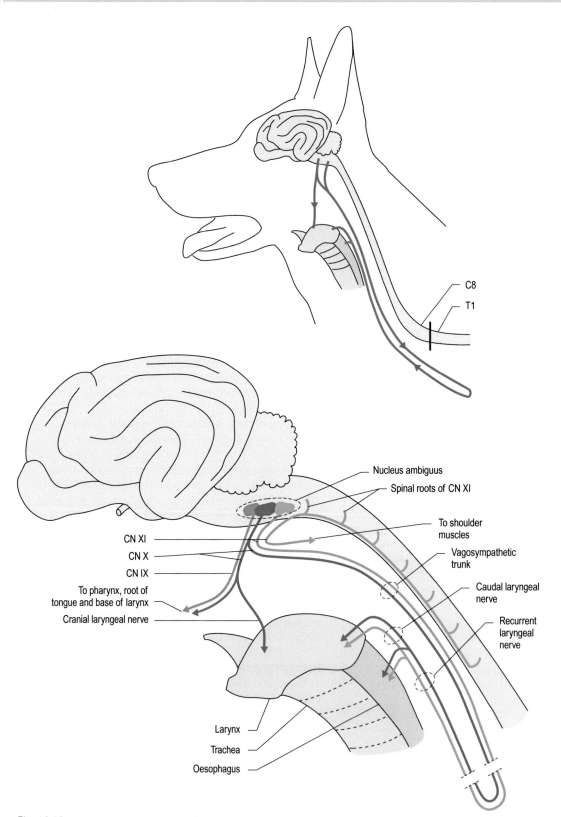

C8
T1

Nucleus ambiguus
Spinal roots of CN XI
To shoulder muscles
Vagosympathetic trunk
Caudal laryngeal nerve
Recurrent laryngeal nerve

CN XI
CN X
CN IX
To pharynx, root of tongue and base of larynx
Cranial laryngeal nerve

Larynx
Trachea
Oesophagus

Fig. 10.19 **Axons and nerves originating in nucleus ambiguus innervate the pharynx, larynx and oesophagus. Note: the sympathetic fibres of the vagosympathetic trunk are not shown.**

■ Axons of the external branch of the accessory nerve (CN XI) originate from the cervical spinal cord and innervate some of the neck muscles and extrinsic muscles of the shoulder.

Striated muscles of the pharynx and larynx are innervated by fibres from the nucleus ambiguus (CNN IX, X, XI). The nucleus ambiguus receives fibres from the nucleus of the

solitary tract (taste and visceral afferents from the body) and participates in reflexes involving the pharynx, larynx and oesophagus such as coughing, swallowing, gagging and vomiting.

The nucleus ambiguus is a long, poorly defined nucleus located ventrolaterally in the medulla oblongata extending from just caudal to the trapezoid body to the level of the pyramidal decussation (see Fig. A27). Additional neurons associated with CN XI (accessory nerve) extend caudally from the nucleus ambiguus into the cervical spinal cord as

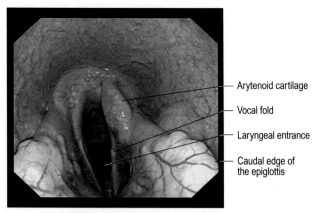

— Arytenoid cartilage

— Vocal fold

— Laryngeal entrance

— Caudal edge of the epiglottis

Fig. 10.20 **Endoscopic view of the larynx of a horse with a neuropathy of the left recurrent laryngeal nerve. The left arytenoid cartilage and vocal fold are adducted (courtesy of Professor Paddy Dixon, University of Edinburgh).**

far as C7. Thus the accessory nerve arises from two sites as follows: (see Figs. A2, A3, A24, A25)

1. Brainstem origin at the caudal end of the nucleus ambiguus. The cranial roots form the internal branch of the accessory nerve. This immediately joins the vagus nerve and ultimately contributes to the recurrent laryngeal nerve innervating the oesophagus and intrinsic muscles of the larynx.
2. The spinal origin (C1–C7) gives rise to the spinal roots that form the external branch of the accessory nerve. This branch innervates some neck muscles and extrinsic forelimb muscles such as the cleidomastoideus, sternomastoideus, cleidocervicalis and the trapezius muscles.

Sensory innervation of the larynx is via the cranial laryngeal nerve (a branch of the vagus nerve) as far as the glottis. Caudal to the glottis it is innervated by the caudal laryngeal nerve, which is the termination of the recurrent laryngeal nerve. Innervation of the intrinsic muscles of the larynx is largely by the caudal laryngeal nerve, although the cranial laryngeal nerve supplies the cricothyroideus muscle. The caudal laryngeal nerve has a long course. The vagus and internal branch of the accessory nerve extend caudally down the neck in the vagosympathetic trunk. The recurrent laryngeal nerve detaches in the cranial thorax, with the right side nerve winding around the right subclavian artery and the left side nerve having a longer course as it passes around the ligamentum arteriosum of the aortic arch. Both nerves travel cranially in the carotid sheath innervating the cervical oesophagus. It terminates as the caudal laryngeal nerve innervating the majority of the intrinsic laryngeal muscles, which are responsible for both abduction and adduction of the vocal folds. Importantly the caudal laryngeal nerve innervates the only muscle that abducts the vocal folds – the cricoarytenoideus dorsalis muscle. Thus damage to the recurrent laryngeal nerve can result in failure of vocal fold abduction, causing narrowing of the glottis and inspiratory difficulties, stridor or changes in phonation. Large dogs and horses are not uncommonly affected by degeneration in these nerves resulting in laryngeal paresis or plegia. In horses, the left recurrent laryngeal nerve seems particularly vulnerable, although lesser changes in other nerves have been noted. The aetiopathogenesis of this degeneration is still unclear (Figs. 10.19 and 10.20).

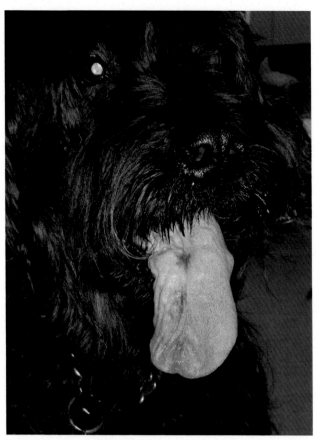

Fig. 10.21 **Atrophy and contracture of the right side of the tongue secondary to loss of hypoglossal innervation (courtesy of Mr. Robert Sawicki IVABS, Massey University).**

The vagus and glossopharyngeal nerves supply both sensory and motor innervation to the pharynx, root of the tongue and base of the larynx.

Tongue function

Key point

- The nucleus of the hypoglossal nerve is located in the caudal medulla oblongata. Its fibres innervate the intrinsic and extrinsic muscles of the tongue.

The hypoglossal nucleus (CN XII) is located in the ventral medulla oblongata near the midline extending rostrally from the pyramidal decussation (A2, A3, A22-24, A28).

Efferent fibres exit the caudal medulla oblongata as a series of rootlets. The rootlets fuse and after emerging from the skull, the nerve becomes prominent due to the addition of connective tissue. It innervates the thyrohyoideus, geniohyoideus, styloglossus, hyoglossus, genioglossus muscles and the intrinsic muscles (m. propria linguae) of the tongue.

Being a LMN, loss of hypoglossal innervation results in atrophy of tongue muscles. In the early stages, a unilateral lesion will present as loss of tone on that side of the tongue, but chronically, due to loss of striated muscle fibres and subsequent fibrosis, the affected side will be shrunken and contracted causing deviation of the tongue (Fig. 10.21).

Sensory input from the tongue is via CNN VII and IX for taste, and CN V (mandibular branch) for touch, mechanoreception and nociception.

Chapter 11
Behaviour, emotion and arousal

Key points

- Behaviour and emotion are associated with the limbic system, which is found at the limbus (border) between the cerebrum and thalamus.
- The limbic system includes a variety of telencephalic gyri and nuclei, and structures of the thalamus.
- Lesions in the limbic system in animals can cause changes in behaviour and emotional responses.
- The ascending reticular activating system (ARAS) of the brainstem determines arousal (consciousness/ awareness) levels and regulates sleep. It is stimulated by collateral axons of most sensory fibres travelling to the thalamus.
- The ARAS functions as a triage system and ranks incoming information in terms of importance.
- The neurotransmitter hypocretin is important in controlling the sleep–wake cycle. Abnormalities can result in signs of narcolepsy-cataplexy.

auditory impulses. It projects to the hypothalamus and the brainstem, especially to those structures influencing visceral activity.

The limbic system includes those regions of the forebrain associated with affective (emotional) behaviour. In humans, this includes emotional experiences, fear, pleasure, memory and sexual activity. Emotional drive ensures that the animal will exert sufficient effort to ensure its own survival and that of its species. Emotion has a major impact on learning and memory and involves autonomic (visceral) responses. The limbic system correlates emotion and behaviour with the autonomic nervous system. This leads to the concept of the visceral brain; that is emotion produces a visceral reaction. In humans it is the part of the brain that is associated with how an individual is feeling – the 'gut reaction'.

Lesions in the limbic system in humans and animals can cause alterations in level of aggression such that docile, or wild animals, may become the opposite. This is the region of the brain specifically targeted by the rabies virus, resulting in behaviour changes in affected animals that are classically described as a 'dumb form' and a 'furious form'. Other signs of limbic lesions include altered cognition, sexual aberrations or altered use of sensory systems, for example, use of oral and olfactory input rather than visual input.

Behaviour and emotion

Normal behaviour in animals depends on complex interactions involving many areas of the brain. The limbic system is the area most commonly associated with behaviour. Phylogenetically, it is part of the archipallium of the cerebrum, which represents a primitive part of the brain. The limbic system is associated with the non-olfactory portion of rhinencephalon (paleopallium). This region originally functioned to correlate olfactory input with other sensory information. During evolution the archipallium has acquired other functions, such as behaviour.

The limbic system curves dorsally around the medial side of the cerebral hemispheres at their borders with the diencephalon. There is no generally accepted classification of its components but it is commonly thought to include the limbic lobe comprising the telencephalic structures such as the hippocampus, parahippocampal, cingulate, subcallosal and dentate gyri, the amygdaloid complex and septal nuclei (Figs. 11.1, A4-6, A13-18). Other components include subcortical, diencephalic structures, such as the mammillary bodies, epithalamus, rostral thalamic area and the interpeduncular nucleus in the midbrain. It receives, and associates, olfactory, visceral, oral, sexual, optic and

Arousal

The ascending reticular activating system (ARAS) and related structures are responsible for arousal (consciousness/ awareness) (Fig. 11.2). The ARAS is part of the reticular formation and extends from the medulla oblongata to the thalamus. It determines the level of arousal. It also filters, and prioritises, the plethora of incoming sensory information, for projection to the cerebrum.

Incoming information in the conscious projection pathways is projected *specifically* to the defined cortical receiving areas via the thalamus, e.g. tactile information projects to the somatosensory cortex. The ARAS receives collateral axons from these sensory/afferent axons travelling to the diencephalon. This includes exteroceptive, interoceptive and proprioceptive information. The collateral axons synapse in the reticular formation and from here the information is projected to the thalamus, from which it is projected *diffusely* to the entire cerebral cortex. Thus incoming information travelling via the ARAS delivers a generalised 'wake-up' call to the cerebral cortices. It keeps the cortex at a general level of alertness ready to receive and process specific, incoming sensory information. Physiologically, sleep is associated with decreased ARAS activity. The ARAS is thought to be the 'seat of consciousness'.

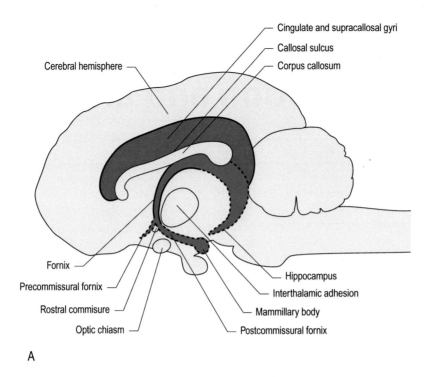

A

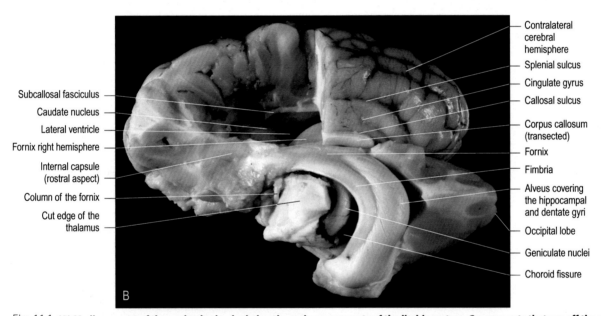

B

Fig. 11.1 **(A) Median aspect of the canine brain, depicting the main components of the limbic system. Components that are off the midline have a dashed outline. (B) Ovine brain, lateral aspect, dissected to display some of the structures of the limbic system. See Appendix glossary for information about limbic system structures.**

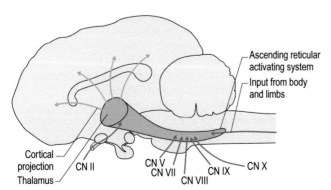

Fig. 11.2 **The ascending reticular activating system.**

Clinically, decreased consciousness can be due to focal lesions involving the reticular formation of the brainstem, or diffuse lesions of the cerebrum (Fig. 11.3). In veterinary medicine, five different levels can be described. Note, the commonly used term 'depressed' is a psychological term and is inappropriate:

1.   Normal – bright, alert and responsive;
2a. Vague
2b. Obtunded – dull, tends to fall asleep if left undisturbed, but can be aroused by non-noxious stimuli;
3.   Stuporous (semicoma) – somnolent; requires a noxious stimulus to arouse it;
4.   Comatose – unconscious; cannot be roused by even a noxious stimulus;
5.   Brain dead – no cerebrocortical electrical activity, no brainstem reflex function.

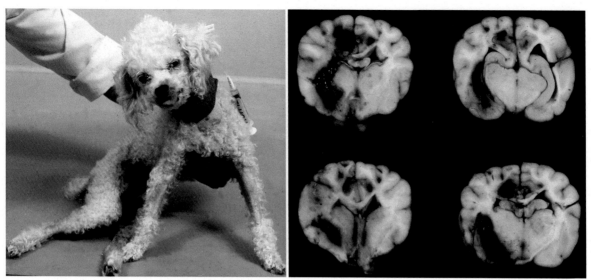

Fig. 11.3 **Stuporous dog after head trauma; the dog is being supported. Post-mortem image of transverse brain slices from this dog, depicting the diffuse left-sided haemorrhage and swelling causing compression of the right side of the forebrain.**

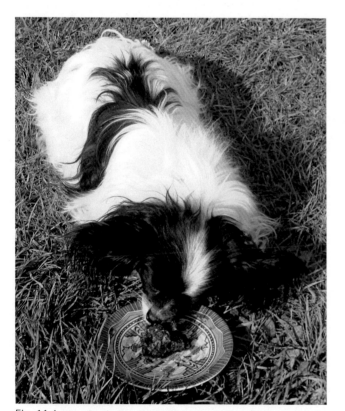

Fig. 11.4 **Narcoleptic dog. Typically excitement, such as associated with feeding, can trigger a narcoleptic attack. This dog's attacks were so frequent that he was having trouble getting sufficient nutrition. Vigorous stroking of the dog would help it to stay awake long enough to eat (courtesy of Dr. Alison Stickney, IVABS, Massey University).**

The brainstem auditory evoked response test (see Fig. 10.18) and brainstem-based cranial nerve reflexes such as the vestibulo-ocular reflex can be used to assess how much brainstem function is still present in comatose animals.

Central to the control of arousal as well as sleep is the neurotransmitter hypocretin (orexin). Hypocretin neurons in the lateral hypothalamus project to areas involved in the sleep–wake cycle, including the ARAS. Hypocretin promotes wakefulness. Hypocretin neurons inhibit the rapid eye movement (REM) stage of sleep by activating brainstem serotonergic and noradrenergic brainstem 'REM-off' neurons, and reduce the activity of pontine cholinergic 'REM-on' neurons. The sleep disorder narcolepsy has been associated with a lack of hypocretin production and, in specific lines of dogs, lack of hypocretin receptors (Fig. 11.4).

The ARAS is also thought to act as a filter, or triage system, for incoming information; it evaluates the different inputs in terms of priority. There is a constant barrage of sensory information coming into the brain. The ARAS filters out information that is not considered important at the conscious level and specifically projects important information to the cerebral cortex. Selective filtration helps minimise stimulation by information that is considered to be unimportant at that time, thereby enabling the animal to focus on a particular activity. For example, a cat watching prey may be relatively oblivious to the owner coming up behind it and may be startled when the owner strokes it.

Chapter 12
The autonomic nervous system

Key points

- The ANS is an involuntary system that preserves a constant internal environment by innervating cardiac muscle, and smooth muscle of blood vessels and visceral structures.
- The system has afferent, central and efferent components.
- It is subdivided into the craniosacral, parasympathetic ('rest and digest'), and the thoracolumbar, sympathetic ('fight or flight') systems.
- Autonomic UMN cell bodies are located in the hypothalamus.
- Efferent presynaptic and a postsynaptic neurons, in series, connect the CNS with the target organ. The presynaptic neuron has its cell body in the CNS and synapses with the postsynaptic neuron in a peripheral ganglion.
- The neurotransmitter at the autonomic ganglia is acetylcholine. The neurotransmitter at the neuromuscular junction is acetylcholine for the parasympathetic system and noradrenaline for the sympathetic nervous system.
- The location of the second neuron is system specific and close to the organ (terminal/intramural) for the parasympathetic system. It is remote from the organ (pre- or paravertebral) for the sympathetic nervous system.

- The presynaptic nerve can pass through a number of ganglia before synapsing, so the terms 'preganglionic' and 'postganglionic' can be misleading. Presynaptic and postsynaptic neurons are the preferred terms.

The ANS is a diffuse system that innervates smooth muscle of visceral structures, glandular myoepithelium, fat and vasculature throughout the body. The system has afferent, central and efferent components. Afferent fibres often use the same pathways as the efferent nerves. Afferent visceral fibres may also travel via somatic spinal nerves to reach the CNS (see also Chapter 1, for introduction to the ANS).

It is an involuntary system in which effects occur in response to both external stimuli and physiological changes within the body and do not require voluntary control. For example, exercise stimulates heart and respiratory rates, blood flow to muscles and sweating. Conversely, eating stimulates increased activity in the gastrointestinal tract, its blood flow and secretions. The ANS aims to preserve a constant internal environment.

Subdivisions of the visceral motor system

The efferent ANS is subdivided both functionally and anatomically. The parasympathetic system, also known colloquially as the 'rest and digest' system, is responsible for processes that conserve and restore energy. It functions in the day-to-day control of viscera for basic 'ticking over' type functions, for example, breathing at rest, digestion and elimination of wastes.

The sympathetic system, also called the 'fight or flight' system, functions when the animal is stressed, that is, when confronted by a need to fight or flee. It enables vigorous physical activity with rapid production of energy (ATP). Thus it is responsible for increasing heart rate, respiration, diverting blood flow to active muscles and pupil dilation for increased vision.

Anatomically, the two systems arise from different areas of the CNS, with the parasympathetic system arising from the brain and sacral spinal cord, and the sympathetic system from the thoracolumbar spinal cord. Hence, they are also known as the craniosacral and thoracolumbar systems, respectively (Fig. 12.1).

Despite the different origins, each organ receives both sympathetic and parasympathetic input. The balance of input from each system determines the organ's function. The motor/efferent component of the ANS is termed the visceral motor system.

The neurotransmitter elaborated at the terminal determines the physiological effect with the parasympathetic

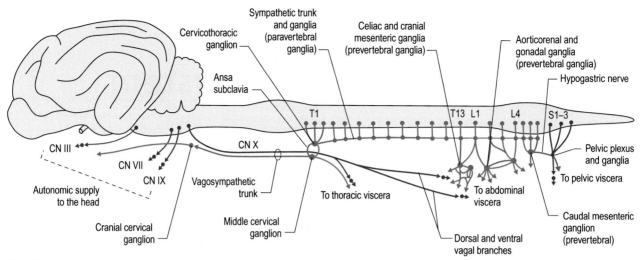

Fig. 12.1 **The two efferent components of the autonomic nervous system. Purple = parasympathetic nervous system; orange = sympathetic nervous system. Note: dots represent ganglia, but fibres may pass through ganglia without synapsing and synapse in a subsequent ganglion. A dot represent neuronal cell bodies/ganglion. If the fibre passes unbroken through the ganglion, then there is no synapse with a second neuron. If the fibre synapses onto a second neuron in the ganglion, this is represented by an arrowhead, space and then another dot.**

system being cholinergic, using acetylcholine, and the sympathetic system being adrenergic, using noradrenaline (norepinephrine). Adrenaline and noradrenaline are also secreted by the adrenal medulla into the circulation enhancing the effect of sympathetic nervous system stimulation.

ANS: Central components and peripheral components

In the CNS, the main control centres for the ANS are located in the hypothalamus; these can be considered to be autonomic UMNs. The rostral hypothalamus influences the parasympathetic system and the caudal hypothalamus influences the sympathetic system. Caudally directed fibres synapse in the brain stem and sacral cord (parasympathetic system) or the thoracolumbar cord (sympathetic system). The cerebrum and limbic system can influence but not command the control centres. For example, emotional states, such as aggression or fear, cause piloerection (raising the 'hackles'). Other parts of the CNS can also influence ANS function as exemplified by olfactory stimulation causing drooling. The hypothalamus integrates autonomic activities associated with temperature regulation, hunger, thirst, sleep, endocrine function and motility of viscera including the gut and urinary bladder. It is also connected to various autonomic brainstem centres that regulate cardiovascular and respiratory function. The cardiovascular centre of the medullary reticular formation can stimulate or depress heart rate. The respiratory centres in the pons and medulla control inspiration and expiration; dysfunction causes abnormal respiration. These areas are regulated by centres in the hypothalamus and the cerebrum.

Afferent and efferent fibres of the ANS travel via the spinal and cranial nerves to connect between the CNS and the target organ.

Two-neuron system in the periphery

The efferent ANS comprises two lower motor neurons in series compared with the single LMN in the somatic nervous system. The cell body of the first neuron is in the CNS and it synapses with the second neuron in a peripheral ganglion. The postsynaptic fibre then synapses

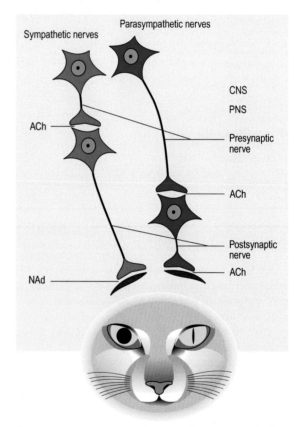

Fig. 12.2 **The two neurons that comprise the sympathetic and parasympathetic nervous systems and their neurotransmitters. The effect of each system on the smooth muscles of the mammalian iris is illustrated. ACh = acetylcholine, NAd = noradrenaline.**

with the target organ. Presynaptic axons are myelinated and postsynaptic are non-myelinated.

The location of the second neuron is system specific. For parasympathetic fibres, the ganglion is terminal or intramural; that is, it lies close to, or within the wall of, the organ being innervated. Therefore it has a long presynaptic neuron and short postsynaptic neuron.

For sympathetic fibres, the ganglion is remote from the organ being innervated. These ganglia are located ventral, or near to the vertebral column in a prevertebral or paravertebral position, respectively. Thus, the sympathetic system has a

Table 12.1 **Summary of key anatomical features of each system**			
Component	**CNS origin**	**Location of ganglion**	**Neurotransmitter released**
Parasympathetic	Craniosacral	Terminal – close to organ	Ganglion – acetylcholine Termination – acetylcholine
Sympathetic	Thoracolumbar	Distant from organ, e.g. pre/para paravertebral near vertebral column	Ganglion – acetylcholine Termination – noradrenaline

shorter presynaptic neuron and longer postsynaptic neuron (Fig. 12.2).

Note that as the presynaptic nerve can pass through a number of ganglia before synapsing, the terms 'pre-ganglionic' and 'post-ganglionic' can be misleading. Presynaptic and postsynaptic neurons are the preferred terms.

A summary of the key anatomical features of each system is given in Table 12.1.

Visceral afferent system
See also Chapter 6.

Key points

- Visceral receptors are stimulated by pressure, stretch and chemical changes.
- Input to the CNS is via cranial nerves (CNN VII, IX, X) and peripheral branches of autonomic and spinal nerves. Input stimulates reflex activity and may stimulate conscious perception.
- The solitary tract and its nucleus in the medulla oblongata receives input from cranial nerves and makes connections with the reticular formation for reflex function.

Receptors located in viscera throughout the body are sensitive to pressure, stretch and chemical changes. Most viscera are not sensitive to touch or cutting. Axons from the head travel via local cranial nerves (CNN VII, IX, X) and from the neck, trunk and limbs via CN X, and branches of sympathetic and spinal nerves. Visceral afferent fibres account for 80% of the proximal vagus nerve (CN X); the fibres originate from the pharynx, larynx, oesophagus, trachea, thoracic and abdominal viscera. Sensory cell bodies are located in specific ganglia such as the geniculate ganglion of CN VII, the proximal and distal ganglia of CN X, and spinal ganglia.

Input via cranial nerves (CNN VII, IX, X) goes to the solitary tract and its nucleus in the medulla oblongata. The efferents from this nucleus go to reticular formation for reflex function (respiratory, cardiac, digestive, elimination). The solitarothalamic tract also conveys information to the thalamus and hence to the somatosensory cortex for conscious perception.

Input via segmental spinal nerves enters the dorsal horn, and may synapse locally for reflex function, or travel cranially via the lateral funiculus (both ipsi- and contralateral) to the thalamus and somatosensory cortex.

Gut function can also occur due to local reflexes that do not involve the CNS. Some visceral afferents from the gut make local connections, in enteric plexi, with visceral motor nerves in the wall of the organ, causing local reflex activity. Most of the smooth muscle contractions such as

segmentation, peristalsis and defecation, can occur in the denervated gut due to activity of local pacemakers found in the intestinal wall.

Visceral efferent system: Sympathetic/thoracolumbar division of the visceral efferent system

Key points

- The sympathetic nervous system originates from the lateral/intermediate horn of the thoracolumbar spinal cord.
- Peripheral ganglia are located in the paired, paravertebral sympathetic trunks, or the median, prevertebral ganglia in the dorsal aspect of the thoracic and abdominal cavities.
- Postsynaptic neurons travel via spinal nerves, or specific named nerves, to their target organ.
- Visceral structures in the head are supplied by postsynaptic neurons originating in the cranial cervical ganglion.
- The thoracic viscera are innervated by neurons primarily originating in the cervicothoracic and middle cervical ganglion.
- The abdominal and pelvic regions are supplied by branches from the thoracic and abdominal sympathetic trunks, and prevertebral ganglia located around the aorta.

Presynaptic fibres originate in the intermediate (lateral) horn of the thoracolumbar spinal cord. Fibres may leave in the ventral root from their spinal cord segment of origin, or they may pass cranially, or caudally, a number of segments within the spinal cord before exiting it. The fibres exit the spinal cord along with the somatic motor neurons using the ventral roots of C8–L4/5 (up to L7) spinal nerves. The ventral roots fuse with the dorsal roots to form proper spinal nerve at the level of the intervertebral foramen (see Fig. 1.1). Lateral to the foramen, the proper spinal nerve splits into epaxial, hypaxial and ventral branches. The ventral branch forms the ramus communicans (ramus – L = branch). The ramus communicans conveys sympathetic efferent and visceral afferent fibres, between the spinal cord and the bilateral, sympathetic trunks that run ventrolaterally on both sides of the vertebral column (Fig. 12.3). The ramus communicans conveys both presynaptic (myelinated) sympathetic efferent fibres that are travelling to the trunk, and postsynaptic (unmyelinated) fibres that return from the trunk to rejoin the spinal nerves. This gives rise to the names of white and grey ramus communicans, respectively. These paravertebral ganglia and trunks are prominent in the thoracic region and extend into the lumbar region (see Fig. 12.4). In the caudal lumbar area, the trunks may fuse and continue caudally, ventral to the sacral and caudal vertebrae. In the abdominal region, nerves leave the paravertebral sympathetic trunks and connect to prevertebral ganglia located ventral to the vertebral column near the large abdominal arteries. From the cranial thorax, sympathetic fibres continue cranially into the cervical region, in conjunction with the vagus nerve forming the vagosympathetic trunk; this is located in the carotid sheath (Fig. 12.5).

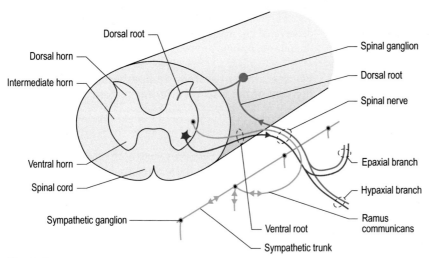

Fig. 12.3 **Sympathetic efferent and visceral afferent fibres connecting between the thoracolumbar spinal cord and the sympathetic trunk.**

A ganglion occurs where each ramus communicans joins the sympathetic trunk. The ganglia are numbered based on the spinal nerve that supplies them. Fibres may pass through several ganglia before synapsing. Thus the sympathetic trunk comprises both pre- and postsynaptic fibres; these are myelinated and unmyelinated, respectively. From the paravertebral ganglia, there are a number of routes that the fibres may take.

(a) Return via the ramus communicans to join spinal segmental nerves to be distributed to somatic targets such as blood vessels or skin (glands).
(b) Travel further ventrally in specific nerves to innervate viscera. For example, fibres from the cervicothoracic ganglion go to the heart via cardiac nerves.
(c) Travel cranially or caudally to other ganglia and then peripherally, via other spinal nerves.
(d) Travel along arteries to supply a distant part of the body. For example, fibres from the cranial cervical ganglion travel rostrally associated with arteries of the head region. Note: sympathetic fibres also supply the walls of these blood vessels and thereby have an important role in circulatory regulation.

Supply to the head and thorax

On each side, ganglia in the caudal cervical and cranial thoracic region have fused to form the cervicothoracic (stellate) ganglion and the more ventrally located, middle cervical ganglion. Sympathetic fibres from T1–T4 (T5) supply the cervicothoracic ganglion, located in the dorsal thorax at the level of the first rib. Some fibres synapse here, but fibres supplying the neck and head pass through it without synapsing. This is the largest autonomic ganglion in the body. Cranial to the cervicothoracic ganglion the sympathetic trunk splits forming the ansa subclavia (*ansa* – L = handle or loop). The ansa subclavia passes ventrally around the subclavian artery and connects with the middle cervical ganglion. Fibres run cranially from each middle cervical ganglion in the vagosympathetic trunk, to supply the neck and head. They synapse in the cranial cervical ganglion near the tympanic bulla. In horses, the ganglion is located in the mucous membrane of the guttural pouch (medial compartment), thus it is susceptible to bystander injury in guttural pouch diseases. In dogs, the postsynaptic neurons pass through the tympano-occipital fissure between the tympanic bulla and the petrosal bone, along with the internal carotid artery. They join the ophthalmic branch of the trigeminal nerve, passing through the orbital fissure to be distributed to the eye. Other axons leave the cranial cervical ganglion and are distributed to the blood vessels and glands of the head, while some fibres may travel with branches of cranial nerves IX–XI to supply the larynx and pharynx.

The sympathetic supply to the head innervates smooth muscle (vascular, ocular and orbital, palpebral including the erector pilae of the eyelashes) and glands (sweat, salivary, nasal).

Sympathetic innervation of the thoracic viscera is derived from the cervicothoracic and middle cervical ganglia. Fibres join with those of the vagus nerve for distribution to thoracic organs.

Supply to the abdomen

Arising from the thoracic and abdominal sympathetic trunk, thoracic and lumbar splanchnic nerves supply pre- and postsynaptic fibres to the abdominal and pelvic regions. These nerves also carry afferent fibres from the viscera. The specific anatomy varies between individual animals. The splanchnic fibres travel to prevertebral ganglia located ventral to the aorta and its branches. These ganglia include the obvious celiac, cranial and caudal mesenteric ganglia, as well as the less obvious adrenal, phrenico-abdominal, renal and gonadal ganglia. Some ganglia are paired and some have contributions from the dorsal branch of the vagus nerve. Hypogastric nerves arising from the caudal mesenteric ganglia are postsynaptic; they supply the pelvic viscera with sympathetic innervation.

Visceral efferent system: Parasympathetic system of the visceral efferent system

> ### Key points
>
> - Presynaptic parasympathetic LMNs originate in the craniosacral CNS, such as from brainstem nuclei and the sacral spinal cord.
> - Postsynaptic nerves originate in ganglia that are situated close to/within the organ they are innervating.
> - Parasympathetic nuclei III, VII, IX and X innervate the head. Additionally the vagus nerve (CN X) also innervates the viscera of the thorax and abdomen. Sacral parasympathetic nerves innervate pelvic viscera.

Table 12.2 **Parasympathetic (PS) innervation of the head**			
Target organ and function	**Origin**	**Ganglion and location**	**Pathway**
Iris and ciliary body Pupillary light reflex and accommodation	PS nucleus of CN III in midbrain	Ciliary ganglion just caudal to the eye	With somatic motor fibres of the oculomotor nerve
Lacrimal gland Smooth muscle of the nasal and oral cavities Tear and mucous membrane secretion	PS nucleus of CN VII in rostral medulla oblongata	Pterygopalatine ganglion located on the pterygoid muscles	With fibres of CN V and CN VII
Sublingual and mandibular salivary glands, glands of the tongue Saliva secretion	PS nucleus of CN VII rostral medulla oblongata	Mandibular ganglion near the mandibular gland	Facial nerve, chorda tympani
Parotid and zygomatic salivary glands Saliva secretion	PS nucleus of IX, (caudal salivatory nucleus), rostral medulla oblongata	Otic ganglion near the origin of the mandibular branch of CN V	With fibres of CN IX; postsynaptic fibres with CN V

The parasympathetic or craniosacral system originates from the cranial end of the CNS (brainstem) in the parasympathetic nuclei of III, VII, IX, X and the intermediate horn of the sacral (S1–S3) spinal cord.

Supply to the head

Cranial nerves III, VII, IX and X supply the head as noted in Table 12.2 and Chapter 10. The vagus nerve, CN X is named for its long, wandering course (*vagus* – L = wandering) as it extends caudally along the neck to supply the viscera of the thoracic and abdominal cavities as far as the transverse colon. Efferent fibres originate from the parasympathetic nucleus of X in the medulla oblongata. The efferent fibres leave the medulla oblongata bilaterally as rootlets in conjunction with somatic fibres of CN IX and CN XI. The caudally directed vagus nerve joins the cranially directed sympathetic trunk, to form the vagosympathetic trunk. The cranial laryngeal nerve exits the vagus at the base of the skull while the recurrent laryngeal nerve exits it in the cranial thorax; they innervate the larynx and oesophagus (see Fig. 10.19).

Supply to the thorax and abdomen

In the thorax, there is a rich vagal innervation to the heart and lungs. Caudal to the root of the lung, the vagus nerve on each side splits into dorsal and ventral branches. The two dorsal branches fuse and the two ventral branches fuse (Fig. 12.4). The fused nerves run dorsally and ventrally to the oesophagus, which they supply, and pass through the diaphragm at the oesophageal hiatus and divide into many smaller branches to supply the abdominal viscera. The vagal fibres are thought to reach as far caudally as the junction between the transverse and descending colon. The remainder of the gut receives parasympathetic innervation from the sacral spinal cord.

Supply to the pelvic viscera

The parasympathetic supply to the pelvic viscera originates from the sacral spinal cord segments. Parasympathetic fibres in the sacral ventral roots fuse to form the pelvic nerve located on the lateral wall of the rectum. These fibres then expand to form the pelvic plexus, which also receives sympathetic fibres via the hypogastric nerve. Both types of autonomic fibres are distributed to the pelvic viscera and reproductive organs. Fibres from the sacral parasympathetic supply have been traced through the length of the large intestine.

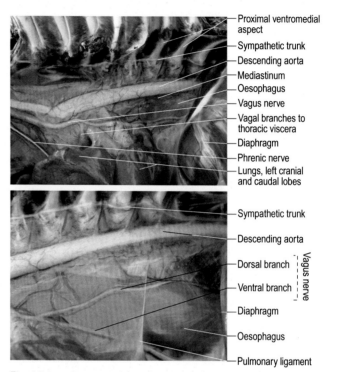

Proximal ventromedial aspect
Sympathetic trunk
Descending aorta
Mediastinum
Oesophagus
Vagus nerve
Vagal branches to thoracic viscera
Diaphragm
Phrenic nerve
Lungs, left cranial and caudal lobes

Sympathetic trunk
Descending aorta
Dorsal branch
Ventral branch
Diaphragm
Oesophagus
Pulmonary ligament

Fig. 12.4 **Dog thorax, left lateral aspect, autonomic innervation. (photo courtesy Mr. Allan Nutman, IVABS, Massey University).**

Autonomic innervation of the eye

> #### Key points
>
> - Parasympathetic LMN innervation to the constrictor muscles of the iris originates in the midbrain, travels with the oculomotor nerve and has its postsynaptic neuron in the ciliary ganglion. It forms the efferent part of the pupillary light reflex.
> - Sympathetic LMN innervation of the dilator muscles of the iris originates in cranial thoracic cord. Presynaptic axons travel cranially in the vagosympathetic trunk, synapse in the cranial cervical ganglion and are distributed to the eye.
> - Loss of sympathetic input to the eye results in 'Horner syndrome' (ptosis, miosis, enophthalmos and protrusion of the third eyelid). It can also affect blood flow and glandular secretion in the head.
> - Lesions of the midbrain can cause 'fixed, dilated pupils' due to damage to the parasympathetic nucleus of III.
> - Denervated smooth muscle is hypersensitive and responds to low concentrations of neurotransmitter. Consequently, dilute concentration of drugs that mimic ANS neurotransmitters, can be used to determine the site of an autonomic lesion.

Parasympathetic innervation of the eye

Bilaterally, the presynaptic neuron originates in the parasympathetic nucleus of III in the midbrain. These parasympathetic fibres mingle with the oculomotor nerve fibres arising from the oculomotor nucleus of the midbrain. The combined fibres emerge from the ventral aspect of the midbrain as CN III, the oculomotor nerve (Fig. A3). The parasympathetic fibres are located superficially on the medial side of the nerve where they are particularly susceptible to compression from any swelling or distortion of the midbrain. The nerve passes through the orbital fissure, into the periorbita and the parasympathetic fibres synapse in the ciliary ganglion close to the eyeball, just ventral to the optic nerve. The short, postsynaptic ciliary nerves travel to the eyeball and primarily innervate the smooth muscle constrictor of the pupil and ciliary body for accomodation.

The parasympathetic fibres of CN III form the efferent component of the pupillary light reflex (see Chapter 10).

Dysfunction of the pupillary light reflex

The clinical signs depend upon where the lesion is located and whether it is in the afferent portion of the reflex arc or the efferent portion. Determining the location is done by applying the primary concept of lesion localisation (see Fig. 13.1) that is by identifying whether other nearby neural pathways are functioning normally or are dysfunctional. Thus, if the lesion is located in the afferent portion of the reflex, then vision may be compromised (uni- or bilaterally). If the lesion is specifically located in the efferent portion of the reflex, then vision may be normal while the oculomotor function may also be compromised, resulting in strabismus (see Tables 13.1 and 13.2).

Sympathetic innervation of the eye

Upper motor neurons travel caudally from the midbrain as the tectotegmentospinal tract to synapse on presynaptic LMNs in the cranial thoracic cord (C8–T5/7). The LMN axons pass through the cervicothoracic and middle cervical ganglia, cranially along the vagosympathetic trunk to synapse in the cranial cervical ganglion near the tympanic bulla. From there they travel with the internal carotid artery and then the ophthalmic branch of the trigeminal nerve to the eye (Fig. 12.5). Sympathetic innervation supplies the smooth muscle of the orbit, the superior eyelid and the iridal dilator muscles. Sympathetically induced, smooth muscle tone keeps the eyeball protruded, the palpebral fissure widened, the third eyelid retracted and pupils dilated. In stressful situations, in which sympathetic nervous system activity is increased, pupillary dilation is stimulated both by the sympathetic innervation and circulating adrenaline; the latter accounts for sustained effects of sympathetic stimulation on the eyes, blood vessels and viscera. Sympathetic stimulation causes increased visual acuity, increased blood flow to postural and locomotory muscles and increased heart and respiratory function.

Clinical signs of sympathetic dysfunction

Loss of sympathetic input to the head results in Horners syndrome due to decreased stimulation of smooth muscle of the eye and periorbita (Fig. 12.6). In dogs, this results in four classical signs – enophthalmos, pupillary constriction, narrowing of the palpebral fissure and prolapse of the third eyelid. The third eyelid prolapses passively due to the enophthalmos and loss of tone in the orbital smooth muscle that attaches to the base of the third eyelid. In

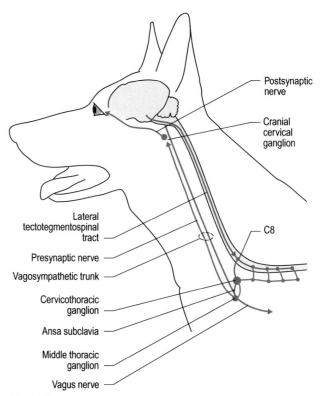

Fig. 12.5 **Sympathetic innervation of the eye.**

horses, the miosis may be subtle but paresis of extensor muscles of the eyelashes results in a prominent decrease in the angle of the eyelashes. Additional signs may also include peripheral vasodilation and warmth. In most species, decreased glandular secretion causes anhydrosis. For example, in cattle, the nasal planum on the affected side may be dry. The exception is in horses in which loss of sympathetic tone can result in sweating due to increased blood flow to sweat glands.

Pupillary function in acute brain disease

Pupil size can be an indicator as to the severity of brainstem damage. Severe bilateral miosis can occur with lesions affecting the forebrain or pretectal area. This may represent increased parasympathetic function due to loss of inhibition of parasympathetic LMNs in the midbrain by UMNs of the forebrain. An expanding lesion in the brainstem can affect CN III function. Experimentally, miosis is caused by compression of the rostral colliculus, whereas mydriasis is caused by compression of the parasympathetic nucleus of CN III, or the proximal portion of CN III as it travels along the floor of the calvarium. Brainstem compression can occur with brain herniation in which neural tissue is forced, rostrally or caudally, under the tentorium cerebelli. Asymmetrical compression can cause unilateral mydriasis, but severe bilateral compression can cause bilaterally, fixed and dilated pupils.

Resolution of the miosis is a favourable prognostic sign but progression from miotic to mydriatic pupils indicates increasing severity of the midbrain lesion.

Pharmacological testing of the pupils

Two principles underlie the use of drugs to determine the site of a lesion in the ANS:

1. Drugs can mimic the neurotransmitters at the synapses. They can stimulate the postsynaptic fibre by mimicking the neurotransmitter in the ganglion

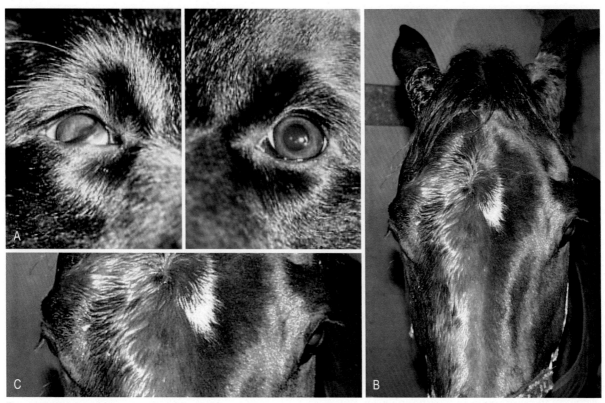

Fig. 12.6 **Horners syndrome affecting: (A) a dog's right eye, (B) the right side of the horse's face. Note the sweating and the drooping of the upper eyelashes (see enlargement, C).**

Table 12.3 **Pharmacological localisation of lesions in ANS innervation of the eye**	
Drug and mechanism	**Effect and lesion localisation**
Phenylephrine (10%) or adrenalin (0.001%) – direct acting sympathomimetic	Pupil dilation (dog) or change in eyelash angle (horse) if postsynaptic sympathetic neuron has been lost. Minimal and delayed effect if the presynaptic neuron has been lost
Hydroxyamphetamine (1%), indirect-acting sympathomimetic that triggers release of adrenaline at neuroeffector junction	Pupil dilation (dog) if presynaptic sympathetic neuron has been lost No effect if postsynaptic sympathetic neuron has been lost
Pilocarpine (2%), direct acting parasympathomimetic	Rapid pupil constriction if postsynaptic parasympathetic neuron has been lost. Reduced and slower effect if presynaptic neuron has been lost
Physostigmine (0.5%), indirect-acting parasympathomimetic that inhibits acetylcholinesterase	Pupil constriction if presynaptic parasympathetic neuron has been lost. No effect if postsynaptic neuron has been lost

where pre- and postsynaptic fibres synapse. Or they can stimulate the effector smooth muscle at the autonomic neuromuscular junction. Cholinergic drugs will stimulate the postsynaptic LMN of both the sympathetic and parasympathetic systems, and the neuroeffector junction in the parasympathetic system. Adrenergic drugs will only act at the sympathetic neuroeffector junction.

2. Denervated tissue is hypersensitive to concentrations of neurotransmitter that normally would not stimulate it. Loss of the presynaptic neuron results in denervation hypersensitivity of the postsynaptic neuron. Loss of the postsynaptic neuron results in denervation hypersensitivity of the smooth muscle.

Using these concepts, the clinician may be able to determine whether the animal's signs are due to loss of either the pre- or postsynaptic fibre (Table 12.3). A dilute concentration of drug that mimics the neurotransmitter at either the interneural synapse or the neuroeffector junction is applied. It will only reverse the signs if denervation hypersensitivity is present.

Elimination systems

> ### Key points
>
> ■ Somatic innervation causes contraction of the external (striated muscle) urethral sphincter (urine retention). Fibres arise in the S1–S3 spinal cord segments and travel via the pudendal nerve.
> ■ Parasympathetic innervation causes contraction of the detrusor muscle of the bladder wall and passive opening of the internal (smooth muscle) urethral sphincter (urination). Fibres arise in the S1–S3 spinal cord segments and travel via the pelvic nerve.
> ■ Sympathetic innervation causes relaxation of the detrusor muscle of the bladder wall and contraction of smooth muscle in the bladder neck (urine retention). Fibres arise in the L1–5 spinal cord segments and travel via the hypogastric nerve.
> ■ Visceral afferent fibres from the urinary bladder and sphincters travel via the pelvic nerve to the sacral spinal cord. They link to efferent fibres for reflex function and also travel to the brain for conscious awareness.
> ■ Reflex arcs for urination are located in the sacral and lumbar spinal cord and are influenced by UMN tracts from brainstem micturition centres, the cerebellum and the cerebrum.

- Urinary and faecal incontinence occur after damage to either UMNs or LMNs, but the clinical signs are distinct for each type of injury.
- Disruption of UMN tracts cranial to the sacral spinal cord can result in an 'upper motor neuron bladder'; this is characteristically full, turgid and difficult to express.
- Disruption of the sacral spinal cord, or the pelvic, or pudendal nerves can result in a 'lower motor neuron bladder'; this is characteristically overdistended, flaccid and easy to express.

Autonomic innervation of the urinary bladder

Receptors in the bladder wall and neck are sensitive to stretch or pressure. Afferent input is via the pelvic and pudendal nerves to the sacral spinal cord (S1–S3 segments).

Neural input from the bladder can stimulate reflex function via synapses in the sacral or lumbar (L1–4 or 5) spinal cord segments. The input is also projected cranially to the brain for coordination of bladder/sphincter function and for conscious perception (Fig. 12.7).

1. Sacral spinal cord (S1–3) connections. Somatic neurons that connect to the striated muscle in the urinary sphincter leave S1–S3 segments and travel via the pudendal nerve to cause contraction of the sphincter and urine retention. This is the most important sphincter for urinary continence. The pudendal nerve supplies the striated muscle of the anal sphincter, thereby forming the efferent arm of the perineal reflex; it also contributes sensory input from the perineum. Parasympathetic innervation originating in the sacral spinal cord travels via the pelvic nerve plexus to the detrusor muscle (smooth muscle) of the bladder wall for contraction. The oblique orientation of the smooth muscle at the bladder neck causes it to passively open when the detrusor contracts. Parasympathetic stimulation functions in bladder contraction and evacuation. The pelvic nerve also supplies parasympathetic fibres to the reproductive organs, rectum and descending colon. The pelvic nerve combines with the hypogastric (sympathetic) nerve to form the pelvic plexus located on either side of the rectum. Cranially directed interneurons connect bladder afferents in the sacral spinal cord to the cranial lumbar sympathetic neurons for reflex function either facilitating

or inhibiting them for urine storage and micturition, respectively.

2. Lumbar cord (L1–4 or 5) connections. Sympathetic fibres leave the lumbar spinal cord segments and travel via the splanchnic nerves to the caudal mesenteric ganglion, synapse and then via the hypogastric nerve to the pelvic plexus. From there they innervate the smooth muscle of the bladder wall inducing relaxation of the detrusor muscle via β-receptors. They also innervate smooth muscle of the bladder neck where they stimulate α-receptors causing contraction. Thus sympathetic stimulation facilitates urine storage. A distinct smooth muscle sphincter in the bladder neck has not been defined anatomically.

3. Brain connections. Cranially directed fibres travel to the brain via the lateral spinothalamic tract and the fasciculus gracilis. They synapse in the following areas:
   (a) Brainstem micturition centres such as the reticular formation of the pons. Reticulospinal tracts carry UMN fibres back down the spinal cord to connect with both visceral and somatic LMNs to stimulate urine storage, or voiding, as appropriate.
   (b) The cerebellum; this has a mainly inhibitory effect on urination.
   (c) The cerebrum, thereby informing the animal of bladder distension. The forebrain controls learned toileting behaviour and connects with the micturition centres of the pontine reticular formation for voluntary control of storage and micturition.

Urinary bladder function

Neural function for urine storage and voiding is summarized in Table 12.4. In the normal animal the distended bladder is located cranial to the pelvic brim and the bladder cavity sits ventral to the urethral outflow; therefore gravity aids urine retention. The position of the bladder relative to the urethra is a key component of urine storage in both the standing and recumbent animal. Changes in the animal's posture cause abdominal compression and may result in urine surging into the neck of the bladder. The distension of the bladder neck stimulates reflex urethral contraction and hence continence. The cause of urine spurting in excited puppies may be due to increased sympathetic tone and abdominal muscle contraction causing urine to surge into the urethra. Reflex urethral contraction may not be sufficiently facilitated by learned behaviour and so the excited puppy urinates

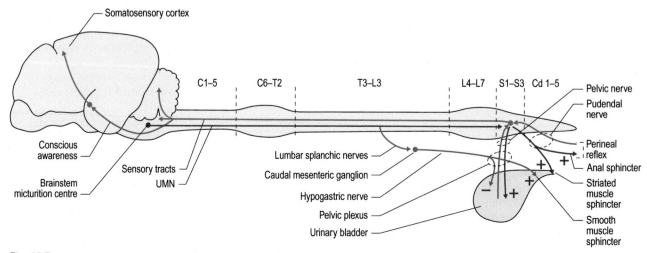

Fig. 12.7 **Innervation of the urinary bladder. Sensory input to the brain travels via the dorsal and lateral funiculi, while UMN fibres travel in the lateral and ventral funiculi (see also figure 13.15). + or – signs mean that neural activity causes muscle contraction or inhibits it, respectively.**

Table 12.4 **Nerve function during urine storage and voiding**				
Storage phase	**Afferent**	**Parasympathetic**	**Somatic**	**Sympathetic**
Storage and bladder filling	Increasing firing rate as bladder distends. Stimulation of brain stem and somatosensory cortex	Minimal, thus bladder wall relaxation	Reflex and voluntary stimulation of striated muscle sphincter contraction	α-adrenergic for contraction of smooth muscle sphincter β-adrenergic for inhibition of bladder wall smooth muscle contraction
Bladder emptying	Initial increase in intravesicular pressure (due to detrusor muscle contraction) causing stimulation, then decreased stimulation as the bladder deflates	Stimulation – bladder wall contraction	Inhibition Striated muscle sphincter relaxation	Inhibition of α-adrenergic fibres (relaxed smooth muscle of sphincter) Minimal β-adrenergic stimulation, so not opposing bladder wall contraction

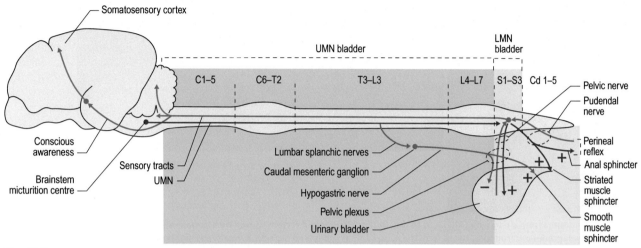

Fig. 12.8 **Lesions in the aqua-highlighted area would result in an UMN bladder (turgid, difficult to express), while lesions in the yellow-highlighted area would result in a LMN bladder (large, flaccid, easy to express).**

inappropriately. Coordination of bladder wall contraction and sphincter relaxation (micturition/voiding), or vice versa (storage), is mediated reflexively in the sacral and lumbar spinal cord and by micturition centres in the pons. Cerebral function modulates reflex activity and toileting behaviour (Table 12.4).

Dysfunction of innervation of the urinary bladder

Urinary incontinence includes signs of inappropriate urination and failure to urinate.

The 'upper motor neuron bladder' occurs when the UMN tracts (central motor neurons) cranial to the sacral spinal cord have been disrupted (Fig. 12.8, aqua region). Loss of UMN input results in loss of inhibition of the somatic outflow, thus striated muscle sphincter contraction is sustained. However, as the parasympathetic innervation to the detrusor muscle is intact, bladder wall tone is maintained. Hence the animal will have a full, turgid bladder that is difficult to express. Note as the overdistended bladder may reflexively trigger parasympathetic outflow and inhibit sympathetic outflow, causing detrusor muscle contraction, urine spurting may occur. Sustained (chronic) bladder overdistension can lead to an irreversible breakdown of the detrusor smooth muscle syncytium and may ultimately lead to decreased tone in the bladder wall.

Normally, detrusor muscle activation causes reflex inhibition of sympathetic outflow, thereby permitting urination. However, lesions between L4 and l7 can block reflex inhibition of sympathetic neurons. Sustained sympathetic outflow facilitates contraction of the smooth muscle in the bladder neck and compounds urine retention.

Spinal cord lesions may also block impulses travelling to the brain and the animal is not aware of having a full bladder; toileting behaviour is not initiated.

If the UMN lesion is chronic, then a so called, 'reflex bladder' may develop after several weeks. Bladder distension triggers reflex parasympathetic stimulation and inhibits somatic and sympathetic outflow. The bladder contracts as the sphincters relax. Mild abdominal pressure may be sufficient to set off reflex micturition. However, micturition may not be complete, leaving a residual volume of urine in the bladder and predisposition to urinary tract infections.

The 'lower motor neuron bladder' occurs with disease affecting the sacral spinal cord, sacral nerve roots, pudendal and/or pelvic nerve (Fig. 12.8, yellow region). Loss of LMN (peripheral motor neuron) function results in the loss of parasympathetic stimulation of detrusor muscle contraction, reduced tone in the bladder wall and overdistension of the bladder. Striated muscle sphincter tone is lost due to damage to the somatic LMNs. The LMN bladder is large, flaccid and easy to express manually. The animal may dribble urine as it moves around due to changing abdominal pressure on the bladder. The bladder is full and there is overflow incontinence, but voiding is not sustained as detrusor muscle contraction is lost. A relaxed urinary sphincter may predispose the animal to ascending urinary tract infections. Sympathetic innervation to the smooth muscle of the bladder neck may lead to partial closure of the urethra but is insufficient to keep the urethra fully closed. The animal may also have a dilated anus as the pudendal nerve also supplies the anal sphincter. This may result in faecal incontinence and loss of the perineal reflex.

Like any LMN lesion, reflex activity is compromised so reflex micturition will not occur. The lesion is also likely to damage afferent input, further compromising reflex function and conscious awareness of bladder distension.

Other sites of dysfunction

Damage to just the pelvic nerve will leave the anal and urinary sphincters intact, but the bladder will be atonic and distended and there will be no perception of filling.

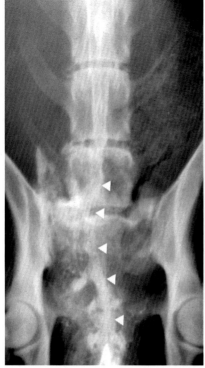

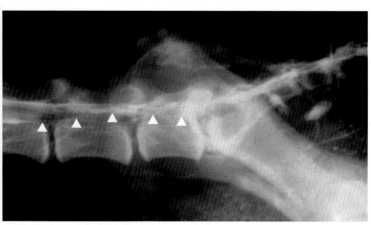

Fig. 12.9 **Radiographs from a dog with LMN signs to the urinary bladder and rectum caused by a tumour affecting the sacral spinal cord and nerve roots. Myelogram-epidurograms, taken from the ventrodorsal and lateral aspects. Arrowheads highlight the deviation of the sacral and caudal spinal cord segments due to the presence of the tumour. At presentation, this dog dribbled urine and had 2 litres of urine in its bladder. It also had no anal tone and was faecally incontinent.**

Brainstem lesions may result in similar signs to UMN bladder.

Cerebellar lesions may result in pollakiuria or increased frequency of urination with spurting and incomplete emptying. This is because the cerebellum usually has an inhibitory effect of urination. Other, more obvious cerebellar signs are likely to dominate the pollakiuria.

Cerebral lesions may result in loss of learned, toileting behaviour, but storage and micturition still occur.

Defaecation

> #### Key points
>
> - Innervation of the rectum is similar to that of the urinary bladder, with visceral afferent and parasympathetic fibres travelling in the pelvic nerve. Somatic afferent (from the anal sphincter and perineum) and efferent fibres to the anal sphincter travel in the pudendal nerve. Both afferent and efferent fibres attach to the sacral spinal cord.
> - UMN and LMN faecal incontinence are differentiated based on tone of the anal sphincter and activity of the perineal reflex (the NeuroRAT).
> - Defecation will still occur with either UMN or LMN disease due to the activity of local neural networks in the bowel/rectal wall causing colonic contraction.

The innervation of the rectum and anal sphincter is similar to that of the urinary bladder. Sympathetic input from L1–L4 or 5 spinal cord segments, via the hypogastric nerves, innervates the descending colon, rectum and internal smooth muscle sphincter of the anus. Originating in the sacral spinal cord, parasympathetic fibres innervate the descending colon and rectum via the pelvic nerve. Somatic fibres from the sacral cord innervate the striated muscle of the well-defined external anal sphincter via the pudendal nerve. The sympathetic innervation inhibits colonic and rectal activity and stimulates contraction of the smooth muscle sphincter for faecal retention. Parasympathetic innervation stimulates colonic and rectal motility for faecal excretion. The somatic innervation is critical for faecal continence by causing contraction of the striated muscle of the external anal sphincter. Afferent fibres from the rectal wall, sphincters and perineum project cranially in the dorsal and lateral funiculi to the brainstem centres for UMN regulation and to the cerebral cortex for conscious perception.

Defecation involves coordinated activity in the parasympathetic, somatic and sympathetic nervous systems. However, as it also involves reflex activity utilising local neural networks in the bowel/rectal wall, contraction of the colonic and rectal walls can still occur in the absence of sacral spinal cord input. Thus defecation may occur in animals with LMN lesions; that is involving LMNs in the sacral spinal cord, pelvic and pudendal nerves. The animal is unlikely to be aware of it due to loss of visceral and somatic afferent input. Damage to LMNs supplying the pudendal nerve would lead to a dilated anus and loss of the perineal reflex (Fig. 12.9).

In animals with lesions cranial to the sacral spinal cord (UMN lesions), then defecation still occurs, due to local reflex activity involving the spinal cord; again the animal may be unaware of the process. Small lesions affecting the dorsal funiculus may affect conscious perception of rectal distension/pressure on the anal sphincter and lead to loss of voluntary defecation with minimal effect on pelvic limb gait.

Chapter 13
The neurological examination and lesion localisation

Key points

- The primary aim of the neurological examination is to localise the lesion.
- The neurological examination assesses behaviour and arousal, sensory systems, motor function, cranial nerve function, spinal reflexes and vertebral column/spinal cord hyperpathia (spinal pain). Methods of examination have to be adjusted according to the species being examined.

In veterinary medicine the primary aims of the clinical neurological examination are to establish whether a neurological disease exists and, if it does, to localise the lesion.

Localising the lesion is done by assessing the results of the neurological examination. Lesion localisation is essential as diseases are often region-specific and determining which region(s) is involved permits the clinician to establish a list of possible causes and then pursue appropriate diagnostic tests.

For example, a different region of their nervous system will need to be evaluated diagnostically in an animal that has proprioceptive deficits, paresis and normal cranial nerve function, compared with one that has proprioceptive deficits, no paresis, but has vision deficits in one eye. The former is probably a spinal cord lesion and the latter is probably a forebrain lesion. To localise the lesion, it is just as important to identify the neural functions that are **normal** as well as those neural functions that are **abnormal**.

To localise the lesion, the clinician observes the animal closely and performs specific, neurological tests that evaluate the function of different neural systems.

Note that a full physical examination including assessment of the ocular fundus must be performed for the clinician to diagnose and treat appropriately the animal's condition. Many neurological conditions are associated with diseases elsewhere in the body. Tumours (multicentric or metastatic), metabolic and nutritional diseases, trauma, intoxications and vascular conditions are just some of the examples of systemic diseases that can cause neurological signs.

The following describes the neurological examination in a domestic cat or dog but the general principles are similar for large animals. Specific comments are given to modify the examination for large animals. This chapter represents the culmination of all the functional neuroanatomy described in chapters 1–12. Please see specific chapters for further details of structure and function.

During the examination, tests are performed that evaluate the following neural functions:

1. Behaviour and arousal;
2. Ascending sensory systems – tactile, proprioception and nociception;
3. Motor function;
4. Cranial nerve function;
5. Spinal cord reflexes;
6. Vertebral column/spinal cord hyperpathia (spinal pain).

From the results of the tests, the clinician determines:

(a) Whether the animal has neurological deficits;
(b) Which parts of the nervous system are functioning normally;
(c) Which parts are functioning abnormally.

Using their knowledge of where those neural functions are situated in the CNS and PNS, the clinician should then be able to localise the lesion. Only when the lesion is localised can the clinician devise a sensible list of differential diagnoses and plan appropriate diagnostic tests. All this has to be done before appropriate treatment can be prescribed.

Note: sometimes it can be quite difficult to localise a lesion and the neurological examination may need to be repeated several times to confirm results.

For example, if an animal is dysmetric and ataxic but is alert with good motor strength and cranial nerve function, then the lesion is unlikely to be in the spinal cord (i.e. no paresis), the forebrain or brainstem (normal arousal and cranial nerve function). However, a cerebellar lesion would account for the dysmetria and ataxia (incoordination) with preservation of the other neural functions.

It matters little where a lesion is located on a pathway (origin, midway along the pathway, or termination), it will still produce similar signs of dysfunction. This is analogous to a battery (origin), connecting wire (the pathway) and a light (end of pathway). Dysfunction in any one of those sections will cause the same outcome (clinical sign), that is, the light will not work. Most regions of the nervous system are associated with a number of functions either because a neural pathway begins or ends in that region, or is passing through it. The key to localising the lesion is based on having knowledge about which neural functions are associated with that region, and, conversely, which functions are not.

If a lesion is in a particular region, then it could damage pathways in that region and cause signs of dysfunction. However if a pathway does not pass through that region, then it will not be affected. Identifying the neural pathways that are functioning normally indicates to the examiner that the lesion is NOT located in the region that those systems occupy.

For example, if the lesion is in the thoracolumbar spinal cord, then pathways passing through that part of the cord may be damaged (see Fig. 13.15), such as proprioception and UMN tracts to the pelvic limbs causing proprioceptive deficits (conscious and subconscious) and either paraparesis or paralysis. But the lesion will not affect the cranial nerves, arousal or the function of the thoracic limbs, as those neural systems are not associated with the thoracolumbar spinal cord (Fig. 13.1).

An applied example of this diagram would be the animal that has conscious proprioception deficits on the right side limbs and blindness in the right eye (see Fig. 4.10). The conscious proprioceptive pathway (e.g. 'B' in Fig. 13.1) begins in the sensory receptors in the forepaw, travels via spinal nerves into the spinal cord, travels cranially in the ipsilateral cervical spinal cord, into the brainstem, crosses

over and passes rostrally on the contralateral side to the somatosensory cortex. The lesion could be anywhere along that long pathway. 'A' represents the cranial nerves that attach to the brainstem (III–XII) and the UMN centres in the brainstem and 'C' represents the visual pathway. As there are no other cranial nerve deficits, or paresis, then the lesion is unlikely to be in region 'X'. But both the right-side visual pathway (C) and right side proprioception are associated with the left side of the forebrain. Thus the lesion is in region 'Y'.

The neurological examination

To find out as much information as possible about a patient requires both keen observation before handling it, and then doing hands-on testing of neural functions. Begin with observation, then move to hands-on testing to assess function of the long tracts (proprioception, motor function), the cranial nerves, spinal cord reflexes, muscle tone and bulk and, finally, vertebral column/spinal cord hyperpathia. This order of testing is from the most benign to the most noxious. A full physical examination must also be performed.

Observation versus hands-on testing
The functioning of the majority of the nervous system can be assessed by close observation (Fig. 13.2). This is particularly useful if the animal cannot be handled; for example if it is fractious or wild. For animals that you can handle, then observation is still critical for getting an overall impression of neural function and is an excellent opportunity to assess arousal and behaviour. Physical contact usually stimulates the animal and subtle deficits in mental alertness may be missed. Assessing the animal's arousal level is done best by observing its interaction with the environment. Answering the following questions provides useful information.

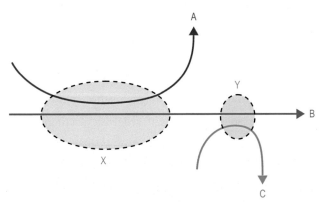

Fig. 13.1 **Consider an animal that presents with clinical signs referable to damage to pathway B. Pathway B is a long pathway, so to determine where the lesion affecting pathway B might be located, the examiner would assess the function of other neural pathways such as A and C. If the animal also has signs referable to damage to pathway C, but not A, then that would suggest that the lesion localises to region Y, not X.**

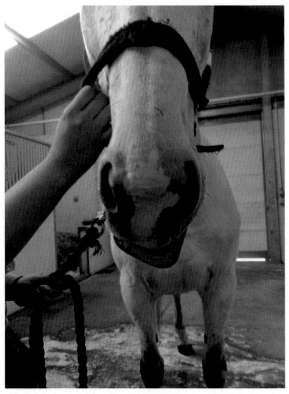

Fig. 13.2 **What neurological deficit can be observed in this picture of a horse? (Answer on next page.)**

Does it respond normally to environmental stimuli? These may include visual, auditory, olfactory, tactile and possibly gustatory stimuli. Does it seem bright, alert and responsive or dull and somnolent? (see Figs. 11.3 and 11.4)

Is the posture of its head, neck, trunk, limbs and tail normal at rest and during locomotion? (See Fig. 6.2) Does it move normally or are there signs of proprioceptive deficits (stumbling, postural abnormalities), ataxia, stiffness, pain or paresis? If so, which limbs and which joints are functioning normally and which are dysfunctional? Is there any change in muscle bulk?

Observe the head closely. Is the head posture normal? Is there any asymmetry of the face (drooping, muscle wasting)? (see Fig. 10.12) Do the ears, eyelids, eyes and nose move normally? Is it blinking? Is it sniffing at objects? Is it observing things or does it bump into them? Do both eyes track in a coordinated manner? Is there any strabismus, anisocoria or nystagmus? Does it respond to auditory stimuli? Is it swallowing normally or is there any evidence of respiratory stridor or change in voice? Is it licking its lips? Does it prehend food or drink normally?

Are there any signs of autonomic dysfunction such as anisocoria, sweating, faecal or urinary incontinence? (see Fig. 12.6) Spinal cord reflexes are difficult to assess by observation, but the animal may show a skin twitch if an insect lands on it, or a perineal reflex after defecating or urinating. If the animal has normal posture and gait, then the spinal cord reflexes are likely to be normal.

The horse in Fig. 13.2 has a left-sided facial nerve paresis. This was due to accidental compression of the facial nerve by the head collar buckle while the horse was recumbent under anaesthesia (see Fig. 10.14B). What do you observe in the horse in Fig. 13.3?

Proprioception and motor function

Normal gait requires both intact proprioception (limbs, trunk, neck and head) and normal motor function (UMN and LMN). Similarly, for an animal to perform normally the proprioceptive tests used in the neurological examination, they require intact motor function. Therefore an animal with a purely motor problem could appear to have faulty proprioception, as it may not have the strength to place the limb in the correct position.

Assessing both proprioception and motor function is done by observing posture (limbs, trunk, neck and head) and gait, and noting where the limbs are with respect to the centre of gravity, both at rest and during locomotion. Are the limbs base-wide or base-narrow? Are the animal's feet placed too far to the side or do they get crossed underneath while ambulating? Note also whether the animal bears weight on the correct part of the foot or whether it has knuckled over and is bearing weight on the dorsal aspect.

If only the subconscious proprioception is compromised, then the limbs are often not placed under the centre of gravity either at rest or during locomotion. This results in base-wide or -narrow stance and ataxia with failure of the limbs to track under the centre of gravity when the animal is walking in a straight line. Deficits are often exaggerated when the animal turns. In horses this is seen particularly by excessive circumduction of the outside pelvic limb during tight turns.

The horse in Fig. 13.3 has proprioceptive deficits when turning in both the thoracic and the pelvic limbs. Note excessive circumduction of the left pelvic limb and the

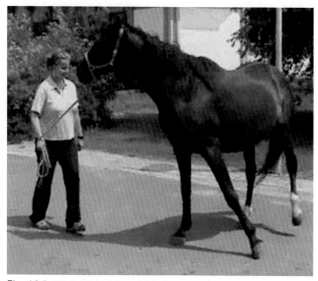

Fig. 13.3 **What obvious type of deficit can be observed in this horse? (Answer in text.)**

Table 13.1 **Observing cranial nerve function**

Testing by observation	CNN being evaluated
Watch as the animal interacts with its environment	Many
Head position – tilted, the eyes are in a different plane compared with lateral rotation (torticollis) in which the eyes are in the same plane	Tilt – CN VIII (a), Vestibular (Torticollis may be due to cervical or forebrain lesions)
Facial symmetry, blinking, nostril and ear movement	CN VII
Blinking – this reflex is due to the stimulus of corneal drying	Ophthalmic nerve of CN V (a), blinking due to CN VII (e)
Pupil size	Parasympathetic CN III (e) for miosis, or sympathetic (e) for mydriasis
Eyeball position	CNN II or VIII (a), CNN III, IV, VI (e)
Olfaction, vision, hearing,	CN I, II, VIII (a)
Masticatory muscle bulk, chewing	CN V (e)
Tongue movement, e.g. licking lips or nose	CN V (a) maxillary branch CN XII (e)
Swallowing	CN IX, X (a) and (e)
Laryngeal noise – phonation and stridor	CN X, XI (e)
(a) = afferent nerve, (e) = efferent nerve.	

delayed movement of the left thoracic limb leaving the foot rotated inappropriately inwards.

If only conscious proprioception is compromised the animal may stand and walk with the limbs placed under the centre of gravity, but it may stand on top of the paw, or scuff the paw along the ground during the protraction phase, resulting in stumbling. Large animals, with their poorly developed corticospinal tracts, may have a remarkably normal gait with a forebrain injury; thus more complex manoeuvres are required to expose any deficit. What do you observe in the animals in Fig. 13.4?

Cranial nerve function

Testing cranial nerve function by observation is outlined in Tables 10.2 and 13.1. Note that as cranial nerves are bilaterally paired, both sides of the head need to be checked (see Chapter 10).

The cat in Figure 13.4, has a dilated pupil in the left eye, subtle ventrolateral strabismus and loss of tone in the superior eyelid. This cat had CN III deficit causing loss of tone in the levator palpebrae superioris muscle (elevator

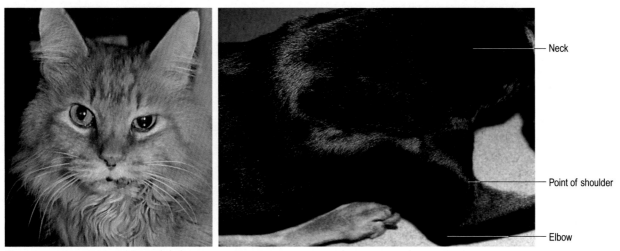

Fig. 13.4 **What neurological deficits can be observed in these animals? (Answer in text.)**

of the superior eyelid), medial and dorsal rectus muscles (strabismus) and the iridal constrictor smooth muscle causing mydriasis. This was due to a tumour in the floor of the cranial vault.

The dog's neurological deficits were readily detectable by observation. Clinically, the dog's gait was ataxic (incoordinated) and paretic. It had marked atrophy of specific shoulder muscles, especially the supraspinatus muscle. In this particular case it was due to hypertrophied ligamentous tissue in the spinal canal compressing primarily the C6 spinal cord segment (see Fig. 5.5 for similar case example.) The C6 spinal nerve arising from this segment is a key component of the suprascapular nerve innervating the supraspinatus muscle. Damage to the C6 segment, LMN cell bodies caused LMN signs, specifically, marked neurogenic atrophy of the supraspinatus (and infraspinatus) muscles (see Table 5.2) (see Fig. 4.7). Loss of supraspinatus muscle function compromises shoulder extension resulting in hypometria (shortened strides) in the thoracic limbs. The lesion also compressed sensory tracts and UMN tracts passing through the region supplying both the thoracic and pelvic limbs (see Fig. 4.8). Clinically the dog's pelvic limb gait was ataxic (incoordinated - 'wobbly') and paretic, while the thoracic limb gait was short-strided and stiff (choppy); there were proprioceptive deficits in all four limbs. This case was an example of 'Wobbler syndrome' (see Fig. 6.3).

Hands-on testing

With respect to the hands-on neurological testing, every clinician has their own approach, but here is an example of an approach that is generically useful for most animals. More detailed information on the neurological examination of large animals is given in books such as *Large Animal Neurology*, by Ian G. Mayhew, Blackwell Publishing, 2009, or *Veterinary Neuroanatomy and Clinical Neurology*, by deLahunta A and Glass E, 3rd edition, Saunders, 2009.

Proprioception and motor function

A key concept to comprehend is that proprioceptive testing also evaluates motor function as the animal has to move the body to perform the test. When evaluating proprioception in a limb, try not to disturb the overall position of the trunk too much as this stimulates proprioceptors throughout the body, rather than just the limb being examined, reducing the specificity of the test.

Hopping

This test is good for evaluating subconscious and conscious proprioception and may be performed, with care, in some large animal e.g. calves. In small animals, one limb is held flexed, e.g. the left thoracic limb, and the animal is pushed gently to the right. As the centre of gravity moves laterally over the right thoracic limb, this changes the subconscious proprioceptive input from the muscle spindles (stretching of muscles), joint angle receptors and Golgi tendon organs. It also changes conscious proprioceptive input by stimulating additional receptors in the feet. In the normal animal, this will induce a lateral hop to replace the limb back under the centre of gravity. In small animals, it is useful to have the animal still bearing weight on the limb girdle that is not being tested. For example, if testing the thoracic limb, let the animal bear weight on its pelvic limbs. Thus the animal pivots in an arc around the supporting limbs; that is around the pelvic limbs when testing the thoracic limbs and vice versa. This makes testing easier for the clinician as they don't have to try to lift the animal clear of the floor. Animals hop better laterally then medially, so only hop them laterally. Count the number of hops the animal makes on that limb, then test the other limb of the same girdle, through a similar size arc. Counting the number of hops, helps the clinician identify asymmetry between the limbs. The number of hops to cover a certain distance will depend on the size of the animal; a tall dog like a Labrador retriever takes bigger steps than a little dog like a Dachshund. In an affected animal, an increase, or decrease, in the number of hops may indicate reduced motor or sensory function, respectively. Thus, the clinician can try to differentiate reduced proprioception from reduced motor function. An animal that has purely motor deficits resulting in reduced motor strength (e.g. myopathy) may not be able to hop properly, even though it has intact proprioception by which it can sense that its feet are not in a good weight-bearing position. Supporting such an animal, by holding one hand underneath it, reduces the motor effort required to move the limb and the animal will move, or attempt to move the limb as soon as it senses abnormal limb position, but being weak, the hops will be shorter. Comparatively, if the animal has a proprioceptive deficit, it will not attempt to move the limb as soon as it is no longer in a good weight-bearing position under the body. The centre of gravity must be shifted further, creating a stronger proprioceptive stimulus to finally induce a hop. Thus the hop, if it occurs, will be bigger.

Paw position response (knuckling)

This test is more specific than hopping for evaluating tactile receptors compared with muscle receptors, thus it is good for conscious proprioceptive testing. The animal's weight is gently pushed to the opposite side, reducing the amount being carried on the leg being tested, then the toes are flipped under (Fig. 13.5). To test for subtle dysfunction, the clinician may just turn under a single toe. The body weight is redistributed back over the limb being tested and the animal is observed to see if it corrects the foot position. To avoid stimulating joint angle and muscle receptors in the proximal limb, the clinician tries to turn the toes under without lifting the limb.

Reflex stepping – the sliding paper test

The following test is more subjective and requires practice and experience to learn to read its results. It is only suitable for small animals, not horses or farm animals. As the name implies, this test consists of placing the animal's foot on a piece of paper and sliding the paper laterally. This alters the relationship between that supporting limb and the animal's centre of gravity. It changes proprioceptive input, especially from the muscle and tendon receptors in the proximal limb (extrinsic muscles), thus it can be good for identifying subconscious proprioceptive deficits. Its principles are similar to hopping. When the limb is no longer in a good weight-bearing position, the normal animal should lift the limb and step it back into a weight-bearing position. The replacing of the limb will be delayed or absent in an animal with proprioceptive dysfunction.

Hopping and paw position response (knuckling) are the two most helpful tests. Interpreting the sliding paper test requires experience, but can help to identify deficits in subconscious proprioception. This latter test and hopping both disturb the position of the props (limbs) with respect to the centre of gravity. Thus both tests may be abnormal with lesions affecting subconscious proprioceptive pathways. The paw position response is most likely to be abnormal if the conscious proprioceptive pathways are affected. Thus in a spinal cord lesion, all three tests may be abnormal. With cerebellar disease, hopping and sliding paper test are likely to be affected, whereas with forebrain lesions, the hopping and paw position response are likely to be affected. In large animals, 'paw position' cannot be reliably assessed and hopping tests can be hazardous. Instead time is spent assessing the gait for evidence of dysmetria (decreased or increased joint movement), particularly when visual and vestibular input is altered. For example, the animal is walked down a slope with its head (see Fig. 8.7). For movements to be performed correctly, conscious and subconscious proprioceptive pathways all have to function normally.

Identifying asymmetry in proprioceptive function

To identify if one side of the body is more severely affected than the other, tests that involve both pelvic limbs or both thoracic limbs are used; this includes the extensor postural thrust test and wheelbarrowing, respectively. For the extensor postural thrust test, the animal is lifted up so that its back feet are dangling. The animal is lowered and when the back feet contact the ground the normal animal will extend/thrust reflexively. However, as the feet contact the ground too far forward to bear weight properly, they will step their feet backwards until the feet are in a weight-bearing position. In an animal with neurological deficits either of proprioception or motor function, that backward stepping can be asymmetrical with reduced stepping on the more affected side. In the wheelbarrowing test, the animal's back feet are lifted just clear of the ground, and the animal is pushed slowly forward (Fig. 13.6). This will exaggerate any paresis and asymmetry of the thoracic limbs.

There are other tests such as hemiwalking, tactile and visual placing and hip sway that may be helpful to confirm subtle lesions. (For details of tests see either deLahunta or Mayhew, cited on the previous page).

Cranial nerves

The function of most cranial nerves can be assessed by observation, but hands-on testing helps to confirm specific functions. Testing cranial nerve function is outlined in Table 10.2 (see also Fig. 10.13). Cranial nerve reflexes are described below and the anatomical basis of the these reflexes is given in Table 13.2.

Note that as cranial nerves are bilaterally paired, both sides of the head must be checked.

(a) Pupillary light reflex. Shining a light into the eye (CN II a = afferent) will cause constriction of the ipsilateral pupil and lesser constriction of the contralateral pupil (CN III, parasympathetic, e = efferent). These reflexes are called the direct and indirect PLR, respectively (see Fig. 10.8).

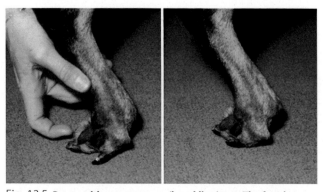

Fig. 13.5 **Paw position response or 'knuckling' test. The foot is turned over so the animal to see if the animal will bear weight on the dorsum of the paw (the knuckles).**

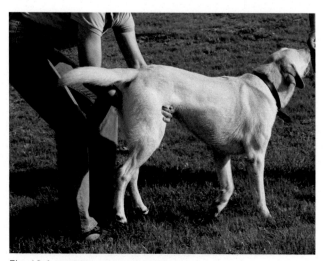

Fig. 13.6 **Wheelbarrowing in a dog.**

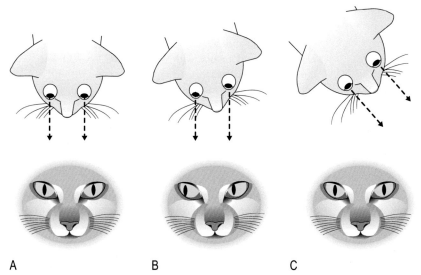

Fig. 13.7 **Vestibulo-ocular reflex. As the head moves, the gaze remains fixed on a position (A to B), so the eyes move slowly in the orbits until they suddenly and rapidly flick in the direction that the head is moving and become centred in orbit once more (C).**

Table 13.2 **The anatomical components of cranial nerve function**

Test	CNS region involved	CNN being evaluated
Palpebral reflex	Brainstem	CNN V (a) and VII (e)
Superior eyelid near medial canthus		CN V ophthalmic nerve
Inferior eyelid near lateral canthus		CN V maxillary nerve
Auriculopalpebral reflex	Brainstem	CNN V (a) mandibular nerve (CN V) and VII (e)
Facial sensation – tactile stimulation	Brainstem and forebrain	CN V (a)
Superior eyelid and nasal mucosa		CN V ophthalmic nerve
Inferior eyelid and muzzle		CN V maxillary nerve
Skin of the chin		CN V mandibular nerve
Masticatory muscle bulk, jaw tone – palpation	Brainstem	CN V (e) mandibular nerve
Olfaction observe the animal sniffing an object	Forebrain	CN I (a)
Menace response – threatening hand movement towards the eye.	Forebrain, brainstem (and cerebellum)	CN II (a), CN VII (e), also CN VI (e) (eyeball retraction)
Vestibulo-ocular reflex and eyeball position	Brainstem	CNN VIII (a), CNN III, IV, VI (e)
Tongue shape and movement	Brainstem	CN XII (e)
Gag reflex	Brainstem	CNN IX, X (a) and (e)
Pupillary light reflex	Forebrain and brainstem	CNN II (a), III (e)
Dazzle reflex	Forebrain and brainstem	CN II (a), VII (e)

(a) = afferent, (e) = efferent.

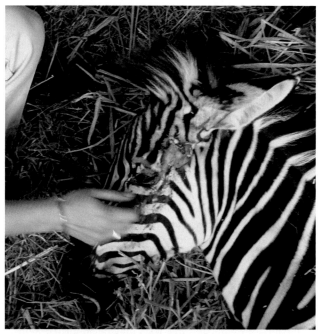

Fig. 13.8 **The menace response test being performed in a zebra that had head trauma. The zebra failed to blink in response to the threatening gesture indicating dysfunction in either CN II (a), the central connections in the brain, or CN VII (e).**

(b) Dazzle reflex. Shining a bright light into the eyes (CN IIa) causes partial narrowing of palpebral fissure (CN VIIe).
(c) Palpebral reflex. Tapping the skin around the eye (CN Va) induces reflex contraction of the orbicularis oculi muscle (CN VII) and closure of the palpebral fissure.
(d) Auriculopalpebral reflex. Lightly stimulating the skin just rostral to the opening of the external ear canal (CN Va) induces contraction of the orbicularis oculi muscle (CN VIIe) and partial closure of the palbebral fissure.
(e) Vestibulo-ocular reflex. Moving the head from side to side, or vertically (CN VIIIa), will induce fast, flicking movements of the eyeballs (CNN III, IV and VIe) in the direction that the head is travelling (Fig. 13.7).

(f) Corneal reflex. This is a noxious and potentially damaging stimulus and only performed if the palpebral reflex is dysfunctional. Gently touching the cornea with a moistened cotton swab (CN Va; ophthalmic nerve) causes closure of the eyelids (CN VIIe).
(g) Gag reflex – Stimulation of the back of tongue and pharynx (CN IX and Xa) with fingers causes gagging with pharyngeal contraction (CN IX and Xe).

A note on the menace response: When a threatening gesture is made to the eye in a normal animal, it will blink and/or pull its head away (Fig. 13.8). The gesture should be made from different positions with respect to the eye so that the temporal and nasal fields of view are tested. This is *not* a reflex however. It is a response as it has to be learnt; it is not hard-wired at birth. In precocial animals, such as foals, it develops 7–10 days after birth whereas in altricial

Table 13.3 **The anatomical components of spinal reflexes in the dog**

Segmental spinal reflexes	Afferent fibres	CNS component (dog)	Efferent fibres
Patellar reflex	Femoral nerve	L4–6 spinal cord	Femoral nerve to quadriceps muscle
Withdrawal reflex pelvic limb	Peroneal or tibial nerve depending on stimulus location (dorsal and plantar aspects of the foot, respectively)	L4–S1/S2 spinal cord	Femoral nerve to rectus femoris muscle +/– lumbar nerves (hip flexion) Sciatic nerve to flexor muscles of the stifle, hock and digits
Withdrawal reflex thoracic limb	Radial, median or ulnar nerve depending on stimulus location (dorsal, palmar or lateral aspect of the foot, respectively)	C6–T2 spinal cord	Axillary, pectoral, thoracodorsal, musculocutaneous, median and ulnar nerves to flexor muscles of the shoulder, elbow, carpus and digits
Perineal reflex	Pudendal nerve	S1–S3 and caudal segments 1–5 of the spinal cord	Pudendal nerve to anal sphincter and caudal nerves to tail depressor muscles
Cutaneous trunci reflex	Dermatomes associated with the L1/L2–T2 spinal nerves	L2/3–C8 spinal cord	Lateral thoracic nerve to the cutaneous trunci muscles
Local cervical and cervicofacial reflexes (horse, cutaneous colli muscle)	Cervical nerves	C1–C6, facial nucleus	Cervical and facial nerves

animals such as puppies, it can take up to 4 months. It primarily utilises sensory input via the optic nerve (CN II) and output via the facial nerve (CN VII) to close the palpebral fissure. It may also utilise a tract (tectospinal tract, see Table 4.3, Fig. 4.5) from the midbrain to the cervical spinal cord to stimulate neck muscle contraction and head movement. The CNS connections involve the entire brain, including forebrain (reception of input) and brainstem (motor output); the cerebellum is also involved (coordination).

The ocular fundus should also be examined as retinal and optic disc lesions may arise in some neurological conditions.

Muscle bulk and tone

After completing the examination of the cranial nerves, the clinician runs their hands over the head, neck, trunk and limbs in the standing animal, checking muscle bulk. Assessing the range of movement in the joints is done in both the standing animal (e.g. vertebral column, pelvis) and recumbent animal (e.g. limbs). Each limb is flexed and extended to test for resistance to movement, which indicates muscle tone. The spinal cord reflexes are assessed. Reduced or no **T**one, and marked muscle **A**trophy are two of the three characteristic signs of LMN disease (remember the Neuro **RAT** see Fig. 5.6).

Spinal cord reflexes

Clinically, the reflexes are tested to evaluate the integrity of the different components of the reflex arc (see Fig. 4.3). Disruption of sensory input, CNS interconnections, or LMN output will result in decrease, or loss of, reflex activity. This is most commonly seen with LMN lesions involving the region of the CNS in which the LMN cell body is housed, or in the LMN itself. A decrease in, or loss of, the reflex is highly localising as it indicates precisely which parts of the PNS and CNS must be compromised (Table 13.3). If the reflex arc is present then the three anatomical components are intact and functioning.

Clinically, an intact reflex, be it normal or exaggerated, tells the clinician that the lesion does not involve that area of the CNS or the PNS. It will be present even if the neuraxis cranial or caudal to the reflex circuit has been severed. Exaggeration of spinal reflexes may occur with lesions affecting UMNs cranial to the reflex; this is because the UMN system has an overall inhibiting influence on LMN (see Chapter 5: Inhibition versus excitation). A UMN lesion in the thoracolumbar spinal cord will compromise

UMNs supplying LMNs in the lumbar intumescence. The patellar reflex may be exaggerated or exhibit clonus in which there is sustained stifle extension with tremor; this is more likely with chronic lesions. Note that increased extension of the stifle during patellar reflex testing can also happen when there is loss of tone in the opposing, hamstring muscles due to LMN disease affecting the sciatic nerve; this is called pseudohyperreflexia.

In affected horses that are still ambulatory, it is technically difficult to assess spinal cord reflexes or motor tone. Signs of UMN dysfunction can be assessed by looking for evidence indicating lack of UMN initiation of voluntary movement, for example, the ability of a horse to resist being pulled to one side by its tail while it is walking (see Fig. 5.7).

Clinically, there are a number of reflexes that can be evaluated in the animal. They include limb and trunk reflexes involving spinal nerves, and head reflexes involving cranial nerves. The anatomical basis of these reflexes is described in Tables 10.2 and 13.3.

The spinal reflexes that can be routinely and reliably tested in companion animals include the withdrawal reflex in the pelvic and thoracic limbs and the patellar reflex in the pelvic limb. These are usually tested in the recumbent animal. The cutaneous trunci and perineal reflexes can be tested either in the recumbent or standing animal.

Pelvic limb

(a) Patellar reflex. The patellar ligament extends from the distal aspect of the patella to the tibial crest. It is the continuation of the quadriceps tendon distal to the patella. With the animal in lateral recumbency, the patellar ligament is tapped with a plexor (hammer). This causes abrupt extension of the quadriceps muscle, eliciting its reflex contraction and extension of the stifle joint. If the animal is tense then the uppermost limb may be too extended to permit the reflex. This upper limb tension may be due to the animal lifting its head to that side, preparing to get up. Head turning will stimulate the vestibular system causing ipsilateral extension, overriding the patellar reflex. In that case, it is useful to test the reflex on the downside limb, as that limb will usually be more relaxed (Figs. 13.9 and 5.1).

(b) Withdrawal (flexor or pedal) reflex. Pinching the toes causes flexion of the limb using all the limb flexor muscles innervated by the sciatic nerve and the femoral nerve innervating the rectus femoris muscle of the quadriceps. Hip flexion may also involve the iliopsoas muscle innervated by lumbar nerves. For the withdrawal

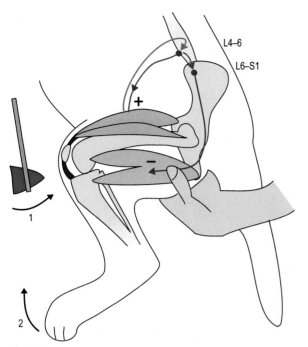

Fig. 13.9 **Testing the patellar reflex in the dog. Tapping the patellar ligament with the plexor (1) results in stifle extension (2) (see section on myotatic reflexes, Chapter 5).**

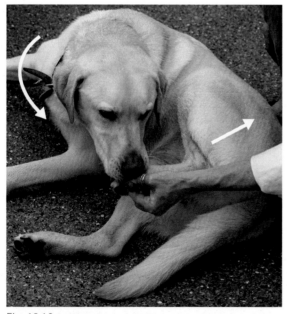

Fig. 13.10 **Testing the pedal/withdrawal reflex in a dog. Barney is reflexively pulling his foot away and showing conscious awareness of the noxious stimulus.**

reflex observe how well the animal can flex each joint in the limb (Fig. 13.10). For example, the hock may not flex well if the animal has a subtle LMN lesion affecting the sciatic nerve.

In ambulant horses the patellar reflexes and withdrawal reflexes cannot be assessed.

Trunk
(a) Perineal reflex. Tactile stimulation of the perineal region will cause reflex contraction of the anal sphincter and flexion of the tail.
(b) Cutaneous trunci reflex. This reflex is elicited by pinching of the dorsal skin, 2–3 cm lateral to the

spinal column, beginning at the iliac crest and moving cranially to the cranial thorax. In the normal animal stimulation of the truncal dermatomes on one side results in twitching of the skin on the lateral aspect of the thorax bilaterally (Fig. 13.11). In horses and cattle the reflex is best elicited by firmly tapping the skin over the trunk with a blunt instrument such as a pair of forceps.
(c) Neck skin reflexes. In horses, pinching/tapping the skin on the lateral aspect of the neck stimulates contraction of the cutaneous colli muscle. This is a local reflex testing the function of cervical nerves (sensory and motor) and the cervical spinal cord.

Thoracic limb
The withdrawal reflex is the main reflex tested in the thoracic limb and is done by pinching the toes. Withdrawal (limb flexion) involves flexor muscles throughout the limb; these muscles are innervated by a variety of nerves from the brachial plexus (see Fig. 4.7).

Nociception
Of clinical importance during the neurological examination is assessing both the reflex action and conscious response of the animal to nociceptive stimuli. The integrity of both the Aδ- (fast- conducting, pin-prick pain) and C-fibres (slow-conducting, acute pain fibres) is evaluated. Both types of fibre synapse in the dorsal horn where they make connections with LMN for a variety of reflex functions, including the withdrawal, cutaneous trunci or perineal reflexes. Input is also transmitted to the brain for conscious perception. Aδ-fibres transmit stimuli from superficial regions (skin) and so stimuli can be localised precisely by the forebrain. From spinal nerves, they travel cranially, primarily in the dorsal funiculus of the spinal cord (fasciculus gracilis and cuneatus). C-fibres are tested using pressure stimuli such as the application of haemostats to the digit. C fibres also convey stimuli from deeply located tissues, e.g viscera, and that maybe only poorly localised by the forebrain. These stimuli travel cranially, in lateral and ventral funiculi on both sides of the spinal cord, in a number of different tracts (see Fig. 6.4). Nociceptive tracts synapse in the brainstem, and pass rostrally to the forebrain (somatosensory cortex and limbic system).

Prognostically, in cases of paralysis, it is essential to determine whether the spinal cord is functionally intact. The last neural function to be lost with increasing severity of spinal cord lesions is nociception from deeply located tissues such as bone. Conveying such nociceptive stimuli are C-type fibres in the PNS and several spinal cord tracts sited in different funiculi (see Chapter 6). To evaluate whether an animal perceives a noxious stimulus requires that a conscious response to the stimulus be observed. A noxious stimulus is applied to the foot by pinching the digit. This stimulus should produce two effects in the normal animal: (a) reflex withdrawal of the foot and (b) conscious perception of the stimulus indicated by the animal turning and looking at the foot, or whining, or pupil dilation due to a response of the sympathetic nervous system (Fig. 13.10). If the animal only demonstrates the withdrawal reflex but no conscious perception of the noxious stimulus, then the clinician knows that the reflex wiring is intact but the animal probably has a functional, or structural, transection of the spinal cord cranial to the region involved with the withdrawal reflex arc. Thus loss of conscious

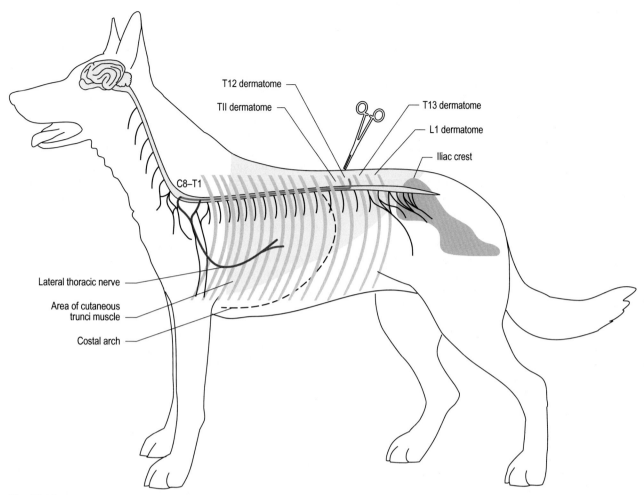

Fig. 13.11 **The cutaneous trunci reflex assesses sensation in dermatomes associated with spinal nerves located from the cranial thoracic region to L1 or L2.**

response to a noxious stimulus usually indicates a guarded or poor prognosis for return of spinal cord function; the outcome for the animal depends on the cause of the lesion and available treatment. Of course, if the LMNs of the withdrawal reflex arc are damaged the withdrawal may be reduced or absent. If the animal shows a conscious response, then that tells the clinician that the spinal cord is not transected (functionally or anatomically). This indicates a better prognosis than if there is no conscious response.

To test nociception in the head, the clinician may stimulate just inside the nares, for example, with the tip of haemostats. This stimulus should result in the animal pulling its head away abruptly. Animals with lesions in the somatosensory cortex may have hypalgesia and not pull the head away when the nostril contralateral to the lesion is stimulated as the pathway to the somatosensory cortex decussates (Fig. 13.12).

Vertebral column and spinal cord hyperpathia

Hyperpathia refers to increased sensitivity, such that a non-noxious stimulus is perceived as a noxious one. Spinal hyperpathia indicates disease in the vertebral column, intervertebral discs, spinal ligaments and/or meninges. It may be focal, as occurs with an extruded intervertebral disc, or extensive as occurs in meningitis. The presence of spinal pain is assessed by palpation and application of focal pressure to the vertebral column or paraspinal muscles. Spinal manipulation, primarily of the neck or lumbosacral region, may also be performed *if appropriate*. Do *not*

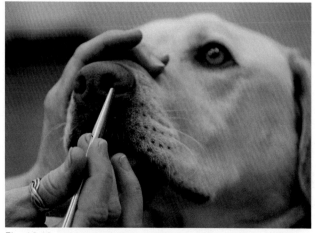

Fig. 13.12 **Testing nociception in the head. The vestibule of the external nares is innervated by the nerve, a branch of the trigeminal nerve; the nasal planum is innervated by the maxillary nerve (CN V) of CN V.**

manipulate, or palpate firmly, the vertebral column in any cases in which spinal instability is suspected, for example in cases of suspected trauma or atlanto-axial subluxation. Neck manipulation in cases of caudal cervical malformation-malarticulation (Wobbler) syndrome may exacerbate compression of the spinal cord. Bending the neck may cause redundant ligament to buckle, increasing spinal cord compression. Firm palpation is also not appropriate in spinal trauma cases as structures may be unstable. Palpation is useful for determining sites of intervertebral disc extrusion, but manipulation is not appropriate as it may exacerbate the extrusion.

To assess for areas of sensitivity along the vertebral column, it is useful to have the animal standing (if it can); it can also be done in the recumbent animal. Placing one hand under the abdomen not only supports the animal, but also can detect tensing of the abdominal muscles. In a more stoic animal, that tensing may help indicate when an area of increased sensitivity is palpated.

When palpating the vertebral column, the clinician gently applies firm pressure to the top or sides of the vertebrae. In the normal animal, this pressure is non-noxious. If the animal has increased sensitivity in the vertebral column already, due to a lesion, then that pressure is perceived as noxious and the animal will indicate that behaviourally by tensing, flinching, whining, snapping, or pulling away.

Beginning at the lumbosacral area and moving cranially to T1, the clinician places their fingers and thumb on opposite sides of the vertebral column and applies downwards pressure to the transverse processes or heads of the ribs (Fig. 13.13). Having done that, it is useful to start caudally again and apply downwards pressure between each dorsal spinous process. The first run is a general survey of the vertebral column, while the second is more specific, testing for precise areas of pain.

For the neck, if no instability is suspected, the animal's head is gently turned laterally to either side, then dorsally and ventrally. The normal animal should be able to look around at its tail, more than 180° upwards and the nose should be able to point ventrally and caudally between its thoracic limbs. For more precise localisation of hyperpathia, a hand is placed on either side of the neck and pressure

applied to the cervical vertebral column from caudal to cranial. Gentle rotational pressure can be applied to the wings of the atlas. Note that the caudal cervical vertebrae are closer to the ventral aspect of the neck than the dorsal. The dorsal aspect of the neck is primarily muscle and nuchal ligament.

Assessing autonomic function

The urinary bladder is palpated for size and tone and, in the incontinent animal, for ease of manual expression. If the animal is incontinent a full, turgid bladder that is difficult to express suggests the presence of an UMN lesion, whereas one that is large, with a flaccid wall and that is easy to express, indicates a LMN lesion involving the urinary bladder (see Fig. 12.8).

In cases of faecal incontinence, the presence or absence of anal tone and the perineal reflex is important in differentiating UMN lesions cranial to the sacral spinal cord from LMN lesions involving the sacral spinal cord or its outflow.

The integrity of the ANS LMNs can also be evaluated by assessing pupil size and response to stimulation by light (pupillary light reflex). The amount of ocular, nasal and oral secretions can be assessed, while warmth and colour of the ears can indicate changes in vascular tone. In horses, changes in cutaneous blood flow may result in sweating (see Fig. 12.6). In animals with dysautonomia, there may also be changes in cardiovascular and gastrointestinal function with altered heart rates and gut motility.

Functional road map of the nervous system

Using a map of the nervous system that depicts the main pathways and functional areas, the clinician can determine what signs the animal will have with lesions in different regions. Conversely, given a set of clinical signs, the clinician will be able to use the map to identify where the lesion is likely to be.

The following is a summary of the location of the functions that are assessed in a neurological examination. From this NeuroMaps of the brain and spinal cord have been drawn (Figs. 13.14 and Fig. 13.15).

Anatomical basis of the neurological examination: key points (see specific chapters for details)
Proprioception (Chapters 4, 6, 7, 8)
(a) The pathways for subconscious proprioception are as follows.
    From the neck, trunk, limbs and tail: muscle and tendon receptors, spinal nerves, dorsal horn of spinal cord, ipsilateral lateral funiculus (mostly), brain stem, ipsilateral cerebellum.
    From the head: Vestibular receptors of the inner ear, vestibular portion of CN VIII, vestibular nuclei of brainstem, cerebellar peduncles (caudal), ipsilateral cerebellum.
(b) The pathways for conscious proprioception are as follows:
    In the neck, trunk, limbs and tail, from tactile, joint, muscle and tendon receptors, to spinal nerves, dorsal horn, ipsilateral dorsal and lateral funiculus, brain stem, decussates, thalamus, contralateral somatosensory cortex.

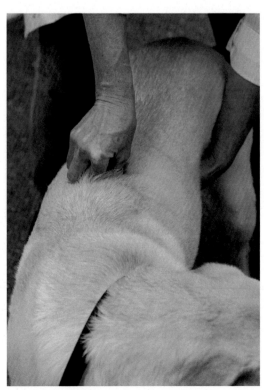

Fig. 13.13 **Testing for increased sensitivity by applying downwards pressure along the vertebral column. Note the supporting hand under the abdomen (see text).**

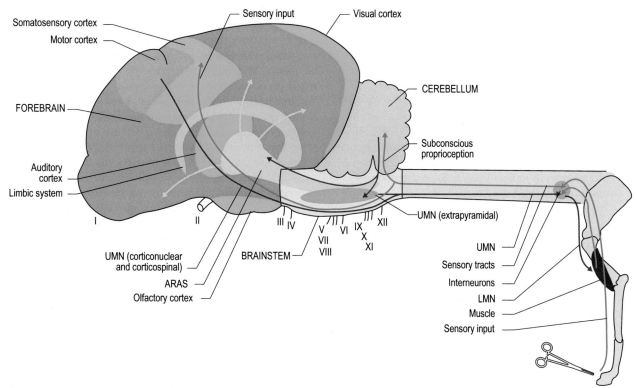

Fig. 13.14 **NeuroMap depicting main neural functions assessed in a neurological examination. If a focal area of the map is covered representing a lesion, then it can be seen which neural functions would be compromised and which would not be affected. The brain is divided into three functional regions – forebrain (orange), brainstem (yellow) and cerebellum (purple) (see also Fig. 4.11 for main functional regions of the brain). Green lines indicate sensory systems and red lines identify motor systems. ARAS = ascending reticular activating system; UMN = upper motor neuron, LMN = lower motor neuron. Note both the corticospinal tract and the sensory projection to the somatosensory cortex, decussate in the caudal brainstem. Thus the motor and somatosensory cortices project to/from the contralateral side of the body.**

From the head: Vestibular receptors of the inner ear, vestibular portion of CN VIII, vestibular nuclei of brainstem, decussates in brainstem, thalamus, contralateral temporal lobe.

Motor function (Chapters 4, 5, 7, 8, 9)
Motor planning centres are located in the forebrain, whereas motor coordination occurs in the cerebellum.

Upper (central) motor neuron (UMN) centres are located in the motor cortex and the brainstem. UMN tracts connect locally to LMN in cranial nerve nuclei of the brainstem. UMN tracts also travel caudally along the spinal cord to influence LMNs of spinal nerves. UMNs in the lateral funiculi, facilitate flexor muscle activity; UMNs in the ventral funiculi facilitate extensor muscle activity.

Lower (peripheral) motor neurons arise in the CNS, but their axons leave it via cranial and spinal nerves and connect with muscles (somatic or visceral (i.e. efferent fibres of the ANS)) at neuromuscular junctions.

For reflex activity, sensory fibres from peripheral receptors connect with LMNs of cranial nerves, or LMNs of spinal nerves in the brainstem or spinal cord, respectively.

Behaviour and memory (Chapter 11)
These functions are associated primarily with the forebrain limbic system (e.g. hippocampus and associated structures).

Arousal (Chapter 11)
Mental awareness is associated with the ascending reticular activating system (ARAS) of the brainstem and diffuse areas of the forebrain. Mental awareness can be decreased with relatively focal lesions in the ARAS of the brainstem or with

diffuse lesions affecting widespread areas of the forebrain. Examples of focal versus diffuse lesions would include a tumour in the brainstem versus hepatic encephalopathy, which globally affects the forebrain.

Cranial nerves (Chapter 10)
The anatomical basis for cranial nerve function is covered in Table 13.2.

Nociception (Chapter 6)
For withdrawal reflex function
For the limbs: Nociceptor, named or spinal nerves, dorsal horn, ventral horns of multiple spinal cord segments in that intumescence, LMNs to flexor muscles of that limb causing flexion of the limb. Additionally, in the standing animal, the other limbs, especially the contralateral one, will be reflexively stimulated to extend, to carry additional weight.

From the head: nociceptor, primarily the trigeminal nerve, CN V (also CNN VII, IX and X from both the oral cavity and external ear), to the spinal nucleus of CN V (medulla oblongata). Reflex connections occur with the motor nucleus of the facial nerve for facial muscle contraction, nuclei of CNN III, IV and VI for eyeball movement and IX and X (nucleus ambiguus) for gagging.

For conscious perception
From the body and limbs: nociceptor, spinal nerves, dorsal horn, dorsal funiculus (for Aδ-fibre input), lateral and ventral funiculi (for C-fibre input). (C-fibre nociception is projected cranially in multiple pathways, some of which are bilaterally represented and may have multiple synapses). Tracts and pathways decussate in the brainstem,

travel to the thalamus and the contralateral somatosensory cortex.

From the head: nociceptor, trigeminal nerve (CN V), spinal tract of V in the medulla oblongata, fibres decussate and travel rostrally (trigeminal lemniscus), to the thalamus and to the contralateral somatosensory cortex.

Vertebral column/spinal cord hyperpathia

The anatomical basis involves sensory receptors in muscles, ligaments, tendon, periosteum and meninges; sensory spinal nerves, especially the C-type fibres, input into the associated spinal cord region and transmission as for nociception to the contralateral somatosensory cortex.

The NeuroMap: Overview of the nervous system

The NeuroMaps are functional road maps of the neuraxis (Figs. 13.14 and Fig. 13.15). They depict the location of the neural functions that are evaluated in the neurological examination. The NeuroMap allows the clinician to see which functions would be compromised, AND which functions would still be normal, if there was a lesion in a particular area. For example, a lesion in the spinal cord

could compromise both conscious and subconscious proprioceptive pathways and UMN pathways, causing gait deficits. However there are no cranial nerves or centres associated with arousal in the cord, so these functions will be normal. The following two key concepts that have been stated previously (see Fig. 13.1 and end of Chap 1); these are fundamental to understanding lesion localisation (1) Noting which neural systems are functioning normally is just as important as noting those that are dysfunctional; (2) It does not matter where the lesion is located on a pathway – origin, midpoint or termination, the clinical signs of dysfunction will be similar. This is analogous to a battery (origin), linked by a wire (midpoint) to a light bulb (termination). The same sign (no light) will be present regardless of where the problem is located (battery, wire, bulb).

Summary of functions in the neuraxis

Table 13.4 has been constructed using the NeuroMap in Fig. 13.14 and can be used in conjunction with it. It tabulates which functions are associated with each region of the brain and the generalised spinal cord. A specific NeuroMap of the spinal cord is given in Figure 13.15 and effects of lesions in different regions are summarised in Table 13.5. From the NeuroMap, it can be predicted

Table 13.4 Summary of neural functions that are associated with the different regions of the neuraxis

Function	Forebrain	Brainstem	Cerebellum	Spinal cord
Proprioception				
a) Conscious	Yes, somatosensory cortex (contralateral projection)	Yes	No	Yes
b) Subconscious	No	Yes, caudal brainstem	Yes	Yes
Nociception	Yes (contralateral projection)	Yes (entire body)	No	Yes (neck, trunk, limbs, tail)
Motor systems	Yes, important for planning motor function and voluntary movement	Yes, major site of UMN nuclei in quadrupeds, important in posture and locomotion	Yes, for motor coordination (not motor strength)	Yes
	Motor cortex (UMN), functions in voluntary motor activity, but has a minor role in gait. No LMNs	Cranial nerves have LMNs innervating head and neck muscles		UMN tracts
				LMNs innervating neck, trunk limbs and tail
Behaviour, emotion and memory	Yes	No	No	No
	Limbic system			
Arousal	Diffuse areas of forebrain	Yes, ascending reticular activating system (ARAS)	No	No
Cranial nerves	CN 1, II (II - mainly contralateral projection)	CN III-XII	CN VIII head and eyeball position[1]	No[2]
Spinal cord reflexes	No	No	No	Yes

[1]the cerebellum has important links with the vestibular nuclei of the brainstem, see Chapter 8
[2]Although the external branch of CN XI arises from the spinal cord, functional deficits in the muscles it innervates are not usually detectable in cervical spinal cord lesions.

Table 13.5 Summary of effect of lesions in different areas of the spinal cord

Location of lesion	Loss of proprioception and sensory input	Presence of UMN signs	Presence of LMN signs to limbs Loss of other reflexes	Loss of urinary and faecal continence
Cervical C1–5	TL, trunk, PL, tail	TL and PL both affected	No LMN signs in TL and PL. Cutaneous trunci and perineal reflexes intact	UMN bladder[a] Faecal incontinence[c]
Cervical intumescence C6–T2	TL, trunk, PL, tail	PL only	TL only, loss of cutaneous trunci reflex if lesion in C8–T1; perineal reflex intact	UMN bladder Faecal incontinence[c] anal sphincter tone intact
Thoracolumbar T3–L3	trunk (caudal to lesion), PL, tail (TL normal)	PL only	No LMN signs in TL and PL Cutaneous trunci reflex lost caudal to lesion; perineal reflex intact	UMN bladder Faecal incontinence[c] anal sphincter tone intact
Cranial lumbosacral L4–S1	PL, tail; (TL normal)	No UMN signs to limbs	LMN signs in PL Cutaneous trunci and perineal reflexes intact	Bladder likely to be UMN Faecal incontinence[c] anal sphincter tone intact
Caudal lumbosacral S1–S3	Perineum, tail; PL probably normal[d]	No UMN signs to limbs	LMN signs to pelvic viscera, loss of perineal reflex; PL probably normal[d]	LMN bladder[b] LMN anal sphincter (dilated anus), faecal incontinence with dropping of faeces
Caudal nerves Cd1-5	Tail	No UMN signs	Tail	Normal continence

TL = thoracic limb, PL = pelvic limb.
[a]UMN bladder – turgid, full, difficult to express.
[b]LMN bladder – flaccid, distended, easy to express, dribbling urine.
[c]Animal will deposit faeces with good emptying of colon, but may not be aware that it is defecating.
[d]May see some proprioceptive deficits or paresis with an S1–S3 lesion as S1 and S2 make variable contributions to the sciatic nerves.
Note: whether or not all signs are present, depends on lesion severity.

which neural functions could be compromised by lesions in the different areas of CNS. For example, by looking at the forebrain in Fig. 13.14 or reading down the column associated with the forebrain in Table 13.4, it can be seen that a forebrain lesion may cause dysfunction in contralateral conscious proprioception, nociception and vision, but the rest of the cranial nerves and gait will be reasonably normal. (It is unusual to detect olfactory or auditory deficits in forebrain disease.) If the animal has reduced alertness, then the lesion involves extensive areas of the forebrain. Decreased voluntary use of the contralateral side of the body may be observed.

Signs of dysfunction in different regions of the neuraxis

Listed in the following text are signs that can occur with lesions affecting different regions of the neuraxis. Note that not all signs may occur depending on the precise location of the lesion and its severity.

Forebrain disease
Abnormal neurological function
- Conscious proprioception (CP) deficits (knuckling and stumbling) on the contralateral side of the body, but ambulation/gait and posture are still quite good indicating retained subconscious proprioception and motor strength. May ambulate in wide circles, usually towards the side of the lesion.
- Could have hypalgesia (decreased nociception) on the contralateral side, this is more readily detected by testing head nociception.
- Decreased voluntary motor function of the contralateral side of the body (e.g. kitten playing with a ball).
- Deficits in vision (contralateral).
- Deficits in olfaction, although it may be difficult to appreciate reduced olfaction.
- Reduced arousal if the lesion involves widespread areas of the forebrain.
- Altered behaviour and emotion and potentially memory (e.g. loss of learned behaviour such as toileting).

Normal neurological function
- It would not affect CNN III–XII, most of the UMN nuclei, subconscious proprioception, motor coordination, therefore gait will be quite good.
- Spinal cord reflexes will be present and vertebral column/spinal cord hyperpathia will not be present.

Brainstem disease
Abnormal neurological function
- Conscious proprioceptive deficits (knuckling and stumbling) as the pathway passes through the brainstem to the forebrain.
- Subconscious proprioceptive deficits (ataxia, base wide/narrow posture) if caudal brainstem disease.
- Nociception (especially superficial, Aδ-fibre input) could be reduced especially from the head and possibly from the trunk and limbs too, as that pathway passes through the brainstem going to the forebrain.
- Decreased motor function – there are many UMN nuclei and UMN axons in this area; this would show up as paresis/gait deficits.
- Decreased arousal due to effect on ascending reticular activating system.

- CNN dysfunction that is specific to the rostral brainstem
  - CNN III–VIII dysfunction.
- CNN dysfunction that is specific to the caudal brainstem
  - CNN IX–XII dysfunction.

Normal neurological function
- It would not affect CNN I or II (forebrain).
- Spinal cord reflexes will be present and vertebral column/spinal cord hyperpathia will not be present.

Cerebellar disease
Abnormal neurological function
- Subconscious proprioceptive deficits causing postural deficits affecting limbs, trunk and head, both at rest and during motion; wide- or narrow-based stance; ataxic gait, truncal sway; circumduction or crossing over of feet during ambulation. Delayed protraction of limbs.
- Tremor due to incoordination of agonist–antagonist muscle function.
- Hypermetria with increased rate, range and force of movement.
- Spasticity due to decreased inhibitory effect of cerebellum on brainstem UMN centres.
- Damage to the vestibulocerebellum/flocculonodular lobe can cause postural disturbances, head tilt and nystagmus.
- The menace response may be decreased with diffuse cerebellar disease.

Normal neurological function
- Conscious proprioception should be normal.
- The animal is not paretic (weak), if anything it tends to spasticity.
- Most cranial nerves function normally (see comments re CN VIII and menace response).
- The animal is bright and alert.
- Spinal cord reflexes will be present and vertebral column/spinal cord hyperpathia will not be present.

Spinal cord disease
See Fig. 13.15. The effects of lesions in different regions of the spinal cord are summarised in table 13.5.

Abnormal neurological function
- Conscious and subconscious proprioceptive deficits occur as both types of proprioceptive pathways travel cranially through the spinal cord. These deficits result in knuckling, stumbling, ataxia and hypometria (reduced rate, range and force of movement).
- Decreased motor function (paresis/paralysis) – due to effects on either UMN tracts or LMNs.
- Spinal cord reflexes may be lost if the lesion affects the spinal cord segments associated with that reflex. Exaggerated spinal reflexes may occur with UMN lesions.
- Hypotonia and atrophy of specific muscles if LMN cell bodies in the spinal cord are damaged.
- Vertebral column/spinal cord hyperpathia may be present and can be quite helpful in localising the lesion.

Normal neurological function
- Behaviour, emotion, memory and arousal would be normal.
- Cranial nerve function would be normal.

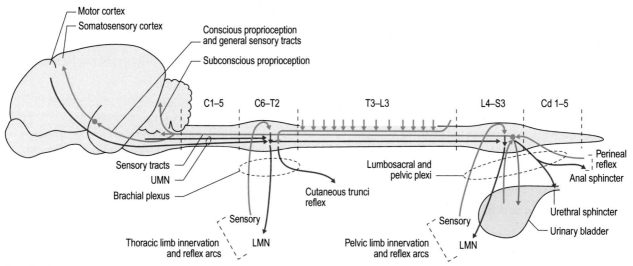

Fig. 13.15 **NeuroMap of the spinal cord. Green indicates sensory systems (conveying tactile, thermal, proprioceptive and nociceptive stimuli), red identifies motor systems and blue identifies autonomic systems. UMN = upper motor neuron, LMN = lower motor neuron**

Spinal nerve disease

Abnormal neurological function

- Loss of afferent (tactile, proprioceptive, nociceptive) input.
- Paresis, (short steps, the animal appears weak) due to loss of LMN output.
- Loss of efferent innervation to muscle may result in LMN signs decreased **R**eflexes, significant muscle **A**trophy and decreased muscle **T**one (the Neuro **RAT** - Fig. 5.6).

Neuromuscular disease

Neuromuscular disease is caused by lesions of the peripheral motor unit. The motor unit involves the LMN cell body, efferent spinal nerve, neuromuscular junction and muscle. Thus the animal could have LMN signs. Marked atrophy and loss of tone may be present if the neuromuscular junction is destroyed, but not if it is maintained as in myasthaenia gravis.

In myopathies, the main signs can include stiffness, paresis (see definition in 'Terminology' section), reduced reflexes and atrophy. Myalgia and changes in muscle bulk may be present, with muscle swelling or atrophy in acute versus chronic cases, respectively.

It the disease purely involves the LMN, NMJ or muscle, then the animal's proprioception should be normal, but it may be too paretic to demonstrate this well.

Multifocal disease

In cases of multifocal disease, a single lesion cannot account for all the signs. For example, an animal with visual deficits and a head tilt has to have a lesion in the eyes, optic nerves or visual pathways in the forebrain, and the inner ear or brainstem to involve the vestibular system. Another example would be an animal with tremor and hypermetria (cerebellar) as well as lower motor neuron signs to the pelvic limbs (LMNs arising from L4–S1 spinal cord). The most common cause of multifocal signs in animals is inflammatory disease. Multifocal neoplasia or generalised neuropathies may also cause multifocal signs.

The NeuroMap: The spinal cord

Lesion localisation along the spinal cord follows the same principles as described earlier. If there is a lesion in a particular area, the NeuroMap of the spinal cord allows the clinician to see which neurological functions could be affected and which neurological functions would not be affected (Fig. 13.15).

If the lesion is constrained to the spinal cord, then the cranial nerves, arousal and behaviour will be normal, indicating that the lesion is not intracranial. From this map, Table 13.5 is generated. Note that UMN signs occur when upper (central) motor neurons are lost, whereas LMN signs occur when lower (peripheral) motor neurons are lost. UMN and LMN signs are differentiated by the Neuro RAT (**R**eflexes, **A**trophy, **T**one) (see Fig. 5.6).

Appendix

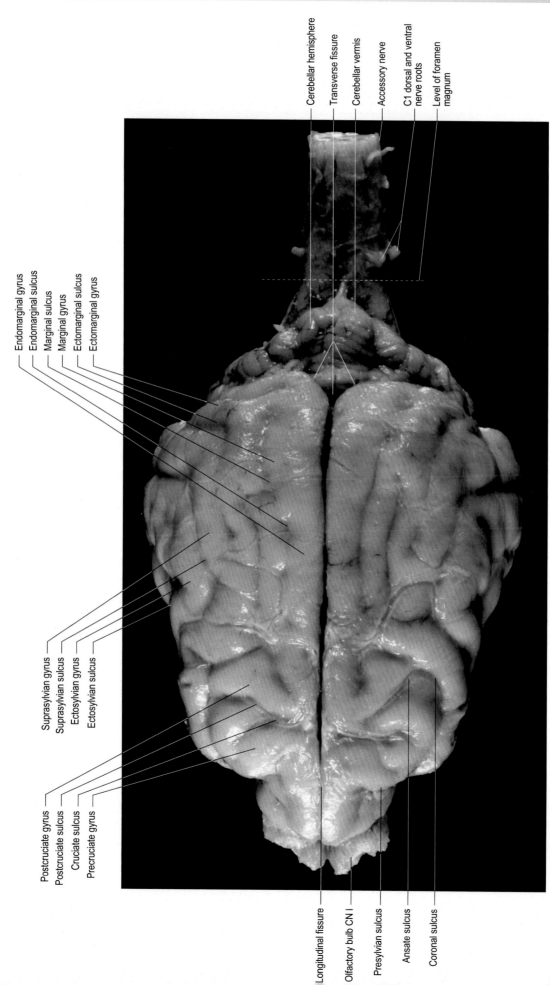

Cerebellar hemisphere
Transverse fissure
Cerebellar vermis
Accessory nerve
C1 dorsal and ventral nerve roots
Level of foramen magnum

Endomarginal gyrus
Endomarginal sulcus
Marginal sulcus
Marginal gyrus
Ectomarginal sulcus
Ectomarginal gyrus

Suprasylvian gyrus
Suprasylvian sulcus
Ectosylvian gyrus
Ectosylvian sulcus

Postcruciate gyrus
Postcruciate sulcus
Cruciate sulcus
Precruciate gyrus

Longitudinal fissure
Olfactory bulb CN I
Presylvian sulcus
Ansate sulcus
Coronal sulcus

Fig. A.1 **Canine brain, dorsal aspect.**

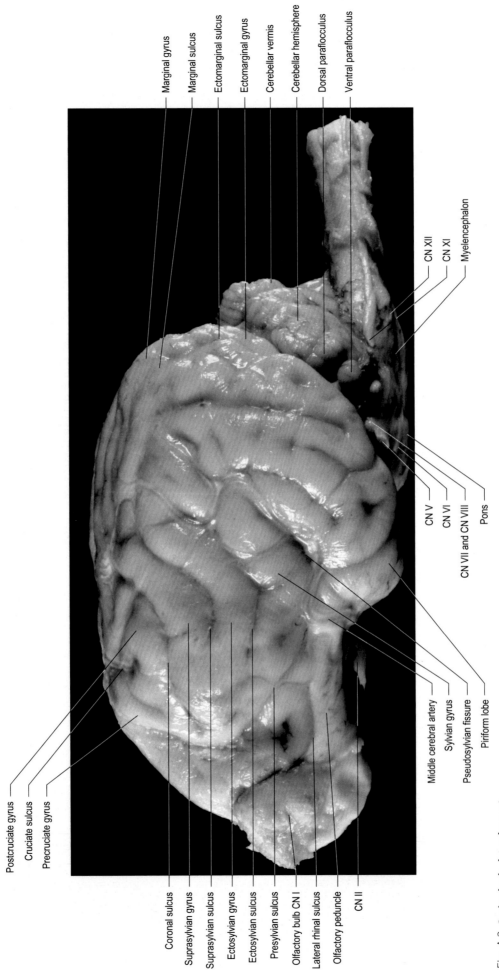

Fig. A.2 **Canine brain, lateral aspect.**

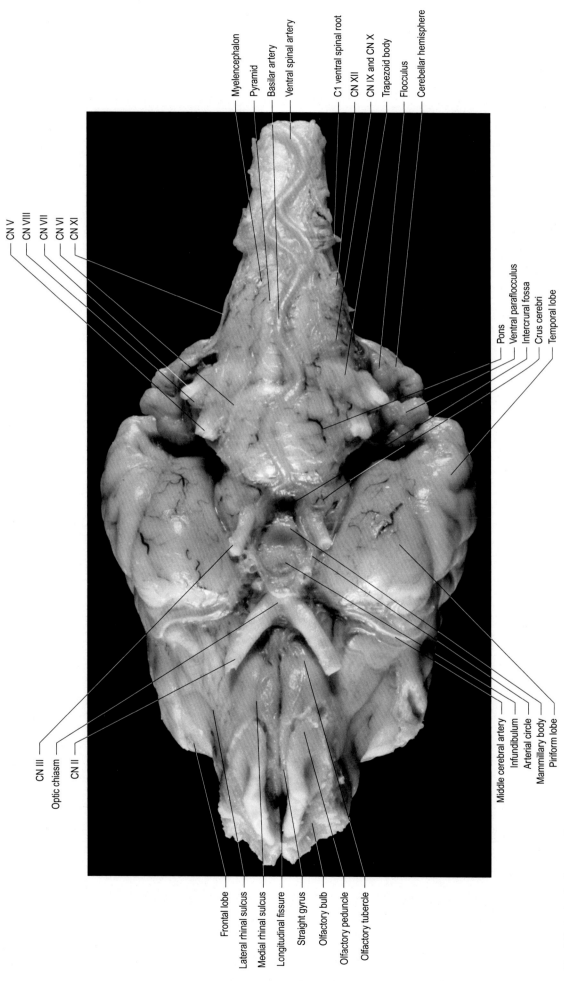

CN V
CN VIII
CN VII
CN VI
CN XI

Myelencephalon
Pyramid
Basilar artery
Ventral spinal artery
C1 ventral spinal root
CN XII
CN IX and CN X
Trapezoid body
Flocculus
Cerebellar hemisphere

Pons
Ventral paraflocculus
Intercrural fossa
Crus cerebri
Temporal lobe

CN III
Optic chiasm
CN II

Middle cerebral artery
Infundibulum
Arterial circle
Mammillary body
Piriform lobe

Frontal lobe
Lateral rhinal sulcus
Medial rhinal sulcus
Longitudinal fissure
Straight gyrus
Olfactory bulb
Olfactory peduncle
Olfactory tubercle

Fig. A.3 **Canine brain, ventral aspect.**

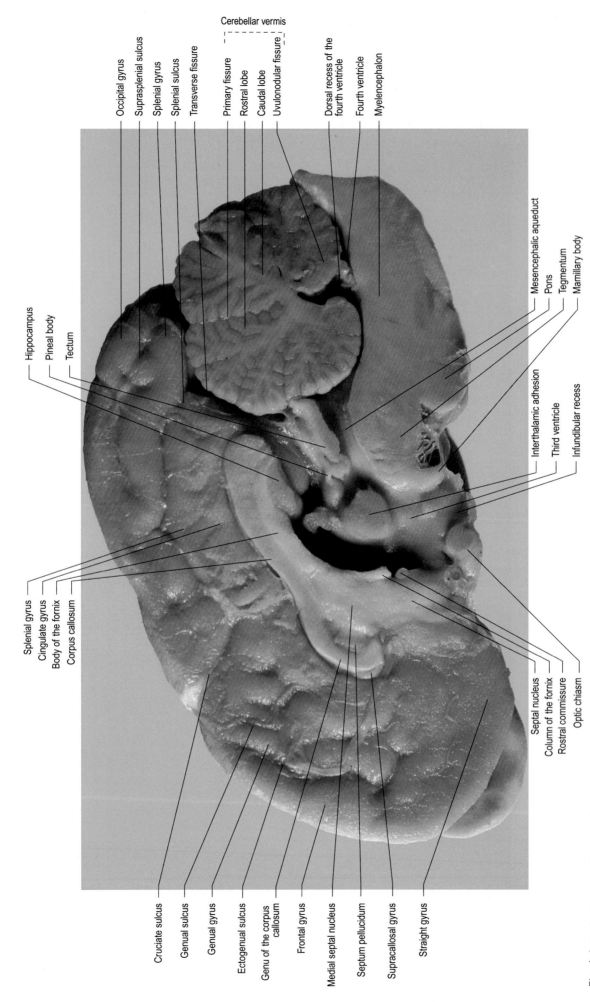

Fig. A.4 **Canine brain, median aspect.**

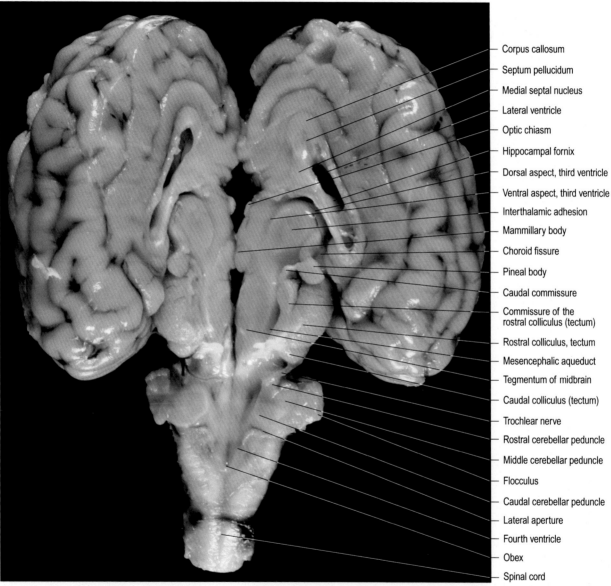

Corpus callosum
Septum pellucidum
Medial septal nucleus
Lateral ventricle
Optic chiasm
Hippocampal fornix
Dorsal aspect, third ventricle
Ventral aspect, third ventricle
Interthalamic adhesion
Mammillary body
Choroid fissure
Pineal body
Caudal commissure
Commissure of the
rostral colliculus (tectum)
Rostral colliculus, tectum
Mesencephalic aqueduct
Tegmentum of midbrain
Caudal colliculus (tectum)
Trochlear nerve
Rostral cerebellar peduncle
Middle cerebellar peduncle
Flocculus
Caudal cerebellar peduncle
Lateral aperture
Fourth ventricle
Obex
Spinal cord

Fig. A.5 **Sheep brain, split dorsally to the level of the fourth ventricle. Forebrain and midbrain viewed from the dorsomedial aspect; medulla oblongata viewed from the dorsal aspect. The bulk of cerebellum has been removed.**

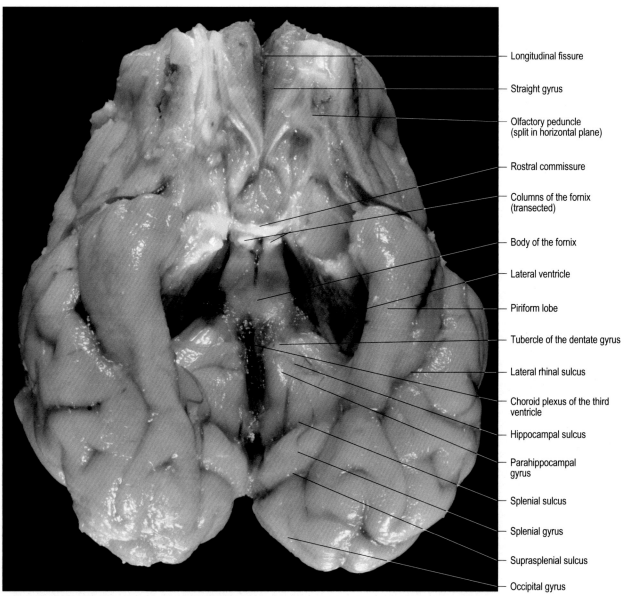

Longitudinal fissure

Straight gyrus

Olfactory peduncle
(split in horizontal plane)

Rostral commissure

Columns of the fornix
(transected)

Body of the fornix

Lateral ventricle

Piriform lobe

Tubercle of the dentate gyrus

Lateral rhinal sulcus

Choroid plexus of the third
ventricle

Hippocampal sulcus

Parahippocampal
gyrus

Splenial sulcus

Splenial gyrus

Suprasplenial sulcus

Occipital gyrus

Fig. A.6 **Sheep cerebral hemispheres, ventral aspect.**

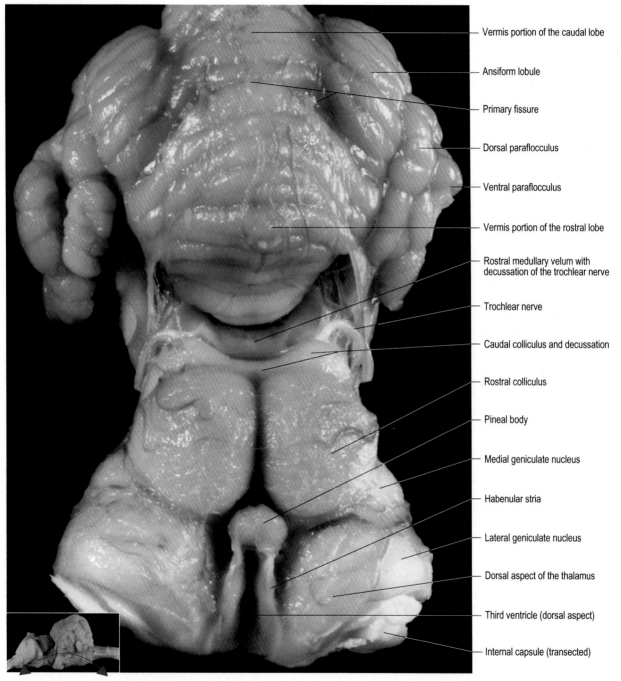

Vermis portion of the caudal lobe

Ansiform lobule

Primary fissure

Dorsal paraflocculus

Ventral paraflocculus

Vermis portion of the rostral lobe

Rostral medullary velum with decussation of the trochlear nerve

Trochlear nerve

Caudal colliculus and decussation

Rostral colliculus

Pineal body

Medial geniculate nucleus

Habenular stria

Lateral geniculate nucleus

Dorsal aspect of the thalamus

Third ventricle (dorsal aspect)

Internal capsule (transected)

Fig. A.7 **Sheep brainstem, dorsal aspect, cerebral hemispheres have been removed. The brainstem has been curved dorsally (see inset) to better display the anatomical features.**

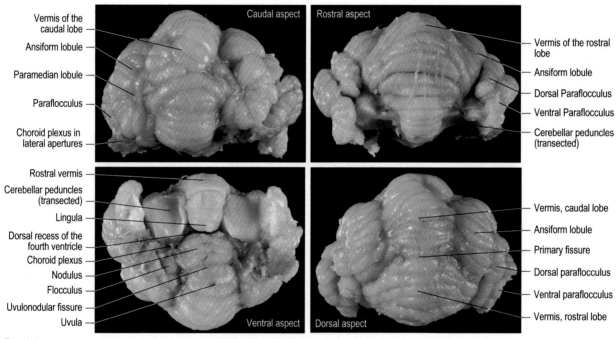

Vermis of the caudal lobe

Ansiform lobule

Paramedian lobule

Paraflocculus

Choroid plexus in lateral apertures

Caudal aspect

Rostral aspect

Vermis of the rostral lobe

Ansiform lobule

Dorsal Paraflocculus

Ventral Paraflocculus

Cerebellar peduncles (transected)

Rostral vermis

Cerebellar peduncles (transected)

Lingula

Dorsal recess of the fourth ventricle

Choroid plexus

Nodulus

Flocculus

Uvulonodular fissure

Uvula

Ventral aspect

Dorsal aspect

Vermis, caudal lobe

Ansiform lobule

Primary fissure

Dorsal paraflocculus

Ventral paraflocculus

Vermis, rostral lobe

Fig. A.8 **Sheep cerebellum, caudal, rostral, ventral and dorsal aspects.**

1. Olfactory bulbs and frontal lobes

2. Olfactory peduncles and frontal lobes

3. Frontal lobes

4. Corpus striatum

5. Corpus striatum and septal nuclei

6. Optic chiasm

7. Rostral thalamus

8. Interthalamic adhesion

9. Geniculate nuclei

10. Rostral mesencephalon

10a. Caudal mesencephalon (rostral aspect)

11. Pons

12. Cerebellar peduncles

13. Rostral fourth ventricle and cerebellar nuclei

14. Caudal fourth ventricle

15. Myelencephalon caudal to the obex

16. Caudal myelencephalon

17. Brainstem-spinal cord junction

18. Cervical spinal cord (dorsal aspect)

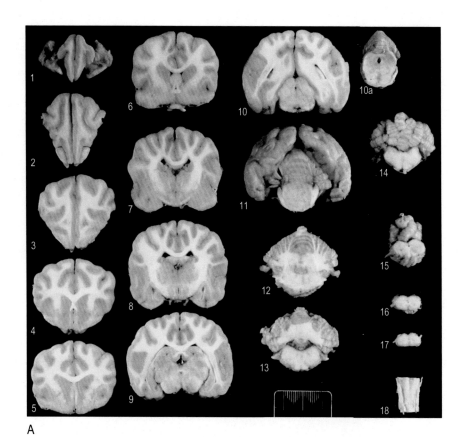

A

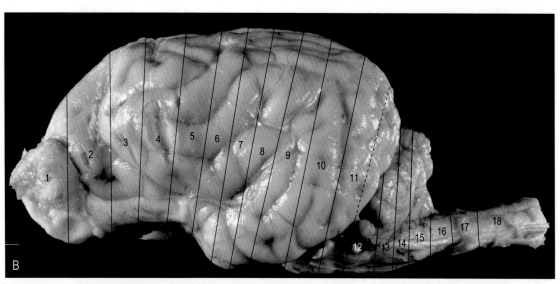

B

Fig. A.9 **(A) Canine brain. The top figure is a general overview of the transverse slices depicted in Figures A10–25. (B) Canine brain lateral aspect depicting the location of the slices labelled in Fig. A9a. Scale ruler is in millimetres.**

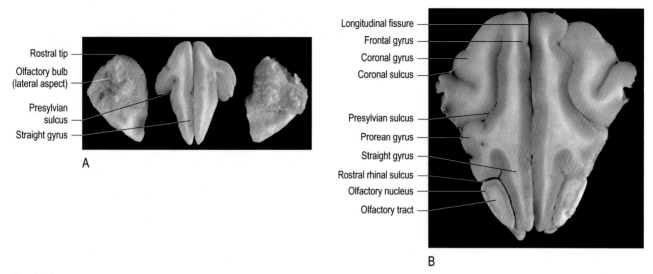

Fig. A.10 **(A) Canine brain, transverse slices at the level of the olfactory bulbs. (B) Canine brain transverse slice through the frontal lobes and olfactory peduncles. (Slices 1 and 2 in Fig. A9a).**

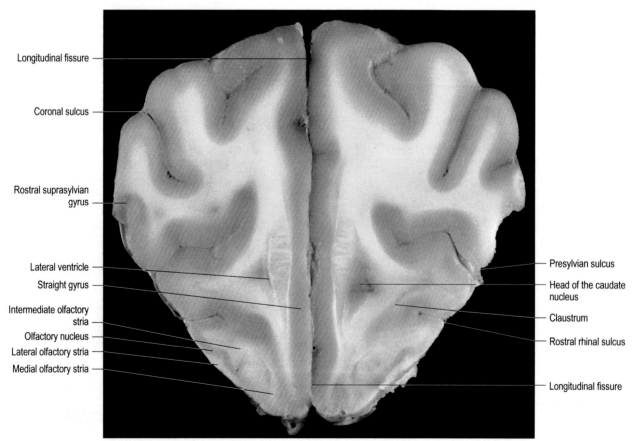

Fig. A.11 **Canine brain, transverse slice at the level of the frontal lobes. (Slice 3 in Fig. A9a).**

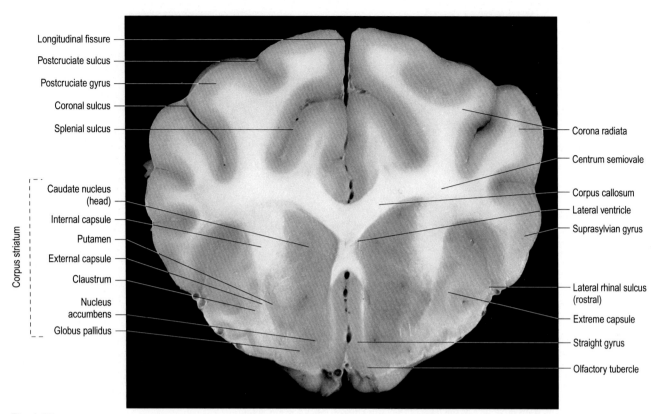

Longitudinal fissure
Postcruciate sulcus
Postcruciate gyrus
Coronal sulcus
Splenial sulcus

Corona radiata
Centrum semiovale
Corpus callosum
Lateral ventricle
Suprasylvian gyrus

Corpus striatum:
Caudate nucleus (head)
Internal capsule
Putamen
External capsule
Claustrum
Nucleus accumbens
Globus pallidus

Lateral rhinal sulcus (rostral)
Extreme capsule
Straight gyrus
Olfactory tubercle

Fig. A.12 **Canine brain, transverse slice at the level of the rostral corpus striatum. (Slice 4 in Fig. A9a).**

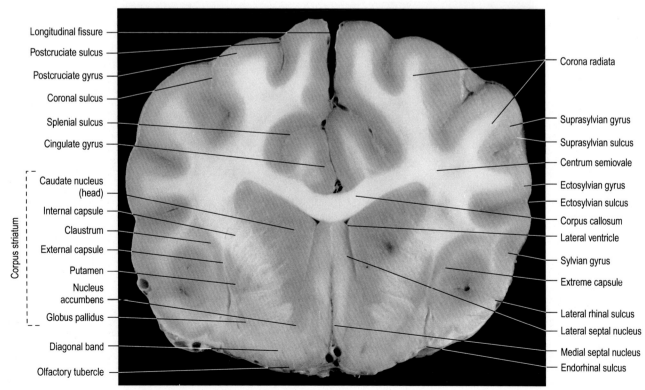

Longitudinal fissure
Postcruciate sulcus
Postcruciate gyrus
Coronal sulcus
Splenial sulcus
Cingulate gyrus

Corona radiata

Suprasylvian gyrus
Suprasylvian sulcus
Centrum semiovale
Ectosylvian gyrus
Ectosylvian sulcus
Corpus callosum
Lateral ventricle

Corpus striatum:
Caudate nucleus (head)
Internal capsule
Claustrum
External capsule
Putamen
Nucleus accumbens
Globus pallidus
Diagonal band
Olfactory tubercle

Sylvian gyrus
Extreme capsule
Lateral rhinal sulcus
Lateral septal nucleus
Medial septal nucleus
Endorhinal sulcus

Fig. A.13 **Canine brain, transverse slice at the level of the septal nuclei. (Slice 5 in Fig. A9a).**

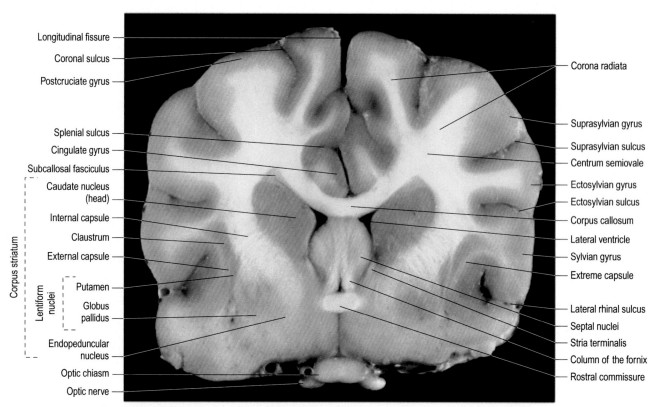

Longitudinal fissure
Coronal sulcus
Postcruciate gyrus

Splenial sulcus
Cingulate gyrus
Subcallosal fasciculus
Caudate nucleus (head)
Internal capsule
Claustrum
External capsule
Putamen
Globus pallidus
Endopeduncular nucleus
Optic chiasm
Optic nerve

Corpus striatum
Lentiform nuclei

Corona radiata
Suprasylvian gyrus
Suprasylvian sulcus
Centrum semiovale
Ectosylvian gyrus
Ectosylvian sulcus
Corpus callosum
Lateral ventricle
Sylvian gyrus
Extreme capsule
Lateral rhinal sulcus
Septal nuclei
Stria terminalis
Column of the fornix
Rostral commissure

Fig. A.14 **Canine brain, transverse slice at the level of the optic chiasm. (Slice 6 in Fig. A9a).**

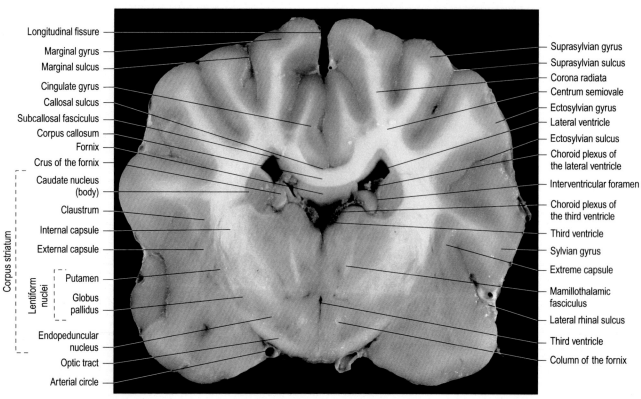

Longitudinal fissure
Marginal gyrus
Marginal sulcus
Cingulate gyrus
Callosal sulcus
Subcallosal fasciculus
Corpus callosum
Fornix
Crus of the fornix
Caudate nucleus (body)
Claustrum
Internal capsule
External capsule
Putamen
Globus pallidus
Endopeduncular nucleus
Optic tract
Arterial circle

Corpus striatum
Lentiform nuclei

Suprasylvian gyrus
Suprasylvian sulcus
Corona radiata
Centrum semiovale
Ectosylvian gyrus
Lateral ventricle
Ectosylvian sulcus
Choroid plexus of the lateral ventricle
Interventricular foramen
Choroid plexus of the third ventricle
Third ventricle
Sylvian gyrus
Extreme capsule
Mamillothalamic fasciculus
Lateral rhinal sulcus
Third ventricle
Column of the fornix

Fig. A.15 **Canine brain, transverse slice at the level of the rostral thalamus. (Slice 7 in Fig. A9a).**

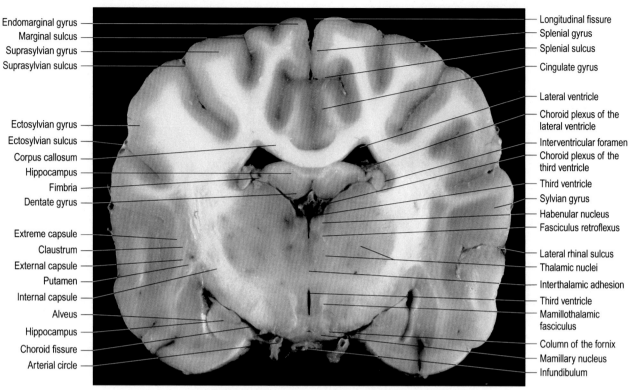

Endomarginal gyrus
Marginal sulcus
Suprasylvian gyrus
Suprasylvian sulcus

Ectosylvian gyrus
Ectosylvian sulcus
Corpus callosum
Hippocampus
Fimbria
Dentate gyrus

Extreme capsule
Claustrum
External capsule
Putamen
Internal capsule
Alveus
Hippocampus
Choroid fissure
Arterial circle

Longitudinal fissure
Splenial gyrus
Splenial sulcus
Cingulate gyrus

Lateral ventricle
Choroid plexus of the lateral ventricle
Interventricular foramen
Choroid plexus of the third ventricle
Third ventricle
Sylvian gyrus
Habenular nucleus
Fasciculus retroflexus

Lateral rhinal sulcus
Thalamic nuclei
Interthalamic adhesion
Third ventricle
Mamillothalamic fasciculus
Column of the fornix
Mamillary nucleus
Infundibulum

Fig. A.16 **Canine brain, transverse slice at the level of the interthalamic adhesion. (Slice 8 in Fig. A9a).**

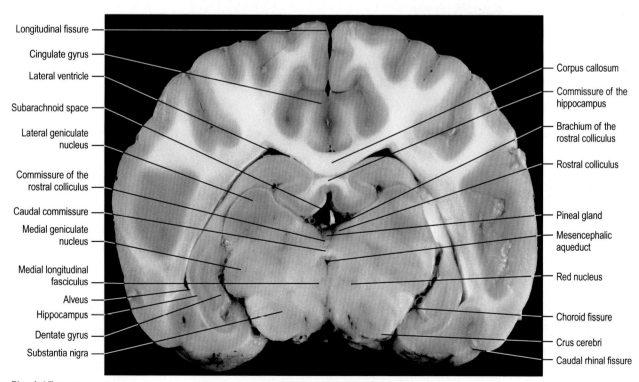

Longitudinal fissure
Cingulate gyrus
Lateral ventricle

Subarachnoid space

Lateral geniculate nucleus

Commissure of the rostral colliculus
Caudal commissure
Medial geniculate nucleus

Medial longitudinal fasciculus
Alveus
Hippocampus
Dentate gyrus
Substantia nigra

Corpus callosum
Commissure of the hippocampus

Brachium of the rostral colliculus

Rostral colliculus

Pineal gland
Mesencephalic aqueduct

Red nucleus

Choroid fissure

Crus cerebri
Caudal rhinal fissure

Fig. A.17 **Canine brain, transverse slice at the level of the geniculate nuclei. (Slice 9 in Fig. A9a).**

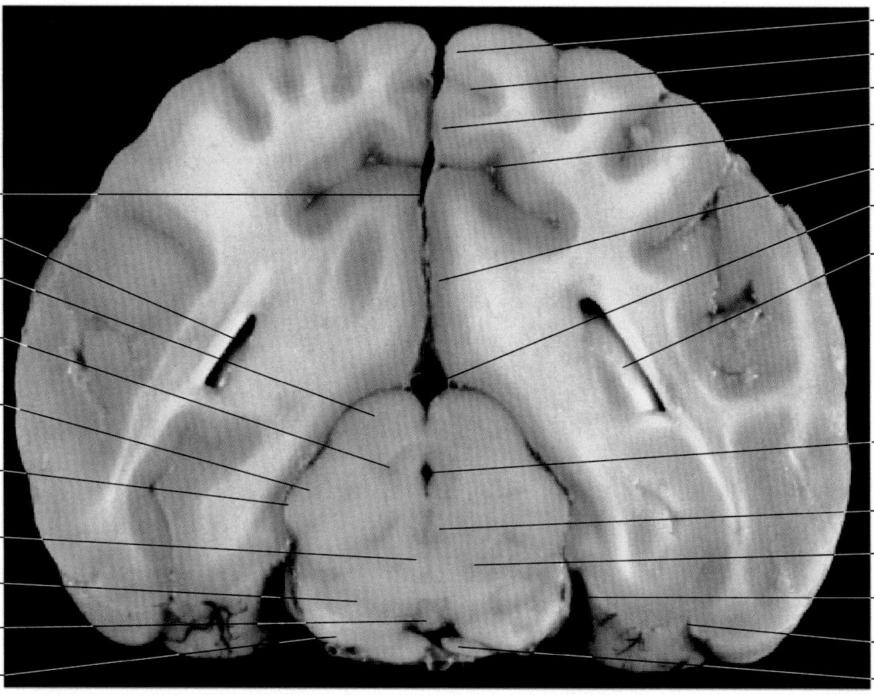
Occipital gyrus
Suprasplenial sulcus
Splenial gyrus
Splenial sulcus
Cingulate gyrus
Quadrigeminal cistern
Hippocampus
Longitudinal fissure
Lateral ventricle
Rostral colliculus
Mesencephalic nucleus of V
Medial geniculate nucleus
Brachium of the caudal colliculus
Medial longitudinal fasciculus
Substantia nigra
Interpeduncular nucleus
Crus cerebri
Mesencephalic aqueduct
Oculomotor nucleus
Red nucleus
Subarachnoid space
Lateral rhinal sulcus
Rostral pons

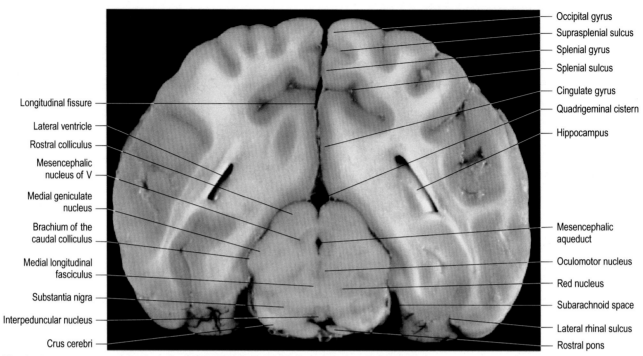

Fig. A.18 **Canine brain, transverse slice at the level of the rostral midbrain. (Slice 10 in Fig. A9a).**

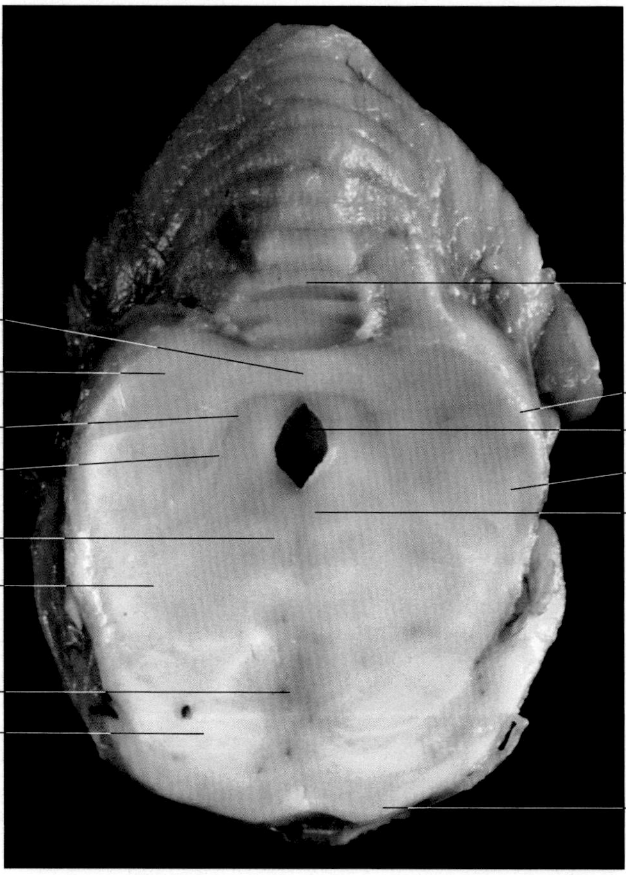
Rostral aspect of the cerebellar vermis
Commissure of the caudal colliculus
Caudal colliculus
Mesencephalic nucleus of V
Mesencephalic tract of V
Medial longitudinal fasciculus
Pontine reticular nucleus
Interpeduncular nucleus
Crus cerebri
Brachium of the caudal colliculus
Mesencephalic aqueduct
Lateral lemniscus
Trochlear nucleus
Transverse fibres of the pons

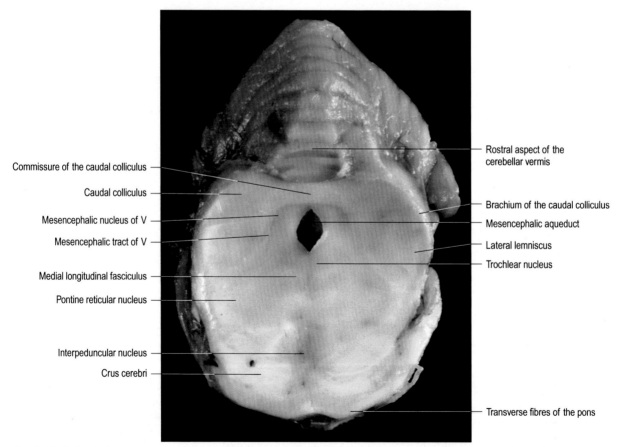

Fig. A.19 **Canine brain, transverse slice at the level of the caudal midbrain, viewed from the rostral aspect. Section is disproportionately enlarged compared with the other transverse sections. (Slice 10a in Fig. A9a).**

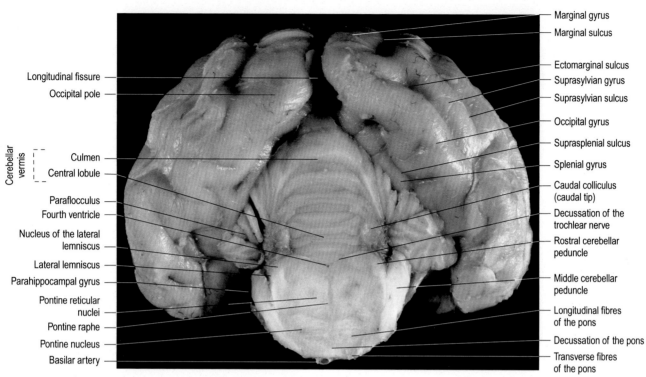

Marginal gyrus
Marginal sulcus

Ectomarginal sulcus
Suprasylvian gyrus
Suprasylvian sulcus

Occipital gyrus
Suprasplenial sulcus
Splenial gyrus

Caudal colliculus
(caudal tip)

Decussation of the
trochlear nerve

Rostral cerebellar
peduncle

Middle cerebellar
peduncle

Longitudinal fibres
of the pons

Decussation of the pons

Transverse fibres
of the pons

Longitudinal fissure
Occipital pole

Cerebellar vermis

Culmen
Central lobule

Paraflocculus
Fourth ventricle

Nucleus of the lateral
lemniscus

Lateral lemniscus

Parahippocampal gyrus

Pontine reticular
nuclei

Pontine raphe

Pontine nucleus

Basilar artery

Fig. A.20 **Canine brain, transverse slice at the level of pons. (Slice 11 in Fig. A9a).**

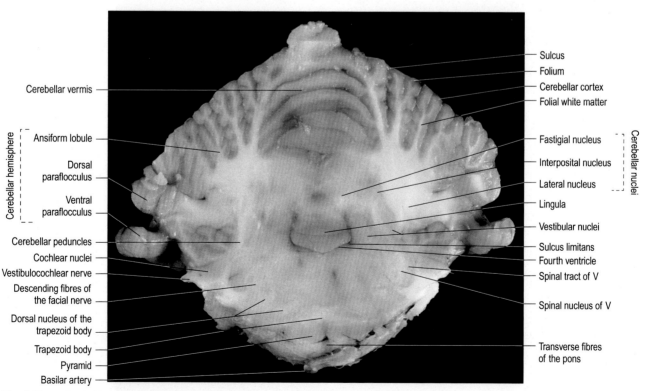

Sulcus
Folium
Cerebellar cortex
Folial white matter

Fastigial nucleus
Interposital nucleus
Lateral nucleus

Cerebellar nuclei

Lingula
Vestibular nuclei
Sulcus limitans
Fourth ventricle
Spinal tract of V

Spinal nucleus of V

Transverse fibres
of the pons

Cerebellar vermis

Cerebellar hemisphere

Ansiform lobule

Dorsal
paraflocculus

Ventral
paraflocculus

Cerebellar peduncles
Cochlear nuclei
Vestibulocochlear nerve
Descending fibres of
the facial nerve
Dorsal nucleus of the
trapezoid body
Trapezoid body
Pyramid
Basilar artery

Fig. A.21 **Canine brain, transverse slice at the level of the cerebellar peduncles. (Slice 12 in Fig. A9a).**

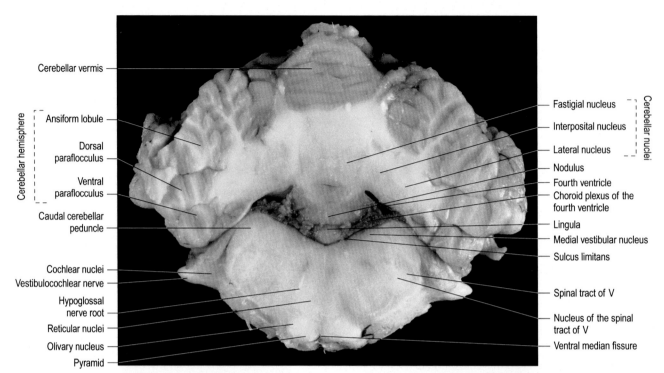

Cerebellar vermis

Cerebellar hemisphere
- Ansiform lobule
- Dorsal paraflocculus
- Ventral paraflocculus

Caudal cerebellar peduncle

Cochlear nuclei
Vestibulocochlear nerve
Hypoglossal nerve root
Reticular nuclei
Olivary nucleus
Pyramid

Cerebellar nuclei
- Fastigial nucleus
- Interposital nucleus
- Lateral nucleus

Nodulus
Fourth ventricle
Choroid plexus of the fourth ventricle
Lingula
Medial vestibular nucleus
Sulcus limitans

Spinal tract of V

Nucleus of the spinal tract of V
Ventral median fissure

Fig. A.22 **Canine brain, transverse slice at the level of the rostral fourth ventricle and deep cerebellar nuclei. (Slice 13 in Fig. A9a).**

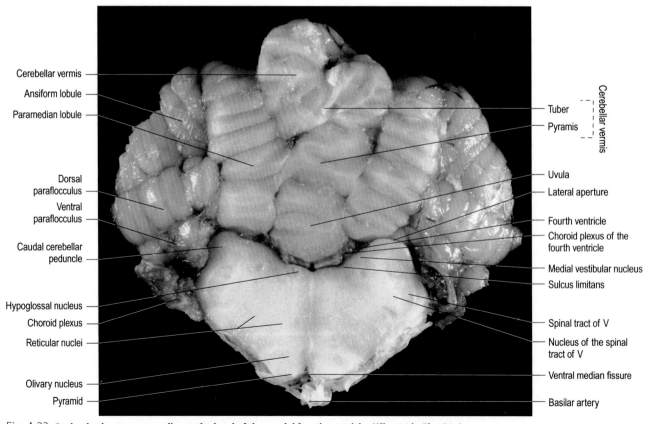

Cerebellar vermis
Ansiform lobule
Paramedian lobule

Dorsal paraflocculus
Ventral paraflocculus

Caudal cerebellar peduncle

Hypoglossal nucleus
Choroid plexus
Reticular nuclei

Olivary nucleus
Pyramid

Cerebellar vermis
- Tuber
- Pyramis

Uvula
Lateral aperture

Fourth ventricle
Choroid plexus of the fourth ventricle

Medial vestibular nucleus
Sulcus limitans

Spinal tract of V

Nucleus of the spinal tract of V

Ventral median fissure

Basilar artery

Fig. A.23 **Canine brain, transverse slice at the level of the caudal fourth ventricle. (Slice 14 in Fig. A9a).**

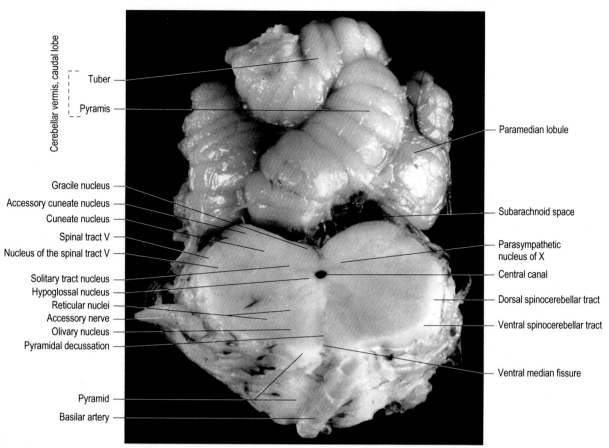

Fig. A.24 **Canine brain, transverse slice at the level of the myelencephalon (medulla oblongata) caudal to the obex. (Slice 15 in Fig. A9a).**

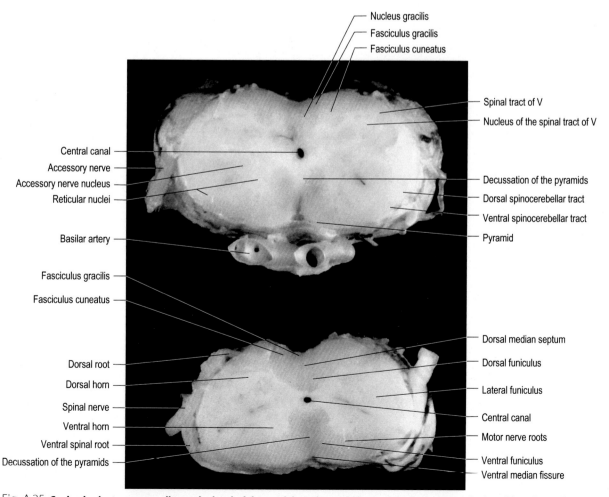

Fig. A.25 **Canine brain, transverse slice at the level of the caudal myelencephalon and the brainstem–spinal cord junction. (Slices 16 and 17 in Fig. A9a).**

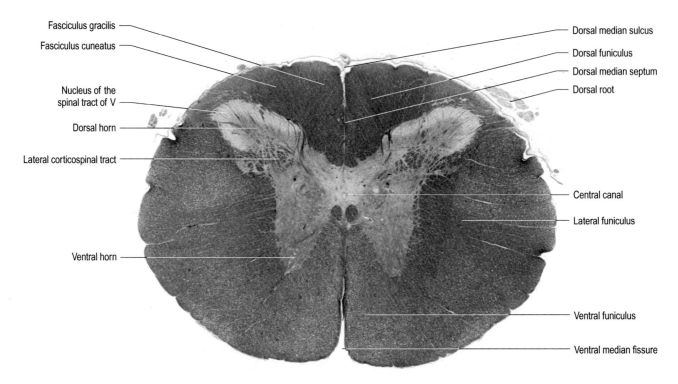

Fasciculus gracilis

Fasciculus cuneatus

Nucleus of the spinal tract of V

Dorsal horn

Lateral corticospinal tract

Ventral horn

Dorsal median sulcus

Dorsal funiculus

Dorsal median septum

Dorsal root

Central canal

Lateral funiculus

Ventral funiculus

Ventral median fissure

Fig. A.26 **Sheep, transverse histological section, C1 spinal cord.**

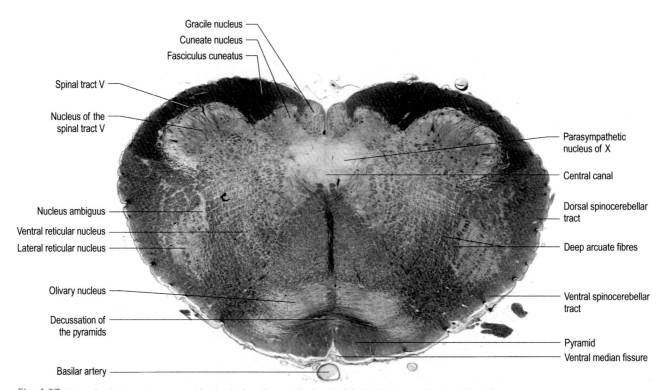

Gracile nucleus

Cuneate nucleus

Fasciculus cuneatus

Spinal tract V

Nucleus of the spinal tract V

Nucleus ambiguus

Ventral reticular nucleus

Lateral reticular nucleus

Olivary nucleus

Decussation of the pyramids

Basilar artery

Parasympathetic nucleus of X

Central canal

Dorsal spinocerebellar tract

Deep arcuate fibres

Ventral spinocerebellar tract

Pyramid

Ventral median fissure

Fig. A.27 **Sheep brainstem, transverse histological section, at the level of the brainstem–spinal cord junction.**

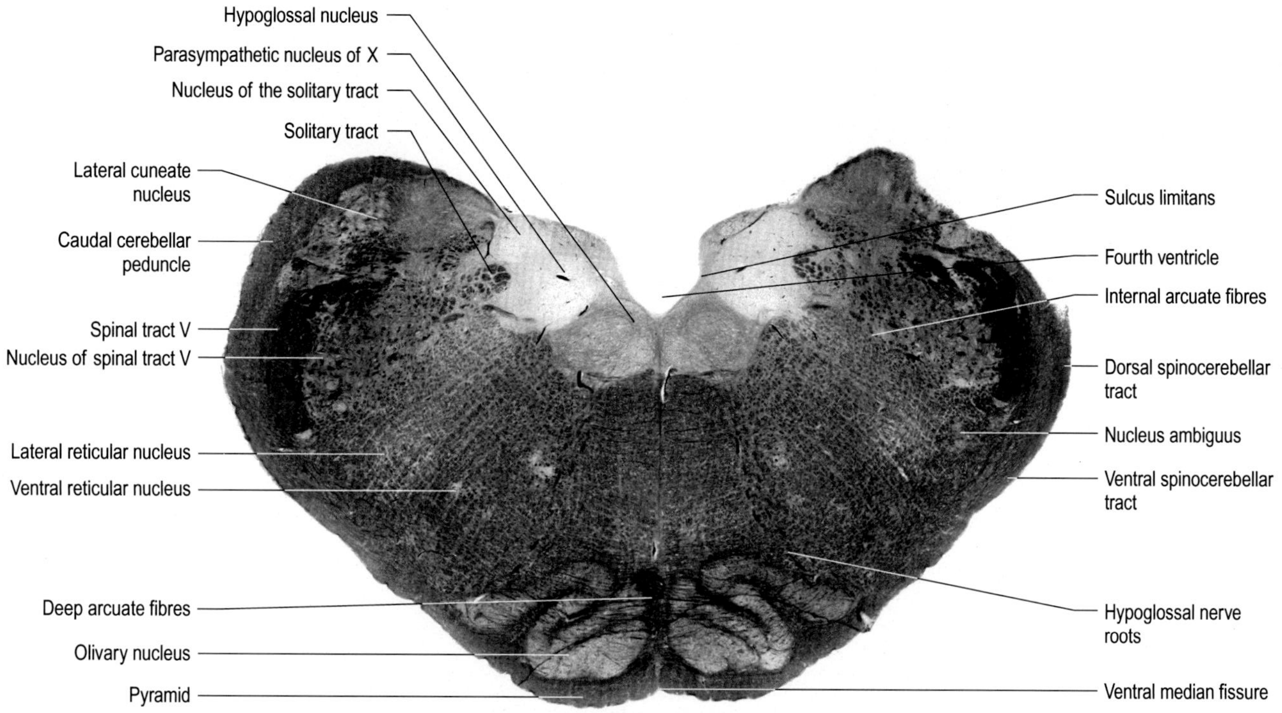
Hypoglossal nucleus
Parasympathetic nucleus of X
Nucleus of the solitary tract
Solitary tract
Lateral cuneate nucleus
Caudal cerebellar peduncle
Spinal tract V
Nucleus of spinal tract V
Lateral reticular nucleus
Ventral reticular nucleus
Deep arcuate fibres
Olivary nucleus
Pyramid
Sulcus limitans
Fourth ventricle
Internal arcuate fibres
Dorsal spinocerebellar tract
Nucleus ambiguus
Ventral spinocerebellar tract
Hypoglossal nerve roots
Ventral median fissure

Fig. A.28 **Sheep brainstem, transverse histological section, at the level of the caudal medulla oblongata.**

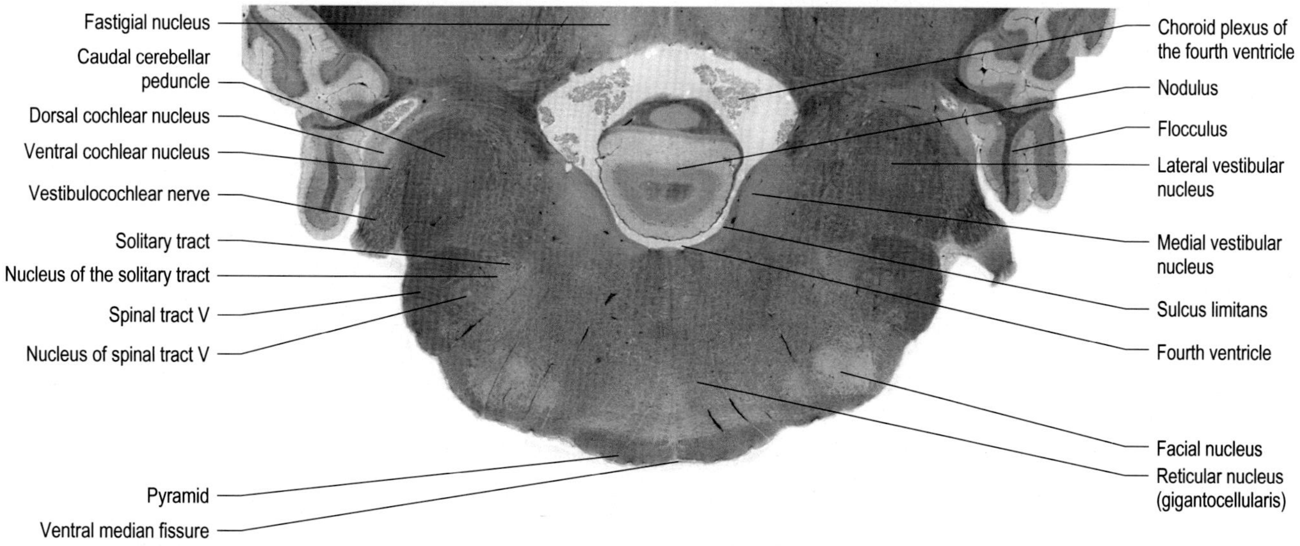
Fastigial nucleus
Caudal cerebellar peduncle
Dorsal cochlear nucleus
Ventral cochlear nucleus
Vestibulocochlear nerve
Solitary tract
Nucleus of the solitary tract
Spinal tract V
Nucleus of spinal tract V
Pyramid
Ventral median fissure
Choroid plexus of the fourth ventricle
Nodulus
Flocculus
Lateral vestibular nucleus
Medial vestibular nucleus
Sulcus limitans
Fourth ventricle
Facial nucleus
Reticular nucleus (gigantocellularis)

Fig. A.29 **Sheep brainstem, transverse histological section, at the level of the rostral medulla oblongata.**

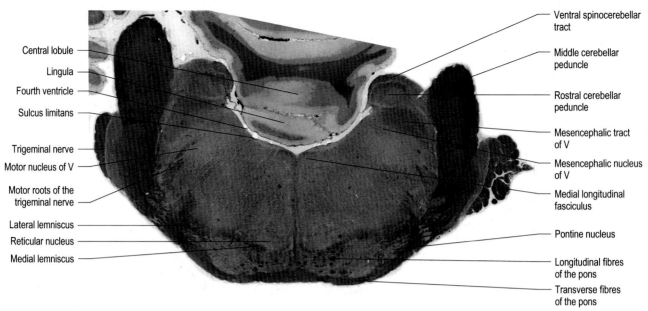

Central lobule

Lingula

Fourth ventricle

Sulcus limitans

Trigeminal nerve

Motor nucleus of V

Motor roots of the trigeminal nerve

Lateral lemniscus

Reticular nucleus

Medial lemniscus

Ventral spinocerebellar tract

Middle cerebellar peduncle

Rostral cerebellar peduncle

Mesencephalic tract of V

Mesencephalic nucleus of V

Medial longitudinal fasciculus

Pontine nucleus

Longitudinal fibres of the pons

Transverse fibres of the pons

Fig. A.30 **Sheep brainstem, transverse histological section, at the level of the pons.**

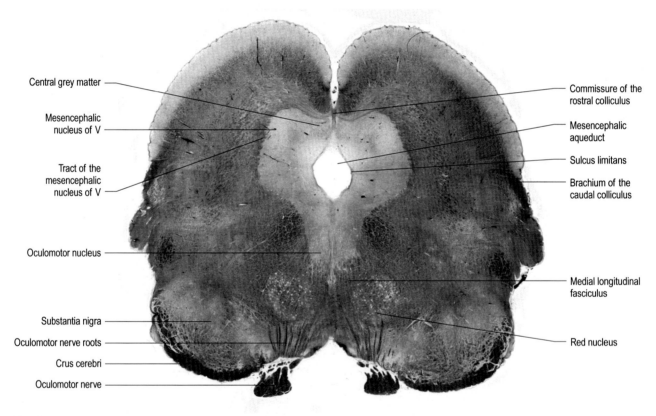

Central grey matter

Mesencephalic nucleus of V

Tract of the mesencephalic nucleus of V

Oculomotor nucleus

Substantia nigra

Oculomotor nerve roots

Crus cerebri

Oculomotor nerve

Commissure of the rostral colliculus

Mesencephalic aqueduct

Sulcus limitans

Brachium of the caudal colliculus

Medial longitudinal fasciculus

Red nucleus

Fig. A.31 **Sheep brainstem, transverse histological section, at the level of the rostral mesencephalon.**

The images of the intact and sliced dog brain were obtained from an adult Bull Terrier bitch weighing 33 kg. This brain was perfusion fixed in situ in the head before removal. The transverse slices are photographed from the caudal aspect, except for Figure A19, depicting the caudal midbrain; this was photographed from the rostral aspect.

The photograph of the dorsal aspect of the sheep brainstem (Figure A7) was obtained after curving the brainstem to open the dorsal aspect for visualisation (see inset).

The black and white images are histological sections from a sheep brain. The sections were prepared in 1959, by Dr. A. Palmer, Cambridge, and were derived from interrupted serial sections of sheep brain, embedded in celloidin, cut at 30 μm width and stained for myelin by the Loyez technique, a haematoxylin lake method.

Glossary of anatomical structures in the Appendix images

Note: as the brain is largely bilaterally symmetrical, the structures are paired, except for when specifically noted.

Accessory nerve – CN XI, attaches to the lateral aspect of the caudal myelencephalon and cervical spinal cord. Cell bodies are located in the caudal part of the nucleus ambiguus and cervical spinal cord. It innervates the larynx (via CN X), some of the lateral neck muscles and some of the extrinsic muscles of the shoulder.

Accessory nerve nucleus – Caudal portion of the nucleus ambiguus in the caudal medulla oblongata, continuous with the motor nucleus of the accessory nerve, which extends through the ventral grey matter of the cervical spinal cord.

Alve(ol)us – Medial aspect of cerebral hemisphere, covering part of the hippocampus. It is white matter comprising efferent fibres arising from the hippocampus and travelling to the fimbria.

Basal nuclei – Collection of deeply located, grey matter in the cerebral hemispheres, lateral and ventral to the lateral ventricles. They function with the extrapyramidal motor system and are primarily concerned with the execution of voluntary posture and movement.

Basilar artery – Artery on the ventral aspect of the brainstem connecting the paired vertebral arteries with the cerebral arterial circle. The direction of blood flow is species-specific.

Body of the fornix – White matter in the ventromedial aspect of the mid region of the lateral ventricles the rostral aspects of the paired, lateral ventricles. The axons from hippocampal neurons form the rostrally-directed, paired crura of the fornix, and meet on the midline to form the body of the fornix between the lateral ventricles.

Brachium of the caudal colliculus – White matter located on the dorsolateral aspect of the midbrain. The brachium conveys auditory afferent fibres from the caudal colliculus of the mesencephalon to the rostral colliculus (origin of the tectospinal tract) and to the medial geniculate nucleus of the diencephalon.

Brachium of the rostral colliculus – White matter of the dorsomedial aspect of midbrain, conveying axons from the optic tract and visual cortex to the rostral colliculus.

Callosal sulcus – The sulcus on the medial aspect of the cerebral hemisphere, at the base of the longitudinal fissure. It separates the corpus callosum from the cingulate gyrus.

Caudal cerebellar peduncle – Bidirectional bundle of fibres connecting the cerebellum to the myelencephalon. They convey proprioceptive information from the dorsal spinocerebellar, cuneocerebellar and cervicospinocerebellar tracts to the cerebellum: also the climbing fibres from the olivary nucleus. Efferent fibres from the fastigial nucleus exit via this peduncle travelling to the vestibular and reticular formation in the medulla oblongata. The medial aspect (juxtarestiform body) connects bidirectionally between the vestibulocerebellum and vestibular nuclei of the myelencephalon.

Caudal colliculus – Protuberance on the caudodorsal mesencephalon (tectum); associated with auditory function and reflex head movement.

Caudal commissure – Caudal diencephalon; connects bilaterally between structures of the caudal thalamus and midbrain; it is associated with the pupillary light reflex.

Caudal lobe of cerebellum – Caudal portion of the cerebellum, separated from the rostral lobe by the dorsally located, primary fissure.

Caudal vestibular nucleus – Medial side of the caudal cerebellar peduncle, see Vestibular nuclei.

Caudate nucleus – Rostral, cerebral hemispheres, with the head and body on the floor of the lateral ventricle while the tail curves ventrally to form the roof of the ventral portion of the lateral ventricle in the temporal lobe. It is one of the basal nuclei and functions in the extrapyramidal system.

Central canal – Remnant of the embryonic neural canal, extending the length of the spinal cord. It is filled with CSF and continuous with the caudal aspect of the fourth ventricle.

Central grey matter of mesencephalon (periaqueductal grey) – Grey matter surrounding the mesencephalic aqueduct. It plays a role in the descending modulation of nociception, and in defensive behaviour.

Centrum semiovale – Cerebral white matter deep to the cerebral cortex at the junction between the corona radiata and the corpus callosum

Cerebellar cortex – Tightly folded external layer of the cerebellum consisting of the granular, Purkinje and molecular cell layers.

Cerebellar hemisphere – Paired lateral portions of the cerebellum. Primarily functions in coordinating muscle activity in the limbs.

Cerebellar hemisphere, ansiform lobule – Lateral lobule of the cerebellar hemisphere.

Cerebellar hemisphere, dorsal paraflocculus – Dorsal component of a lobule on the ventrolateral aspect of the cerebellar hemisphere.

Cerebellar hemisphere, paramedian lobule – lobule just lateral to the vermis of the caudal lobe.

Cerebellar hemisphere, ventral paraflocculus – Ventral component of a lobule on the ventrolateral aspect of the cerebellar hemisphere, just dorsal to the flocculus.

Cerebellar nuclei – Lateral, interpositial and fastigial nuclei are located in the cerebellar white matter, just dorsal to the fourth ventricle. They receive collateral branches from the afferent fibers entering the cerebellum, and Purkinje neurons of the cerebellar cortex; efferent fibres project to extrapyramidal upper motor neurons.

Cerebellar peduncle – White matter bundles connecting bidirectionally between the cerebellum and the rostral medulla oblongata. The caudal, middle and rostral peduncles converge at the confluence of the cerebellar peduncles.

Cerebellar vermis – Midline portion of the cerebellum. It primarily functions in coordinating axial musculature. It comprises lobules of the rostral lobe (lingula, central, culmen), the primary fissure on the dorsal aspect, caudal lobe (declive, folium, tuber, pyramis, uvula), uvulonodular fissure on the caudoventral aspect and the nodulus.

Cerebellar white matter – Deep to the cerebellar cortex, forms the white laminae of the folia (arbor vitae) and the central medulla, which contains the cerebellar nuclei.

Cerebral arterial circle – Anastomotic circle of arteries on the ventral aspect of the forebrain and midbrain, supplying blood to these regions. Input to, and direction of flow from, the circle is species-specific.

Cerebral peduncle – The region of the mesencephalon ventral to the tectum and mesencephalic aqueduct that includes the tegmentum, substantia nigra and crus cerebri.

Choroid fissure – Subarachnoid space surrounding the diencephalon and separating it from the hippocampus. Dorsally it extends rostrally under the fornix. It is separated from the dorsal aspect of the third ventricle by a thin roof plate, which forms the site of attachment of the choroid plexus.

Choroid plexus – Vascular structures in the ventricles of the brain comprising modified ependymal cells and clustered capillaries forming villi; the plexi are the main site of cerebrospinal fluid production.

Cingulate gyrus – Medial aspect of cerebral hemispheres, dorsal to corpus callosum. It is part of the limbic system. It has connections with the parahippocampal gyrus, neocortex and rostral thalamus.

Claustrum – One of the basal nuclei, lateral to the putamen.

Cochlear nuclei – Collections of neurons on the lateral aspects of the rostral medulla oblongata where CN VIII attaches. They receive input from the cochlear nerve, conveying auditory information from the cochlear of the inner ear. Many efferent fibres from the cochlear nuclei decussate forming the trapezoid body and then project rostrally via the lateral lemniscus to synapse in the caudal colliculus and medial geniculate nucleus. From there they project to the auditory cortex. Other efferent fibres make multiple connections in the brainstem for reflex function.

Columns of the fornix – Medial aspect of the rostral cerebral hemispheres, ventral to the genu of corpus callosum. The columns originate from the body of the fornix and descend ventrally to split at the rostral commissure forming the smaller, pre- and larger, post-commissural fornix. These columns pass into the septal area or the mamillary bodies, respectively.

Commissure – Join between two related structures (*commissura* – Latin = a meeting or joining together).

Commissure of the fornix – Transverse fibres connecting the left and right fornix of the hippocampus.

Commissure of the rostral colliculus – Axons connecting the left and right rostral colliculi.

Corona radiata – These are the white matter laminae that are surrounded by cerebral cortex. They are in the center of all the gyri.

Coronal sulcus – Sulcus on the dorsolateral aspect of the rostral third of the cerebral cortex. It is the rostral extension of the marginal sulcus and may be considered to separate the motor and somatosensory cortices.

Corpus callosum – At the base of the longitudinal fissure of the telencephalon. It is the principal, white matter commissure joining the left and right cerebral hemispheres. It is only present in placental mammals.

Corpus striatum – Located deep in the telencephalon, ventrolateral to the lateral ventricles. It comprises most of the basal nuclei and intervening white matter; that is caudate nucleus and its ventral extension, the nucleus accumbens, the lentiform nuclei (putamen and the globus pallidus) and claustrum with the internal and external capsules of white matter. The name refers to the striated appearance produced by connected bands of grey substance alternating with the intervening white matter. It is involved in voluntary posture and movement and selectively inhibits and controls motor output from the forebrain.

Cruciate sulcus – Major sulcus in the dorsal frontal lobe. On the dorsal aspect, it forms a cross with the longitudinal fissure. It extends ventrally on the medial surface of the cerebral hemisphere. It is found in some mammals and is the equivalent of the central sulcus in primates. The motor cortex surrounds the cruciate sulcus.

Crus cerebri – Longitudinal bulges that extend along the ventral aspect of the midbrain. They comprise the corticospinal, corticopontine, corticonuclear and corticoreticular fibres. They continue rostrally as the internal capsule, and caudally as the longitudinal fibres of the pons.

Crus of the fornix – These are rostrally directed bands of white matter that arise from the fimbria on the lateral side of each hippocampus.

Decussation of the pons – Region on the ventral midline of the pons where axons from the pontine nuclei decussate, before ascending through the middle cerebellar peduncle to the cerebellum. It is part of the corticopontocerebellar pathway.

Decussation of the pyramids – Crossing over of corticospinal tracts at the spinomedullary junction on the ventral aspect.

Decussation of the trochlear nerve – CN IV is the only cranial nerve that emerges from the brainstem dorsally, and the only cranial nerve that decussates to innervate the contralateral side. The decussation occurs in the rostral medullary velum, which is located, caudal to the caudal colliculi under the rostral aspect of the cerebellum.

Deep arcuate fibres – Efferent fibres arising from the gracile and medial cuneate nuclei of the caudal, dorsal medulla oblongata. These fibers decussate to form the medial lemniscus and convey sensory information from the neck, trunk, limbs and tail to the thalamus and then onto the somatosensory cortex.

Dentate gyrus – Medial aspect of the telencephalon. It caps the free edge of the hippocampus, which is part of the limbic system functioning in learning, memory and emotion.

Diagonal band – This is the lamella diagonalis, which is located within the gyrus diagonalis and gyrus parsterminalis. The axons in this band join the median forebrain bundle to convey information from olfactory nuclei to the hypothalamus.

Dorsal cochlear nucleus – Lateral, rostral medulla oblongata. See Cochlear nuclei.

Dorsal funiculus – Dorsal white matter of the spinal cord, medial to the dorsal horns. Main tracts are the funiculus gracilis and cuneatus. It principally consists of primary afferent projection neurons to nuclei in the brainstem involved in conscious proprioception.

Dorsal horn of the spinal cord – Grey matter in the dorsal spinal cord categorised variously into nuclei and laminae. It receives afferent information from the body and limbs, including impulse generated by tactile, proprioceptive nociceptive and interoceptive stimuli.

Dorsal median septum of the spinal cord – Longitudinal sheet of glial tissue in the median plane of the spinal cord that partitions the dorsal part of the spinal cord into right and left halves.

Dorsal median sulcus of the spinal cord – Shallow longitudinal groove in the dorsal midline of the spinal cord.

Dorsal paraflocculus of cerebellum – see Paraflocculus.

Dorsal root – Afferent root of a spinal nerve. They convey sensory information, and there is one pair per spinal cord segment. At the lateral end of the dorsal root is the spinal ganglion, which contains the neuronal somata of the nerve fibres conveyed by the root.

Dorsal spinocerebellar tract – White matter tract at the periphery of the dorsolateral spinal cord. It transmits subconscious proprioceptive information from spinal nerves caudal to the thoracic limb, via the caudal cerebellar peduncle to the ipsilateral cerebellar cortex.

Ectomarginal sulcus – Sulcus lateral to the similarly named gyrus on the dorsocaudal aspect of the brain. The caudal third of the ectomarginal gyrus extends into the occipital lobe.

Ectosylvian gyrus – Curved gyrus on the lateral side of the brain, principally in the temporal cortex.

Ectosylvian sulcus – Curved sulcus on the lateral side of the brain making up the ventral border of the ectosylvian gyrus.

Endomarginal gyrus – Gyrus bordering the longitudinal fissure on the dorsal aspect of the cerebrum.

Endomarginal sulcus – Lateral margin of the endomarginal gyrus.

Endopeduncular nucleus – Relatively large grey matter area in the ventral diencephalon (subthalamus), between the optic tract ventrally and the internal capsule dorsolaterally. It connects between the globus pallidus and the dorsal thalamus.

Endorhinal suclus – Ventral aspect of the olfactory peduncle of the telencephalon. It separates the olfactory tubercle from the lateral olfactory tract.

External capsule – Ventrolateral telencephalon, white matter tract separating the the lentiform nuclei and the claustrum. It connects motor areas of the telencephalon with the basal nuclei.

Extreme capsule – Ventrolateral telencephalon, white matter tract separating the claustrum from the cortex of the temporal lobe.

Facial nerve – Cranial nerve VII, the nucleus is located in the ventral, rostral medulla oblongata. Its principal function is innervation of muscles of facial expression but it also sends efferent fibres to the stapedius muscle of the inner ear, the rostral digasticus muscle and parasympathetic fibres to palatine and lacrimal salivary glands. Afferent fibres convey taste from the rostral two-thirds of the tongue.

Fasciculus cuneatus – Large white matter tract in dorsal funiculus of the spinal cord, lateral to fasciculus gracilis. It comprises axons from primary afferent neurons, which enter the fasciculus without synapsing in the dorsal horn. They convey conscious proprioceptive information from the neck, thoracic limbs, and cranial half of the trunk to the medial cuneate nucleus in the caudal medulla oblongata. Fibres that enter the caudal portion of the tract are located medially.

Fasciculus gracilis – Medially located tract in the dorsal funiculus of the spinal cord. It is organised like the fasciculus gracilis and conveys the same type of

information but from the caudal trunk and pelvic limbs to the nucleus gracilis in the caudal medulla oblongata.

Fasciculus retroflexus (habenulointerpeduncular tract) – Dorsomedial thalamus. This is a compact bundle of fibres arising in the habenula nuclei and passing ventrally to the interpeduncular nucleus between the crus cerebri. This primitive tract carries negative feedback from forebrain caudally onto midbrain reward cells. In humans, drug abuse specifically results in degeneration of fibres in this tract.

Fastigial nucleus of cerebellum – The most medial of the three, paired cerebellar nuclei in the medulla of the cerebellum. It receives input from the vermis and its efferent fibres project to the vestibular and reticular nuclei of the brainstem.

Fimbria – Medial aspect of the caudal telencephalon, extending along the lateral edge of the hippocampus between the alveus and the crus of the fornix. It comprises myelinated axons originating from the hippocampus and continues rostrally as the fornix.

Flocculus of cerebellum – Small lobule of the ventrolatereral cerebellum at the caudal border of the middle cerebellar peduncle. It is part of the vestibulocerebellum.

Folia of cerebellum – Folds of cerebellar cortex with central laminae of white matter.

Fornix of the hippocampus – Medial aspect of the cerebral hemispheres, ventral to the corpus callosum. It comprises the efferent white matter of the hippocampus continuing rostrally and consists of crura, body and columns. It connects to the opposite side by commissural fibres.

Fourth ventricle – The most caudal of the four, connected, fluid-filled cavities within the brain. It extends from the mesencephalic aqueduct to the obex in the caudal medulla oblongata, and is filled with cerebrospinal fluid.

Frontal gyrus – Most rostral gyrus on the medial side of the frontal lobe of the telencephalon. It is dorsal to the straight gyrus and olfactory bulb.

Genual gyrus – Gyrus rostral to the genu of the corpus callosum, medial aspect of the rostral telencephalon.

Genual sulcus – Caudal margin of the genual gyrus.

Globus pallidus – Ventrolateral to the head and body of the caudate nucleus, on the ventrolateral aspect of the lateral ventricles of the telencephalon. It is the ventral nucleus of the lentiform nuclei and a component of the basal nuclei. It facilitates activity in extrapyramidal nuclei.

Habenular nuclei (medial and lateral) – Part of the epithalamus of the diencephalon, situated on the dorsomedial surface of the thalamus. They are involved in many functions, including processing of nociception, behavioural and stress responses, and learning.

Hippocampus – Paleontologically ancient, internal gyrus of the telencephalon, forming the medial wall and roof of the caudal half of the lateral ventricle. It arches dorsally, medially and rostrally. Afferent and efferent axons of the hippocampus form the alveus and combine to form the fimbria continuing rostrally as the fornix of the hippocampus. It is part of the limbic system and is associated with emotion, learning and memory. The hippocampal formation comprises the hippocampus proper, the subiculum and the dentate gyrus.

Hypoglossal nerve roots – CN XII axons arising from the hypoglossal nucleus that course ventrolaterally through the caudal medulla oblongata to form the cranial nerve supplying tongue muscles.

Hypoglossal nucleus – Nucleus of CN XII in the dorsal, caudal medulla oblongata, ventromedial to the parasympathetic nucleus of CN X.

Infundibular recess – Ventral extension of the third ventricle of the diencephalon. It forms a funnel-shaped recess extending into the infundibulum.

Infundibulum – A funnel-shaped, ventral extension of the hypothalamus connecting the caudal pituitary gland with the hypothalamus.

Intermediate olfactory stria – See Olfactory tract.

Internal capsule – Prominent white matter tract ventrolateral to the lateral ventricles of the telencephalon that connect bidirectionally between the brainstem and the cerebral cortex.

Interpeduncular nucleus – An unpaired, ovoid cell group lying between the cerebral peduncles on the ventral aspect of the midbrain. It receives information from the habenula nuclei and projects to the raphe nuclei and periaqueductal gray substance of the midbrain. It may have a role in the regulation of rapid eye movement sleep.

Interpositus nucleus – Middle of the three cerebellar nuclei in the white matter of the cerebellum. It receives fibres from the paravermal cerebellar cortex and its efferent fibres exit via the rostral cerebellar peduncle to connect with contralateral brainstem nuclei.

Interthalamic adhesion – Flattened band of grey matter connecting the medial walls of the left and right thalami. It contains neurons and axons, but very few appear to cross the mid-line, and humans lacking this structure appear to suffer no consequences.

Interventricular foramen – Channels that connect the paired lateral ventricles of the telencephalon with the third ventricle on the midline of the diencephalon. Cerebrospinal fluid produced in the lateral ventricles connects via the foramens to the third ventricle. Choroid plexus from the lateral ventricle is continuous with that of the third ventricle through this foramen.

Lateral aperture – Opening of the fourth ventricle at the level of the cerebellar peduncles, allowing CSF to flow into the subarachnoid space. In non-primates, this is the only brain connection between the ventricular system and the subarachnoid space.

Lateral cuneate nucleus – Lateral to the medial cuneate nucleus on the dorsal aspect of the caudal medulla oblongata. It receives proprioceptive information from muscle spindles and Golgi tendon organs receptors from the neck, cranial trunk and thoracic limbs. Axons from the lateral cuneate nucleus enter the adjacent caudal cerebellar peduncle and pass into the cerebellum (subconscious proprioception).

Lateral funiculus – Large region of white matter in spinal cord located laterally and bounded by the dorsal and ventral roots. It contains cranially projecting sensory and caudally projecting motor tracts, specifically those that influence flexor muscle activity.

Lateral geniculate nucleus – Dorsolateral aspect of the caudal diencephalon (metathalamus), caudal to the thalamus. It is part of the visual pathway.

Lateral lemniscus – White matter tract of the auditory system, in the brainstem, extending from the cochlear

nuclei and trapezoid body to the caudal colliculi of the midbrain.

Lateral nucleus of the cerebellum – The most lateral of the three, paired cerebellar nuclei in the white matter of the cerebellum. It receives fibres from the cerebellar hemisphere and its efferent fibres exit via the rostral cerebellar peduncle to connect with contralateral brainstem nuclei.

Lateral olfactory stria – See Olfactory tract.

Lateral reticular nucleus – See Reticular nuclei.

Lateral rhinal sulcus – Dorsal margin of the rhinencephalon, located on the ventrolateral aspect of the cerebrum.

Lateral septal nucleus – see Septal nuclei.

Lateral ventricle – Fluid-filled, C-shaped cavity oriented longitudinally in each cerebral hemisphere. It is the most rostral part of the ventricular system.

Lateral vestibular nucleus – Medial to the caudal cerebellar peduncle in the medulla oblongata. See Vestibular nuclei.

Lentiform nuclei – Putamen plus globus pallidus; a component of basal nuclei.

Lingula – see Cerebellar vermis.

Longitudinal fibres of the pons – Contains axons projecting from the cerebral cortex, via the internal capsule and crus cerebri. Some longitudinal fibres synapse on pontine nuclei, decussate and travel to the contralateral cerebellum via the middle cerebellar peduncle. Other fibres project to other brainstem nuclei (corticonuclear tract) or via the pyramids to the spinal cord (corticospinal tract).

Longitudinal fissure – Fissure separating the two hemispheres of the vertebrate brain.

Mamillary body – Caudal and ventral hypothalamus, forming bulges on the ventral aspect of the forebrain. It has links with the hippocampus (via the fornix), the thalamus and midbrain tegmentum. The mammillary nuclei are associated with the limbic system.

Mamillothalamic tract – Connects the mamillary body to the rostral group of thalamic nuclei. The mamillotegmental tract connects the mamillary body with midbrain tegmental nuclei.

Marginal gyrus – Gyrus lateral to the endomarginal gyrus on the dorsal aspect of the cerebrum.

Marginal sulcus – Lateral border of the marginal gyrus.

Medial cuneate nucleus – Nucleus on the dorsal aspect of the caudal medulla oblongata. It receives information from specialised touch, pressure, vibration and joint receptors from the thoracic limbs and cranial trunk. Efferent axons from this nucleus decussate in the deep arcuate fibres and travel rostrally as part of the medial lemniscus to the thalamus and somatosensory cortex (conscious proprioception).

Medial geniculate nucleus – Lateral aspect of the caudal diencephalon caudal to the thalamus, a component of the metathalamus. It is part of the auditory pathway.

Medial lemniscus – Sensory pathway travelling rostrally through the substance of the brainstem to the thalamus. It conveys the majority of information from the mechanoreceptors that mediate tactile discrimination and proprioception, from the nucleus gracilis and medial cuneate nuclei to the thalamus. Fibres arising from the trigeminal nuclear complex (which receives sensory input from the head) also travel with it (quintatothalamic tract).

Medial longitudinal fasciculus – Median brainstem, ventral to the ventricular system. It conveys fibres rostrally from the vestibular nuclei to synapse on the motor nuclei of cranial nerves III, IV and VI; this connection functions in the vestibulo-ocular reflex. This fasciculus also projects to the reticular formation (basis of motion sickness) and extends caudally into the spinal cord reaching cranial thoracic level; this part of the fasciculus is involved in maintaining head position.

Medial olfactory stria – see Olfactory tract.

Medial rhinal sulcus – Ventromedial aspect of the rostral telencephalon. It forms the medial boundary of the olfactory peduncle and meets with the rostral aspect of the lateral rhinal sulcus dorsal to the peduncle, thereby separating the peduncle from the frontal cortex.

Medial septal nucleus – see Septal nuclei.

Medial vestibular nucleus – Medial to the caudal cerebellar peduncle in the medulla oblongata. See Vestibular nuclei.

Mesencephalic aqueduct – Portion of the ventricular system reduced to a small tube extending through the midbrain. It connects the third and fourth ventricle.

Mesencephalic nucleus of V – Thin column of large neurons on the lateral border of the central grey matter of the mesencephalon. Afferent fibres are proprioceptive from the mouth, including the teeth, and muscles of mastication. Their cell bodies are located in this nucleus, hence the nucleus is the equivalent of a ganglion. Efferent fibres project to the motor nucleus of V (mastication) or via the medial lemniscus to the thalamus and somatosensory cortex for conscious perception. The nucleus is absent in lampreys and hagfishes (the only vertebrates without jaws).

Mesencephalic tract of V – Narrow tract on the periphery of the mesencephalic nucleus of V. It contains axons travelling between the trigeminal nerve and the nucleus.

Middle cerebellar peduncle – Neuronal processes on each side of the fourth ventricle connecting the transverse fibres of the pons with the cerebellum. It conveys afferent fibres only, from the pons (part of the corticopontocerebellar pathway).

Motor nerve roots – Efferent fibres within the brainstem or spinal cord travelling towards the peripheral nervous system.

Myelencephalon – Medulla oblongata.

Nodulus – see Cerebellar vermis. This ventrocaudal portion of the vermis is associated with the vestibulocerebellum.

Nucleus accumbens – Rostro-ventral telencephalon, located between the head of the caudate nucleus and the septal nuclei. It is a ventral extension of the caudate nucleus, which is a component of the basal nuclei.

Nucleus ambiguus – Poorly defined, elongated nucleus in the ventrolateral substance of the caudal medulla oblongata. Efferent fibres form the glossopharyngeal (CN IX), vagus (CN X) and the cranial roots of accessory nerve (CN XI), to innervate the striated muscle of the pharynx, larynx and oesophagus.

Nucleus gracilis – Nucleus on the dorsal aspect of the caudal medulla oblongata, medial to the medial cuneate nucleus. It receives proprioceptive information from specialised touch, pressure, vibration and joint receptors from the pelvic limbs and caudal trunk. Axons from neurons in the nucleus gracilis decussate in the deep arcuate fibres and travel rostrally as part of the medial lemniscus to the thalamus and somatosensory cortex.

Nucleus of the lateral lemniscus – Prominent mass of grey matter dorsal to the trapezoid body in the rostral medulla oblongata. It receives afferent fibres from the cochlear nuclei (audition) and projects to the caudal colliculus via the lateral lemniscus.

Nucleus of the solitary tract – Nucleus dorsal to the sulcus limitans of the fourth ventricle in the caudal medulla oblongata. It receives afferent fibres carrying visceral sensation including taste from the facial (VII), glossopharyngeal (IX) and vagus (X) cranial nerves.

Nucleus of the spinal tract of V – Prominent sensory nucleus located in the dorsal brainstem extending from the pons to the cranial cervical spinal cord. It receives input from the trigeminal, facial, glossopharyngeal and vagus nerves especially associated with noxious and thermal stimuli. It is continuous with the substantia gelatinosa of the spinal cord. Efferent fibres are involved in reflex cranial nerve activity and project to the somatosensory cortex.

Occipital gyrus – Most caudal gyrus of the occipital lobe, caudal telencephalon.

Occipital pole – Caudal portion of the occipital lobe, caudal telencephalon.

Oculomotor nerve – CN III, exits the ventral aspect of the midbrain. It conveys somatic motor fibres to the majority of the extraocular muscles (ventral, medial, and dorsal rectus and ventral oblique muscles), as well as parasympathetic fibres to the ciliary ganglion and smooth muscles of eye. It is the efferent arm of the pupillary light reflex.

Oculomotor nerve roots – CN III axons within the parenchyma of the midbrain tegmentum.

Oculomotor nucleus – Nucleus of CN III in the midbrain, ventral to the mesencephalic aqueduct. It comprises somatic motor neurons that innervate the striated, extraocular muscles. Just rostral to this nucleus is the separate parasympathetic nucleus of III; fibres from this nucleus innervate the smooth muscle of the pupillary constrictor muscle of the iris.

Olfactory bulb – Ventral and most rostral part of the telencephalon, expanded rostral aspect of the olfactory peduncle. Olfactory bulb neurons receive input from olfactory cells in the olfactory epithelium, and project via the olfactory tract (see Olfactory tract).

Olfactory nucleus – Grey matter in the olfactory peduncle, ventro-rostral telencephalon. It is one of the relay stations in the olfactory pathway from the olfactory bulb to the piriform lobe.

Olfactory peduncle – Longitudinal bulge on the ventral and rostral aspect of the telencephalon extending from the olfactory bulb to the olfactory tubercle. The peripheral grey matter layer is the olfactory nucleus and the central white matter is the olfactory tract.

Olfactory tract – The tract conveys axons from neurons in the olfactory bulb. It divides into the medial, intermediate and lateral olfactory stria. The lateral olfactory stria axons synapse in the olfactory tubercle and then continue to the primary olfactory cortex in the piriform lobe. Fibres in the intermediate olfactory stria decussate via the rostral commissure and project to the contralateral olfactory bulb. Fibres from the medial olfactory tract connect to the septal nuclei and from there, via the medial forebrain bundle, to the hypothalamus or reticular formation for olfacto-visceral reflexes. Note: the terms 'olfactory tract' and 'olfactory stria' seem to be used somewhat interchangeably.

Olfactory tubercle – Ventral and rostral forebrain, forms a bulge at the caudal end of the olfactory peduncle. It is one of the relay stations in the olfactory pathway travelling between the olfactory bulb to the piriform lobe.

Olivary nucleus – Prominent nuclear complex within the ventrocaudal medulla oblongata on the dorsolateral border of the pyramids. Afferent fibres are mostly travelling between the extrapyramidal motor system and the cerebellum. Efferent fibres form the climbing fibres that decussate and ascend into the contralateral cerebellum via the caudal cerebellar peduncle.

Optic chiasm – Single structure rostral to the infundibulum on the ventro-rostral aspect of the forebrain. It is the site of attachment of the optic nerves, part of the visual pathway and where the majority of optic nerve fibres decussate.

Optic nerve – CN II originating in the optic retina, conveys axons from retinal ganglion cells to the brain. The left and right optic nerves join at the optic chiasm ventral to the hypothalamus. Although referred to as a cranial nerve, it is similar to a CNS tract as it develops as an outgrowth of the embryonic prosencephalon, and is myelinated by oligodendroglial cells.

Optic tract – Part of the diencephalon, continuation of retinal ganglion cell axons caudal to the optic chiasm. The tract projects caudally and dorsally to the lateral geniculate nucleus of the thalamus and to the midbrain.

Paraflocculus of cerebellum – Lobule on the ventrolateral aspect of the cerebellar hemisphere. It has dorsal and ventral components.

Parahippocampal gyrus – Cerebrocortical gyrus on the ventromedial surface of the temporal lobe that extends caudally from the piriform lobe and borders the hippocampus; it is continued dorsally by the cingulate gyrus. This gyrus connects to the hippocampus proper by the subiculum.

Paramedian lobule of cerebellum – Lobule lateral to caudal portion of cerebellar vermis.

Parasympathetic nucleus of X – Nuclear column in the caudal medulla oblongata, dorsolateral to the hypoglossal nucleus, and lateral to the sulcus limitans of the fourth ventricle. Efferent axons form the vagus nerve that provides presynaptic, parasympathetic innervation to the thoracic and abdominal viscera.

Pineal gland – Small endocrine gland that projects caudally from the dorsal aspect of the third ventricle, on the midline between the cerebral hemispheres. It produces serotonin and its derivative melatonin, a hormone that modulates wake/sleep patterns and seasonal functions.

Piriform lobe – Cerebral cortex on the ventrolateral aspect of the telencephalon. It is the primary receiving area for olfactory stimuli and is involved in olfaction and the limbic system. It contains the amygdaloid nucleus.

Pons (metencephalon) – Portion of the brainstem between the midbrain and medulla oblongata. Important components include the motor nucleus of the trigeminal nerve (CN V), the transverse fibres of the pons, pontine nuclei.

Pontine nucleus – Scattered nuclei in the ventral pons. Afferent fibres are from the cerebral cortex. Efferent fibres form the transverse fibres of the pons, which decussate and ascend via the contralateral middle cerebellar peduncle to the cerebellum; it is part of the corticopontocerebellar pathway.

Pontine raphe – Nucleus consisting of a small number of serotonergic neurons in the midline of the pons; it also extends into the medulla oblongata.

Pontine reticular nuclei – Diffuse network of neurons in the substance of the pons. They are important in regulating consciousness or wakefulness and are part of the upper motor neuron system. See Reticular nuclei.

Postcruciate gyrus – Gyrus on dorsal surface of the rostral cerebrum, immediately caudal to the cruciate sulcus. It is part of the motor cortex.

Presylvian sulcus – Sulcus on the rostrolateral aspect of the cerebrum rostral to the pseudosylvian fissure. It forms the border between the lateral rostral composite gyrus and the more rostral prorean gyrus.

Primary fissure of cerebellum – Transverse sulcus on the dorsal cerebellum. It separates the body of the cerebellum into rostral and caudal lobes.

Prorean gyrus – Rostral gyrus on the ventrolateral aspect of the rostral telencephalon rostral to the presylvian sulcus and dorsolateral to the olfactory peduncle.

Pseudosylvian fissure – Lateral aspect of the telencephlon, in the temporal lobe. Situated around this fissure are both the primary auditory cortex and the area for conscious perception for the vestibular system.

Putamen – Component of the basal nuclei, lateral to the internal capsule in the substance of the rostral telencephalon. It, and the globus pallidus, comprise the lentiform nuclei.

Pyramid – Prominent longitudinal bulge on the mid-ventral surface of the medulla oblongata. It comprises caudally directed corticospinal fibres, which facilitate voluntary motor function especially of skilled activities.

Pyramidal decussation – Ventrocaudal medulla oblongata at the spinomedullary junction. It is the site where the pyramids become less prominent as they cross to project to the contralateral side and a more dorsolateral position in the spinal cord.

Pyramis – see Cerebellar vermis.

Red nucleus – Prominent upper motor neuron nucleus in tegmentum of midbrain, ventrolateral to the oculomotor nucleus. It is named such because of its rich vascularisation. Afferent fibres are from the lateral nucleus of the cerebellum, which are projected onto the thalamus (dentatorubrothalamic pathway) as a major feedback route to the cerebrum from the cerebellum. Efferent fibres decussate immediately and project to brainstem nuclei (CNN V, VII, IX–XI) and to the spinal cord. It is involved in semi-automatic movements such as swallowing, chewing and sucking, and flexor activities such as sitting.

Reticular nuclei – Form a complex, poorly defined network extending through the core of the brainstem. It includes the gigantocellular and parvocellular nuclei of the medulla oblongata. The lateral area receives afferent fibres from the spinal cord, cerebellum and forebrain. Efferent fibres arise from the medial area and have diverse functions including modulating respiration, heart rate and blood pressure, protective reflexes (coughing and vomiting) and maintenance of consciousness via connections to the cerebrum (ascending reticular activating system). It is involved in regulating rhythmical activities, and is also the origin of the UMN of reticulospinal tracts; different reticulospinal tracts stimulate, or inhibit, motor activity of the body and limbs.

Rostral cerebellar peduncle – Connects the cerebellum with the midbrain. It contains mainly efferent processes from the interposital and lateral cerebellar nuclei exiting the cerebellum and travelling to contralateral brainstem nuclei. It also conveys afferent fibres from the craniospinocerebellar, ventral spinocerebellar and rubrocerebellar tracts.

Rostral colliculus – Prominent dorsal protrusion on the tectum of the midbrain. It functions as a reflex centre for visual pathways receiving afferent fibres from the optic tract, visual cortex, caudal colliculus and spinal cord (spinomesencephalic tract). Efferent fibres (tectobulbar and tectospinal) influence movement of the eyes, ears and head in response to visual and auditory stimuli.

Rostral commissure – Small commissure in the rostral, ventral telencephalic substance around which the columns of the fornix split. The commissure connects the olfactory bulbs on each side.

Rostral lobe of cerebellum – Separated from caudal lobe by the dorsally located, transverse, primary fissure. It is especially inhibitory to extensor muscles.

Rostral rhinal sulcus – Rostral extension of lateral rhinal sulcus making up the dorsal margin of the olfactory peduncle.

Rostral suprasylvian gyrus – Rostral extent of the suprasylvian gyrus on the lateral aspect of the rostral cerebrum.

Rostral vestibular nucleus – Pons, at the level of the rostral cerebellar peduncle. See vestibular nuclei.

Rubrospinal tract – UMN axons extending from the red nucleus of the midbrain tegmentum, caudally through the brainstem into the lateral funiculus of the spinal cord, medial to the dorsal spinocerebellar tract. It is important in facilitating flexor motor function for voluntary and postural activities.

Sensory roots of the trigeminal nerve – Pontine–medullary junction. Axons coursing dorsomedially from the trigeminal nerve to the sensory nucleus of the trigeminal nerve.

Septal nuclei (medial and lateral) – Located rostral to the rostral commissure on the medial aspect of the rostral telencephalon. They form the medial wall of the rostral aspect of the lateral ventricle, and attach dorsally to the corpus callosum. It receives input from the medial olfactory stria and has reciprocal connections with the hippocampus and hypothalamus. The septal nuclei, along with the nucleus accumbens, play a role in reward and reinforcement.

Septum pellucidum – A midline, fibrous lamina that connects between the septal nuclei and the corpus callosum, separating the rostral aspect of the lateral ventricles.

Solitary tract – Dorsal medulla oblongata, ventral to the floor of the fourth ventricle. It conveys afferent fibres carrying visceral sensation and taste from the facial (VII),

glossopharyngeal (IX) and vagus (X) cranial nerves to the adjacent solitary nucleus.

Solitary tract nucleus – see Nucleus of the solitary tract.

Spinal nerve – The nerve that is formed by the union of dorsal roots and ventral roots that attach to the spinal cord. The nerve emerges from the vertebral column at the level of the intervertebral foramen. These are mixed nerves conveying sensory, motor and, in the thoracolumbar and sacral regions, autonomic fibres.

Spinal tract of V – Tract in the dorsolateral pons and medulla oblongata, dorsolateral to its nucleus. It conveys general somatic afferents from the trigeminal ganglion (CN V), geniculate ganglion of CN VII and the distal ganglion of CN X.

Splenial gyrus – Gyrus on the caudal aspect of the medial cerebral hemispheres. It is bordered by splenial sulcus ventrally and the supraspenial sulcus dorsally.

Splenial sulcus – Rostral border of the splenial gyrus on caudal and medial aspect of the cerebral hemispheres.

Straight gyrus – Rostral telencephalon, the gyrus on the ventral aspect of the longitudinal fissure. It is medial to the olfactory peduncle and the lateral ventricle.

Stria terminalis – Medial cerebrum, in the angle between the thalamus and the caudate nucleus. It conveys efferent fibres from the amygdala (basal nuclei) to the rostral hypothalamus and septal area. The amygdala influences behaviour, autonomic activity and movement.

Subarachnoid space – CSF-filled space between the arachnoid mater and pia mater surrounding the CNS. It is criss-crossed by fine arachnoid trabeculae. On the lateral aspect of the spinal cord, the space is traversed by paired denticulate ligaments, formed from thickenings of the pia mater and which attach the spinal cord to the spinal dura mater. The subarachnoid space collapses at death due to lack of CSF pressure.

Subcallosal fasciculus – Bundle of axons running longitudinally in the dorsolateral aspect of lateral ventricles of the cerebral hemisphere, beneath the lateral angle of the corpus callosum. It has similar connections to the cingulate gyrus (part of the limbic system) and also connects to the caudate nucleus.

Substantia nigra – Longitudinal nuclei, producing dopamine, on the ventral aspect of the mesencephalon, dorsal to the crus cerebri. It may be pigmented, especially in older animals. It is associated with the basal nuclei and the extrapyramidal motor system.

Sulcus limitans – Sulcus in the lateral wall of the central canal of the spinal cord, fourth ventricle and mesencephalic aqueduct; it is only grossly visible in the fourth ventricle. Embryologically, it divided the neural tube into the dorsal/sensory alar plate and the ventral/motor basal plate.

Supracollosal gyrus – Small gyrus sited dorsal to the rostral corpus callosum on the medial side of the cerebrum. It is part of the small, supracallosal portion of the hippocampal formation.

Supraspenial sulcus – Sulcus forming the rostral margin of the occipital gyrus on the caudomedial border of the cerebrum.

Suprasylvian gyrus – Elongated, curving gyrus on lateral aspect of the cerebrum. It is bounded ventrally by the suprasylvian sulcus and dorsally by the marginal sulcus.

Suprasylvian sulcus – Ventral to the suprasylvian gyrus on the lateral side of the cerebrum.

Sylvian gyrus – Gyrus surrounding the pseudosylvian fissure on the lateral side of the cerebrum. It comprises the auditory cortex.

Tectum – Dorsal part of the midbrain. It is formed primarily by the paired rostral and caudal colliculi, which together, make up the corpora quadrigemina. It primarily functions in visual and auditory reflexes.

Tegmental fasciculus – Fibre bundle passing longitudinally through the central mesencephalic and pontine tegmentum, lateral to the medial longitudinal fasciculus. It contains fibres from the mesencephalic tegmentum and regions surrounding the central gray substance travelling caudally to the olivary nucleus; and fibres travelling rostrally from more caudal reticular formation to the diencephalon.

Tegmentum – Ventral part of the midbrain. It includes the oculomotor and red nuclei as well as the substantia nigra and crus cerebri.

Thalamic nuclei – Part of the diencephalon on the medial aspect of the forebrain. The thalamic nuclear group comprises numerous nuclei that are divided into major groups by medullary lamina. The thalamic nuclei act as a relay between a variety of subcortical areas and the cerebral cortex and form numerous bidirectional links with the cerebral cortex.

Third ventricle – CSF-filled, ring-shaped cavity, vertically oriented around the interthalamic adhesion of the diencephalon; part of the ventricular system.

Transverse fibres of the pons – Prominent fibres on the ventral aspect of the pons. They consist of axons arising from the pontine nuclei, which decussate and ascend into the cerebellum via the middle cerebellar peduncles.

Transverse fissure – Located between the caudal poles of the cerebrum and the rostral face of the cerebellum. It contains the fibrous tentorium cerebelli, an extension of the dura mater, which arises from the osseous tentorium.

Trapezoid body – Large band of transverse fibres on the ventral surface of the rostral medulla oblongata. It is formed by fibres of the ventral cochlear nucleus and is part of the pathway projecting auditory stimuli rostrally.

Trochlear nucleus – Nucleus of the fourth cranial nerve, situated in the midbrain tegmentum caudal to the oculomotor nuclei. Uniquely, its fibres exit the brainstem dorsally and decussate. They innervate the dorsal oblique, extraocular muscles.

Tuber – See Cerebellar vermis.

Uvula of cerebellum – See Cerebellar vermis.

Uvulonodular fissure of cerebellum – Ventrocaudal aspect of the cerebellum, separates the large body of the cerebellum from the small flocculonodular lobe.

Ventral cochlear nucleus – Lateral aspect of the rostral medulla. See Cochlear nuclei.

Ventral funiculus – Ventral region of white matter of the spinal cord between the ventral median fissure and the ventral root. Principally consists of caudally directed, upper motor neuron tracts that facilitate extensor muscle function.

Ventral horn of the spinal cord – Ventral grey matter of the spinal cord, contains somata of lower motor neurons supplying the neck, trunk and limbs.

Ventral median fissure – Longitudinal groove in the midline of the ventral aspect of the spinal cord and the medulla oblongata.

Ventral paraflocculus of cerebellum – see Paraflocculus of the cerebellum.

Ventral reticular nucleus – see Reticular nuclei.

Ventral spinal root – Efferent/motor root of a spinal nerve. See Spinal nerve.

Ventral spinocerebellar tract – Tract conveying subconscious proprioceptive fibres from the caudal half of the trunk, the pelvic limbs and tail, to the cerebellum via the rostral cerebellar peduncle. The tract decussates in the spinal cord and then again in the cerebellum.

Vestibular nuclei – Four pairs (rostral, medial, lateral and caudal) located in the dorsal aspect of the rostral medulla oblongata, adjacent to the cerebellar peduncles and the lateral aspect of the fourth ventricle. They receive input from the vestibular nerve (head proprioception), the cerebellum and the spinal cord. Their axons project to the cerebellum (subconscious proprioception), the cortex of the temporal lobe (conscious proprioception), motor nuclei of the extraocular muscles (head and eyeball position – vestibulo-ocular reflex), the spinal cord (postural adjustments to accommodate changes in head position) and the reticular formation (basis of motion sickness).

Vestibulocochlear nerve – CN VIII, attaches to the brainstem laterally at the pontine–medullary junction. It conveys afferent axons from vestibular and cochlear receptors in the inner ear.

Index

The index comprises topics discussed in the main text of the book. For anatomical structures illustrated in the Appendix, readers should refer to the Appendix Glossary.

Page numbers followed by "f" indicate figures, "t" indicate tables, and "b" indicate boxes.

Printed in the United States
By Bookmasters